Neuroradiology Cases

Neuroradiology Cases

Clifford J. Eskey, MD, PhD

Associate Professor of Radiology
Director, Division of Neuroradiology
Department of Radiology
Dartmouth-Hitchcock Medical Center
Lebanon, New Hampshire

Clifford J. Belden, MD

Associate Professor of Radiology
Department of Radiology
Dartmouth-Hitchcock Medical Center
Lebanon, New Hampshire

David A. Pastel, MD

Associate Professor of Radiology
Department of Radiology
Dartmouth-Hitchcock Medical Center
Lebanon, New Hampshire

Arastoo Vossough, MD, PhD

Assistant Professor of Radiology
Children's Hospital of Philadelphia and
Hospital of the University of Pennsylvania
Philadelphia, Pennsylvania

Albert J. Yoo, MD

Instructor, Harvard Medical School
Staff, Interventional Neuroradiology
Massachusetts General Hospital
Boston, Massachusetts

OXFORD
UNIVERSITY PRESS

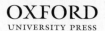

Oxford University Press, Inc., publishes works that further
Oxford University's objective of excellence
in research, scholarship, and education.

Oxford New York
Auckland   Cape Town   Dar es Salaam   Hong Kong   Karachi
Kuala Lumpur   Madrid   Melbourne   Mexico City   Nairobi
New Delhi   Shanghai   Taipei   Toronto

With offices in
Argentina   Austria   Brazil   Chile   Czech Republic   France   Greece
Guatemala   Hungary   Italy   Japan   Poland   Portugal   Singapore
South Korea   Switzerland   Thailand   Turkey   Ukraine   Vietnam

Copyright © 2012 by Oxford University Press, Inc.

Published by Oxford University Press, Inc.
198 Madison Avenue, New York, New York 10016
www.oup.com

Oxford is a registered trademark of Oxford University Press

Library of Congress Cataloging-in-Publication Data

Neuroradiology cases / Clifford J. Eskey . . . [et al.].
   p. ; cm. — (Cases in radiology)
  Includes bibliographical references and index.
  ISBN 978-0-19-973598-3
I. Eskey, Clifford J. II. Series: Cases in radiology.
  [DNLM: 1. Nervous System Diseases—radiography—Case Reports.
  2. Diagnostic Techniques, Neurological—Case Reports. WL 141]
  616.8047572—dc23
                                            2011039719

This material is not intended to be, and should not be considered, a substitute for medical or other professional
advice. Treatment for the conditions described in this material is highly dependent on the individual
circumstances. And, while this material is designed to offer accurate information with respect to the subject
matter covered and to be current as of the time it was written, research and knowledge about medical and
health issues is constantly evolving and dose schedules for medications are being revised continually, with
new side effects recognized and accounted for regularly. Readers must therefore always check the product
information and clinical procedures with the most up-to-date published product information and data sheets
provided by the manufacturers and the most recent codes of conduct and safety regulation. The publisher
and the authors make no representations or warranties to readers, express or implied, as to the accuracy
or completeness of this material. Without limiting the foregoing, the publisher and the authors make no
representations or warranties as to the accuracy or efficacy of the drug dosages mentioned in the material.
The authors and the publisher do not accept, and expressly disclaim, any responsibility for any liability, loss or
risk that may be claimed or incurred as a consequence of the use and/or application of any of the contents of
this material.

9 8 7 6 5 4 3 2
Printed in China
on acid-free paper

Preface

The cases in this book represent much of the neuroradiology material which one should master as a diplomat of the American Board of Radiology. The format of each case is designed to provide an easy-to-read summary of the most important information on each condition. We seek to emphasize information that is most relevant to patient care, i.e., the expertise that the referring physicians will need from the imaging studies. We include challenging examples of common diseases and typical examples of less common ones.

The cases are organized into the three major areas of the ABR examination—brain imaging, spine imaging, and head & neck imaging. Within each of these areas, the cases are randomly ordered.

We hope that you will enjoy challenging yourself and learning from these cases.

Acknowledgments

Many stellar radiologists contributed to the cases in this book. We would particularly like to thank the following physicians for preparing cases for inclusion:

Ali R. Sepahdari, MD of UCLA for cases of venous thrombosis and infarction, gliomatosis cerebri, giant cell astrocytoma, pineoblastoma, and colloid cyst.

Amit A. Raheja, MD of Mass General Hospital for arterial dissection, vasospasm, glioblastoma multiforme, pleomorphic xanthoastrocytoma, choroid plexus carcinoma/papilloma, and dermoid.

Gaetano T. Pastena MD, MBA of Mass General Hospital for border-zone infarction, oligodendroglioma, and subependymoma.

Jerry C. Lee, MD of Mass General Hospital for perfusion diffusion mismatch, subarachnoid hemorrhage, fibrillary astrocytoma, ependymoma, lymphoma, and hypothalamic hamartoma.

John P. Kim, MD of Mass General Hospital for fibromuscular dysplasia and moyamoya.

Mara M. Kunst, MD of L&M Radiology for HIE, ICH, leptomeningeal carcinomatosis, radiation necrosis, DNET, and craniopharyngioma.

Michael T. Preece, MD of Mass General Hospital for brainstem glioma, medulloblastoma, and epidermoid.

Ronil V. Chandra, MBBS, FRANZCR of Mass General Hospital for aberrant carotid artery and carotid cavernous fistula.

Thabele M. Leslie-Mazwi, MD of Mass General Hospital for RCVS and mycotic aneurysm.

Zeshan A. Chaudhry, MD of Mass General Hospital for central neurocytoma and pituitary adenoma.

The Publisher thanks the following for their time and advice:

Mark Anderson, University of Virginia
Sanjeev Bhalla, Mallinckrodt Institute of Radiology, Washington University
Michael Bruno, Penn State Hershey Medical Center
Melissa Rosado de Christenson, St. Luke's Hospital of Kansas City
Rihan Khan, University of Arizona
Angela Levy, Georgetown University
Alexander Mamourian, University of Pennsylvania
Stacy Smith, Brigham and Women's Hospital

Contents

Part 1   Brain

History

▶ 33-year-old woman presenting to the ED with headaches, nausea, and vomiting

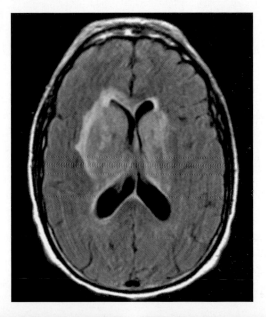

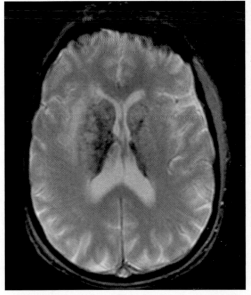
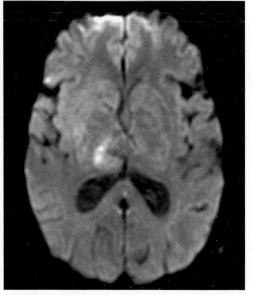

Case 1 Cerebral Venous Thrombosis and Infarction

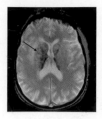 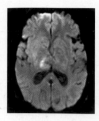 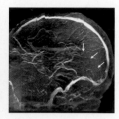

Findings

▶ There is T2/FLAIR hyperintensity and mass effect within the deep gray nuclei and adjacent white matter.
▶ T2*-weighted GRE sequence demonstrates susceptibility-related signal loss consistent with hemorrhage or venous congestion (black arrow).
▶ DWI reveals focal restricted diffusion in the right thalamus, with normal or elevated diffusion elsewhere.
▶ 2D time-of-flight MR venogram demonstrates absence of flow-related enhancement in the deep venous structures, including the internal cerebral veins, vein of Galen, and straight sinus (white arrows).

Differential Diagnosis

▶ Viral encephalitis
▶ Lymphoma
▶ Glioma
▶ Basilar artery/artery of Percheron occlusion
▶ Acute disseminated encephalomyelitis

Teaching Points

▶ Cerebral venous thrombosis (CVT) is a rare cause of stroke and predominantly affects young women. Risk factors include oral contraceptive use, dehydration, malignancy, and underlying hypercoagulable state.
▶ CVT can be difficult to recognize due to variable clinical presentation. Imaging is critical for early diagnosis and initiation of therapy.
▶ Imaging clues to CVT include regional edema with or without hemorrhage, not corresponding to an arterial territory. Unlike arterial infarction, venous infarction is surrounded by areas of elevated diffusion (i.e., vasogenic edema).
▶ Knowledge of venous territories can suggest the diagnosis.
  ▪ Symmetric deep gray and white matter: deep cerebral veins
  ▪ Parasagittal frontoparietal: superior sagittal sinus
  ▪ Posterolateral temporal: vein of Labbé
▶ Venous thrombus appears hyperdense on noncontrast CT. On contrast CT and CT venography the clot produces a filling defect within the veins or dural sinuses.
▶ The thrombosis may be visible as uniform hyperintense or iso-intense signal on T1-weighted images filling a dural sinus. MR venography demonstrates absence of flow-related enhancement within the involved veins. Isolated cortical vein thrombosis may be identified as serpiginous susceptibility artifact on T2* sequences.

Management

▶ Anticoagulation is advisable even if substantial intracerebral hemorrhage is present.
▶ Catheter-directed thrombolysis or clot extraction should be considered in cases of further deterioration.

Further Reading

Bentley JN, Figueroa RE, Vender JR, et al. From presentation to follow-up: diagnosis and treatment of cerebral venous thrombosis. *Neurosurg Focus.* 2009;27:E41-47.
Leach JL, Fortuna RB, Jones BV, et al. Imaging of cerebral venous thrombosis: current techniques, spectrum of findings, and diagnostic pitfalls. *Radiographics.* 2006; 26:S19-S41.

History

▶ 9-year-old boy with headache

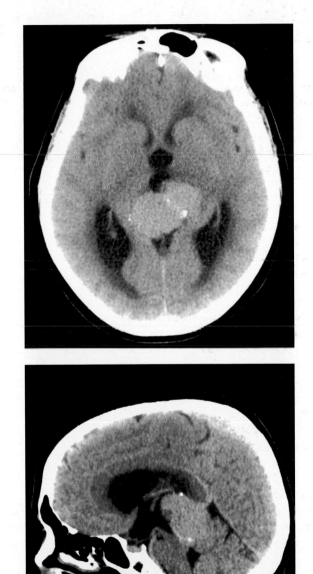

Case 2   Pineoblastoma

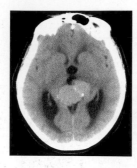 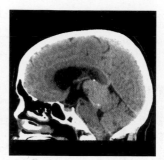

Findings

► There is a large pineal region mass.
► The mass has peripheral calcification and generally higher attenuation than cerebral parenchyma.
► There is moderate obstructive hydrocephalus due to deformation of the tectum and compression of the cerebral aqueduct with transependymal edema at the occipital horns of the lateral ventricles.

Differential Diagnosis

► Germ cell tumor
► Pineocytoma
► Meningioma
► Astrocytoma of the tectum, thalamus, or corpus callosum

Teaching Points

► Pineoblastomas are malignant (WHO grade IV) primitive neuroectodermal tumors. They are less common than germ cell tumors and unlike germ cell tumors demonstrate no sex predilection. Prognosis is poor, with median survival less than 2 years.
► Masses of the pineal region may present with signs of hydrocephalus or with Parinaud syndrome from mass effect upon the tectum.
► Patient demographics and key imaging features are helpful for constructing an appropriate differential diagnosis.
► Pineoblastomas are hyperdense on CT scan. If physiologic calcifications are present, they are typically "exploded" by the tumor (as in this case). Pineoblastomas tend to be larger and more irregular in shape than germinomas or pineocytomas at the time of diagnosis, and they frequently invade adjacent structures or spread via the CSF. They may demonstrate internal cystic/necrotic change, particularly when they are large. On MRI, they frequently demonstrate restricted diffusion.
► CSF dissemination and drop metastases are common.
► Pineocytoma is a benign, well-differentiated pineal parenchymal tumor that is uncommon in children. It may have a similar appearance to pineoblastoma and should be included in the differential of a solid pineal region mass.

Management

► Treatment of hydrocephalus is often the first step. It is important to obtain MR imaging of the brain and spine to detect tumor dissemination through the CSF prior to surgery. Treatment includes surgical resection with craniospinal radiation and chemotherapy.

Further Reading

Smirniotopoulos JG, Rushing EJ, Mena H. Pineal region masses: differential diagnosis. *Radiographics*. 1992;12:577-596.
Tien R, Barkovich AJ, Edwards MS. MR imaging of pineal tumors. *AJR Am J Roentgenol*. 1990;155:143-151.

History

▶ 46-year-old man with a 1-week history of fever, fatigue, and myalgia. He presents to the ER with confusion, memory impairment, and speech difficulty

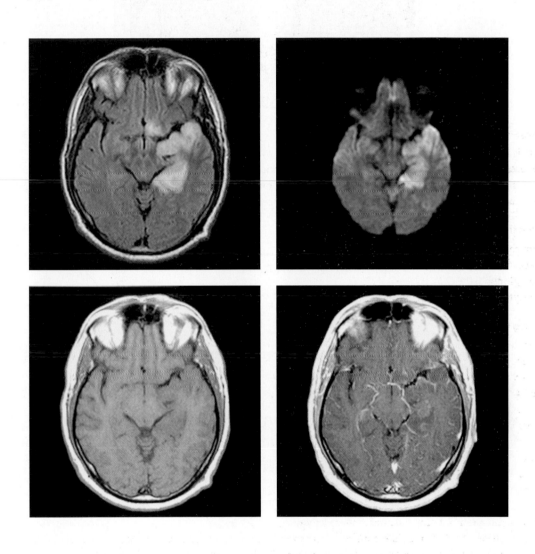

Case 3 Herpes Encephalitis

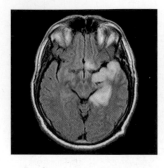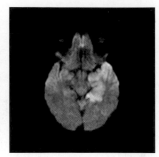

Findings

▶ The FLAIR sequence demonstrates hyperintense signal involving cortex and adjacent subcortical white matter of the medial and anterior left temporal lobe as well as the posterior aspect of the left gyrus rectus.
▶ Most of these areas are hyperintense on DWI.
▶ There is subtle cortical enhancement on the postcontrast T1-weighted sequence.

Differential Diagnosis

▶ Other viral encephalitis
▶ Limbic encephalitis
▶ Cerebral infarction
▶ Glial or glioneuronal neoplasm
▶ Seizure edema in status epilepticus

Teaching Points

▶ Herpes encephalitis results from primary infection or reactivation of HSV-1. This virus, which causes oral herpes, may lie dormant in the trigeminal ganglion for decades.
▶ Patients present with fever, headache, rapidly progressive cognitive decline, and focal neurologic deficits. When left untreated, this disease results in severe morbidity and mortality.
▶ The areas typically involved include the medial temporal lobe, inferior frontal lobe, insula, and cingulate gyrus. Initially unilateral, the infection can rapidly spread to similar areas on the other side of the brain. There is a predilection for the cortex over white matter.
▶ Early MRI findings include hyperintensity on FLAIR and T2-weighted sequences, hypointensity on T1-weighted sequences, and the presence of restricted diffusion on DWI.
▶ Later findings include gyriform cortical hyperintensity on T1-weighted images and postcontrast enhancement of the cortex.
▶ Features that differentiate this entity from its mimics include:
  ▪ Clinical picture and the classic distribution of signal changes differentiate it from acute infarction. HSV crosses vascular boundaries.
  ▪ The paucity of mass effect, presence of restricted diffusion, and predilection for gray matter distinguish it from most neoplasms.

Management

▶ The diagnosis may be corroborated by CSF sampling with PCR analysis for HSV DNA.
▶ Immediate treatment with such antivirals as acyclovir and gancyclovir will limit the extent of injury.

Further Reading

Bulakbasi N, Kocaoglu M. Central nervous system infections of herpesvirus family. *Neuroimaging Clin North Am.* 2008;8:53-84.

History

► 55-year-old man who fell down eight stairs

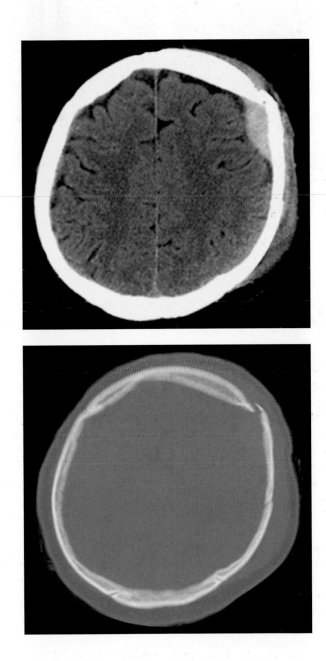

Case 4 Epidural Hematoma

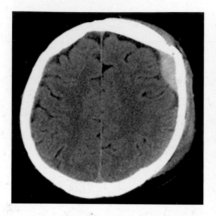 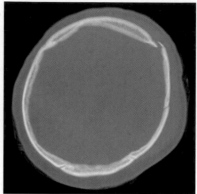

Findings

- A biconvex, hyperdense collection is present in the left frontal extra-axial space.
- The brain is displaced away from the inner table of the skull.
- There is an adjacent depressed frontal bone fracture.

Differential Diagnosis

- Subdural hematoma
- Meningioma

Teaching Points

- Epidural hematomas are the result of arterial bleeding in 90% of cases (typically the middle meningeal artery) and are usually associated with an adjacent skull fracture (85% to 95% of the time). Unlike subdural hematomas, epidural hematomas occur on the side of impact.
- The epidural space is located between the skull periosteum and dura. Epidural hematomas, which are most commonly found in the temporoparietal region, typically have a biconvex shape and their extent is limited by the cranial sutures.
- Small epidural hematomas are sometimes difficult to distinguish from a subdural hematoma. MRI can show the displaced dura, confirming the diagnosis of an epidural hematoma.
- In the acute phase epidural hematomas are hyperdense. A low-density "swirl" can be seen, indicating active bleeding.
- Venous epidurals are much less common than arterial ones and are usually due to laceration of a dural sinus from bony fragments. The posterior fossa and middle cranial fossa are the most common locations for venous epidural bleeds.
- The classic presentation of an epidural hematoma is a "lucent period" after an initial loss of consciousness. This is followed by nausea, vomiting, seizures, and focal neurologic deficits. It is important to recognize epidural hematomas promptly because they can rapidly increase in size, resulting in brain herniation. Overall mortality is 5%.

Management

- All but the smallest epidural hematomas are managed surgically with evacuation.

Further Reading

Hardman JM, Manoukian A. Pathology of head trauma. *Neuroimaging Clin North Am.* 2002;12:175-187.

History

▶ Child with a prior history of myelomeningocele repair, now with vomiting

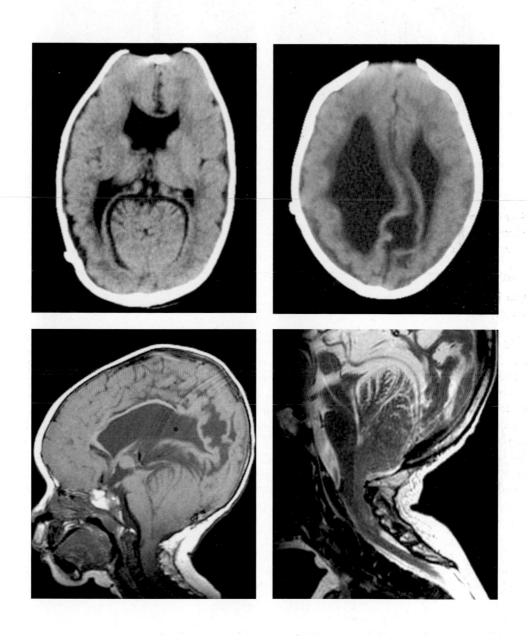

Case 5 Chiari II Malformation

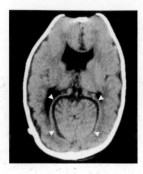 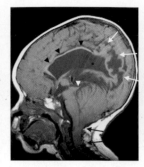 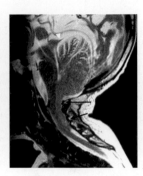

Findings

▸ Axial CT images demonstrate a towering cerebellum through a gaping tentorial incisura (white arrows), absence of the septum pellucidum, deficient falx cerebri, and narrow gyri with shallow sulci posteriorly.

▸ Sagittal T1- and T2-weighted MR images show a low-lying torcula herophili with a small posterior fossa and downward displacement of the cerebellum into the upper cervical canal (black arrows in Fig. 5F and 5G), a small fourth ventricle, a beaked tectum (white arrowhead in Fig. 5F and 5G), narrow gyri posteriorly (white arrows), and a thin dysgenetic corpus callosum (black arrowheads).

Differential Diagnosis

▸ Chiari I malformation
▸ CSF hypotension

Teaching Points

▸ Chiari II malformation (Arnold-Chiari malformation) is a complex congenital malformation of the brain, virtually always associated with a neural tube defect, most commonly a lumbar myelomeningocele.

▸ Manifestations of Chiari II include a small posterior fossa, low-lying torcula herophili, downward displacement of the cerebellum into the upper cervical canal, narrow fourth ventricle, tectal beaking, deficient falx cerebri with interdigitation of medial hemispheric gyri, stenogyria (narrow gyri with shallow sulci) posteriorly, kinking of the brain stem, and a large massa intermedia.

▸ Many other abnormalities are commonly associated with Chiari II malformation, including neural tube defects (virtually always), dysgenesis of the corpus callosum, gray matter heterotopia, absent septum pellucidum, syringohydromyelia, and other vertebral anomalies.

▸ Most patients with Chiari II malformation will develop hydrocephalus, requiring shunting or diversion. Many of the symptoms are related to the myelomeningocele, but bulbar symptoms and signs of hydrocephalus (headache, vomiting, increasing head size) are also common. Degree of disability depends on severity of associated malformations.

Management

▸ Myelomeningocele repair is undertaken at the time of birth. Most patients will require CSF shunting/diversion. Sometimes they undergo Chiari decompression at the craniocervical junction for improvement of bulbar symptoms or syringohydromyelia.

▸ Folate supplementation in the mother decreases the risk of neural tube defects.

Further Reading

Juranek J, Salman MS. Anomalous development of brain structure and function in spina bifida myelomeningocele. *Dev Disabil Res Rev.* 2010;16:23-30.

Miller E, Widjaja E, Blaser S, et al. The old and the new: supratentorial MR findings in Chiari II malformation. *Childs Nerv Syst.* 2008;24:563-575.

History

▶ 35-year-old woman with hyperemesis gravidarum and confusion

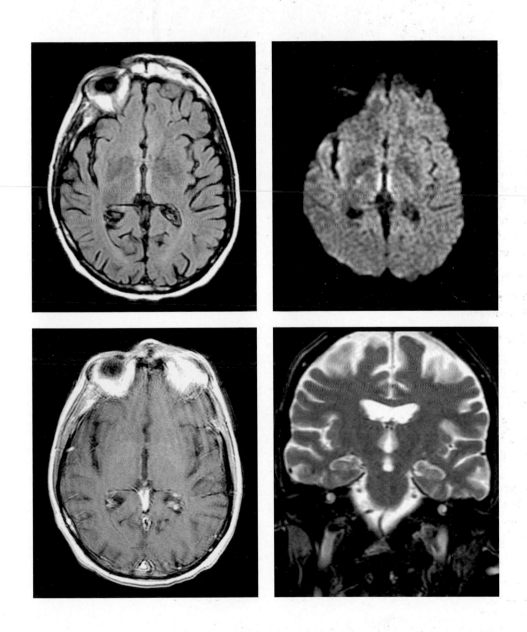

Case 6 Wernicke Encephalopathy

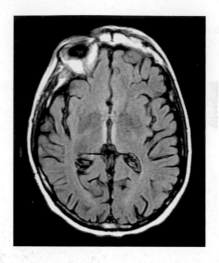

Findings

▶ There is hyperintense signal on FLAIR, T2-weighted, and DWI images in the bilateral medial thalami along the walls of the third ventricle with restricted diffusion.
▶ No abnormal enhancement

Differential Diagnosis

▶ Artery of Percheron infarction
▶ Internal cerebral vein thrombosis
▶ Viral encephalitis

Teaching Points

▶ Wernicke encephalopathy (WE) is a rare but acute neurologic emergency caused by thiamine (vitamin B1) deficiency.
▶ It most commonly occurs in alcoholics but is found in other conditions producing thiamine depletion, including hyperemesis gravidum, starvation, anorexia nervosa, and bariatric surgery.
▶ The classic clinical presentation is the triad of ophthalmoplegia, ataxia, and confusion. The most common presentation is diminished consciousness.
▶ Early MRI is helpful in confirming the diagnosis in suspected cases. MRI shows hyperintense signal on T2-weighted images in the medial thalami, mammillary bodies, periaqueductal gray matter, and tectum.
▶ Enhancement and diffusion-weighted abnormalities are variable. Enhancement of the mammillary bodies may be the only abnormality.
▶ In chronic or repeated thiamine deficiency, atrophy of the mammillary bodies predominates. This scenario presents most commonly in alcoholics with WE.

Management

▶ The disorder is reversible in the early stages with intravenous administration of thiamine. If left untreated, Korsakoff psychosis or death may ensue.

Further Reading

Zuccoli G, Pipitone M. Neuroimaging findings in acute Wernicke's encephalopathy: Review of the literature. *AJNR Am J Neuroradiol.* 2009;192:501-508.

History

▸ 74-year-old man with frequent falls

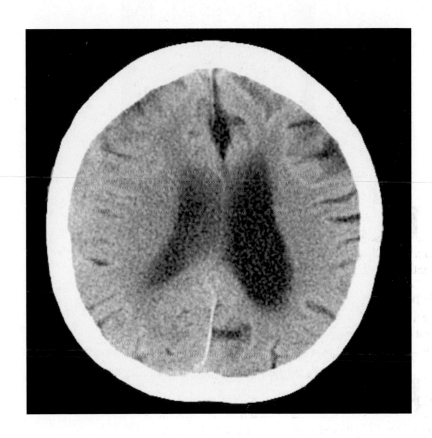

Case 7 Isodense Subdural Hematoma

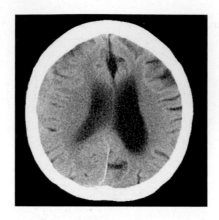

Findings

▶ Axial CT shows a crescentic extra-axial collection along the right cerebral convexity. The collection is iso-attenuating to cerebral gray matter.

▶ Note that the sulci along the right hemisphere do not reach the inner table of the skull.

Differential Diagnosis

▶ Subdural empyema

▶ Subdural effusion

▶ Thickened dura (intracranial hypotension, sarcoid, tuberculosis)

▶ Extra-axial neoplasm (meningiomas, lymphoma metastasis)

Teaching Points

▶ Trauma, with tearing of the bridging cortical veins, is the most common cause of subdural hematoma. The trauma may be mild, especially in older patients.

▶ The density and signal intensity of subdural hematomas vary with age. Acute (1 to 3 days) subdural hematomas are hyperattenuating relative to cerebral cortex. With resorption of the blood products, the collections become isodense to hypodense over time.

▶ In the subacute phase (3 days to 3 weeks), subdural hematomas may become difficult to see when the blood is isodense to cortex. Secondary signs, including displacement of the cortex away from the inner table of the skull and sulcal effacement, can be helpful in diagnosing small isodense subdural hematomas.

▶ In the chronic phase, subdural hematomas become hypodense and are easy to distinguish from the adjacent cortex.

▶ Contrast-enhanced studies can display enhancing membranes and inward displacement of enhancing vessels.

▶ On MRI, subacute subdural hematomas are usually iso-to hyperintense on T1-weighted images and have variable signal intensity on T2-weighted images. On T2*-weighted (gradient-echo) sequences the hematoma will demonstrate susceptibility-related signal loss.

Management

▶ Conservative management with follow-up CT scans for smaller collections

▶ Surgical evacuation for large or symptomatic collections

Further Reading

Lee KS, et al. The computed tomographic attenuation and the age of subdural hematomas. *J Korean Med Sci.* 1997;12:353-359.

History

▸ 54-year-old woman with headache and obtundation

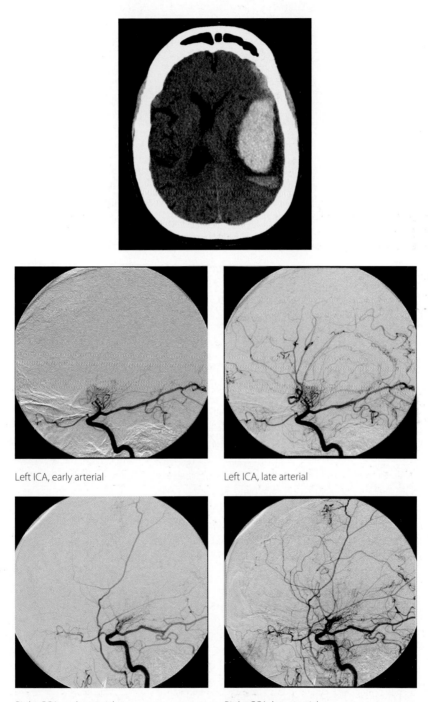

Left ICA, early arterial

Left ICA, late arterial

Right CCA, early arterial

Right CCA, late arterial

Case 8 Moyamoya Disease

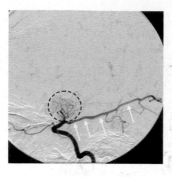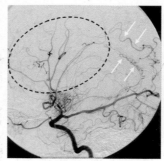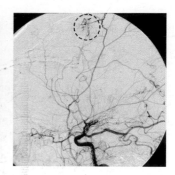

Findings

▶ Noncontrast CT demonstrates an intraparenchymal hemorrhage in the left frontal lobe.

▶ Catheter angiography reveals severe narrowing of the distal left internal carotid artery (ICA) with formation of small-vessel collaterals that have a "puff of smoke" appearance (dotted circle, left). There is delayed flow into cortical branches of the left anterior (ACA) and middle (MCA) cerebral arteries (dotted oval, middle) and posterior cerebral artery (PCA) collaterals to the anterior circulation (arrows).

Differential Diagnosis

▶ Vasculitis

▶ Atherosclerosis

▶ Arterial dissection

Teaching Points

▶ Moyamoya disease is a noninflammatory cerebrovascular disorder of unknown cause, characterized by progressive stenosis of the intracranial ICA and often the proximal ACA and MCA. The pathologic findings include vascular smooth muscle hyperplasia and luminal thrombosis.

▶ The term "moyamoya disease" is reserved for idiopathic bilateral involvement. Moyamoya syndrome is invoked in the setting of a similar angiographic pattern but when the involvement is unilateral or occurs in the setting of known causes of vasculopathy (e.g., radiotherapy, Down syndrome, NF-1, and sickle cell disease).

▶ It occurs most frequently in East Asians. There are two age peaks: early childhood and the fifth decade.

▶ Infarction is the most common presentation in children. Intracerebral hemorrhage (ICH) is more common in adults and is thought to arise from the extensive fragile pial collaterals.

▶ The large vessel steno-occlusive disease is visible on MR or CT angiography. The prominent lenticulostriate collaterals may be visible on conventional MR imaging.

▶ Angiographic findings of vascular narrowing in the distal ICA and proximal ACA/MCA accompanied by prominent (net-like) small vessel collaterals at the base of the brain are diagnostic of moyamoya.

Management

▶ Imaging assessment of regional cerebrovascular reserve (with SPECT, CT perfusion, etc.) can show areas of greatest risk and predict which patients are most likely to benefit from surgical intervention.

▶ Surgical bypass techniques (e.g., STA-MCA bypass, encephaloduroarteriosynangiosis) augment cerebral blood flow and have been shown to reduce stroke risk.

Further Reading

Ortiz-Neira CL. The puff of smoke sign. *Radiology.* 2008;247:910-911.
Scott RM, Smith ER. Moyamoya disease and moyamoya syndrome. *N Engl J Med.* 2009;360:1226-1237.

History

▶ 18-year-old man with headache, nausea, and double vision

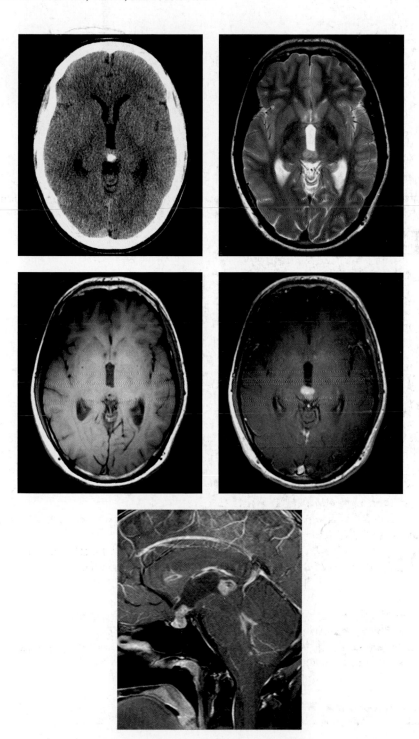

Case 9 Germinoma

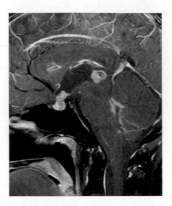

Findings

▶ Noncontrast CT shows a small mass surrounding the pineal calcification. Its attenuation is slightly greater than that of gray matter.
▶ A small enhancing pineal mass surrounds the coarse pineal calcification.
▶ There is a separate enhancing mass of the posterior pituitary, infundibulum, and floor of the third ventricle.
▶ There is nodular subependymal enhancement along the fourth ventricle, consistent with CSF dissemination.

Differential Diagnosis

▶ Pineoblastoma
▶ Non-germinomatous germ cell tumor
▶ Glioblastoma multiforme
▶ Metastasis

Teaching Points

▶ Germinoma is the most common intracranial germ cell tumor (65%) and the most common solid pineal mass, followed by pineal cell tumors. Peak incidence is in the second decade, with a strong male predominance.
▶ Clinical signs include obstructive hydrocephalus and dorsal midbrain compression (paralysis of upward gaze, mydriasis, and convergence abnormality [Parinaud syndrome]). Germinomas may also occur in the suprasellar region (30%), where they can produce hypopituitarism and diabetes insipidus.
▶ Characteristic imaging findings of germinoma reflect its dense cellularity (CT hyperattenuation, signal that is iso-intense to gray matter on T2-weighted images, and restricted diffusion). If physiologic pineal calcifications are present, they are typically "engulfed" by the tumor. Synchronous pineal and suprasellar masses strongly suggest the presence of germinoma. This neoplasm has a propensity for CSF dissemination and invasion of the adjacent parenchyma.
▶ Pineoblastomas may have a similar imaging appearance to germinoma. Findings suggestive of pineoblastoma include:
  ▪ A large (>3 cm), lobulated mass
  ▪ "Exploded" pineal calcification along the tumor periphery
  ▪ Cystic or necrotic change
▶ Non-germinomatous germ cell tumors include teratoma (second most common), choriocarcinoma, embryonal carcinoma, and endodermal sinus tumors. Teratomas have a heterogeneous appearance, with foci of fat, coarse calcification, and cystic change. Serum tumor markers are helpful for diagnosing particular germ cell tumors, and for monitoring therapeutic response.

Management

▶ Imaging of the craniospinal axis is mandatory to detect CSF tumor dissemination.

▶ Localized tumor is treated with radiation therapy and has an excellent prognosis, with a 10-year survival of 90%.

▶ Disseminated or recurrent tumor is treated with chemotherapy.

Further Reading

Kyritsis AP. Management of primary intracranial germ cell tumors. *J Neurooncol.* 2010;96:143-149.

Smith AB, Rushing EJ, Smirniotopoulos JG. Lesions of the pineal region: radiologic–pathologic correlation. *Radiographics.* 2010;30:2001-2020.

History

▶ 14-year-old boy with chronic headache

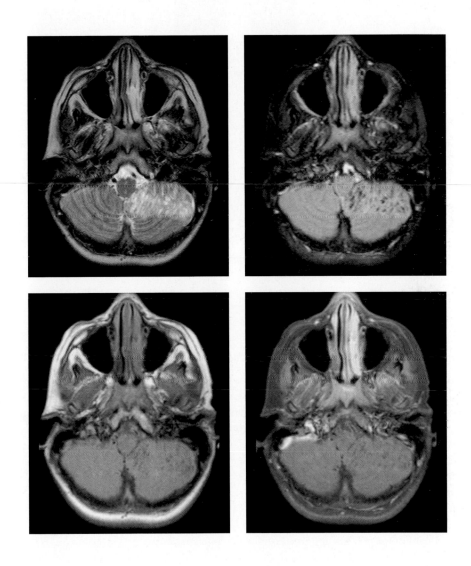

Case 10 Lhermitte-Duclos Disease (Dysplastic Gangliocytoma of the Cerebellum)

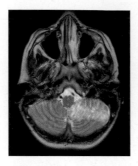

Findings

▶ There is a lesion in the left cerebellar hemisphere, hyperintense on T2-weighted images and iso- to hypointense on T1-weighted images. There is mild mass effect.
▶ The T2-weighted images show a striated or gyriform pattern within the lesion.
▶ It shows no postcontrast enhancement.

Differential Diagnosis

▶ Medulloblastoma
▶ Diffuse or pilocytic astrocytoma
▶ Cerebellar infarct
▶ Cerebellitis
▶ Ganglioglioma

Teaching Points

▶ Lhermitte-Duclos disease is a rare mass-like lesion in the cerebellar hemispheres, also called dysplastic cerebellar gangliocytoma. It is thought to be hamartomatous, and lesions do not grow or grow very slowly.
▶ The disease may be discovered in infancy but is more often discovered later in life. Many are found incidentally, but patients may present with headache, mild cerebellar dysfunction, or cranial nerve palsy. They occasionally cause sufficient mass effect to produce hydrocephalus.
▶ Most patients with Lhermitte-Duclos disease have Cowden syndrome, which is a multiple hamartoma-neoplasia syndrome with mutation of the PTEN tumor suppressor gene. These patients are prone to a variety of neoplasms, including thyroid, breast, GI, and GU tumors.
▶ The lesions are well circumscribed and hyperintense on T2-weighted images. They produce mass effect but no surrounding edema. Enhancement and calcification are rare.
▶ One key to the identification of Lhermitte-Duclos and differentiation from aggressive neoplasms is the presence of a parallel striated or gyriform architecture to the thickened folia, usually best demonstrated on T2-weighted images.
▶ On DWI, they are hyperintense because of "T2 shine-through."

Management

▶ Patients need to be screened for Cowden syndrome and its associated potential neoplasms. Surgical resection can be performed in symptomatic patients. The tumor may recur after surgery.

Further Reading

Buhl R, Barth H, Hugo H, et al. Dysplastic gangliocytoma of the cerebellum: rare differential diagnosis in space-occupying lesions of the posterior fossa. *Acta Neurochir (Wien).* 2003;145:509-512.
Patel S, Barkovich AJ. Analysis and classification of cerebellar malformations. *AJNR Am J Neuroradiol.* 2002;23:1074-1087.

History

▶ 59-year-old with flu-like illness brought to hospital after being found unresponsive and febrile in bed at home

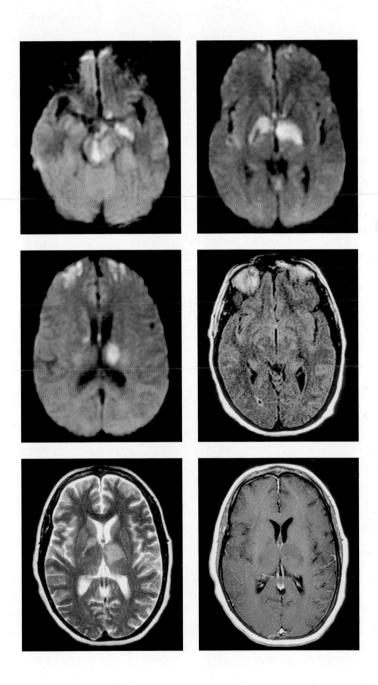

Case 11 Infarcts Secondary to Meningitis

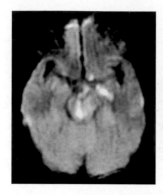 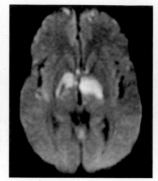 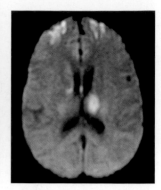

Findings

► There are areas of decreased diffusion and hyperintense signal on T2-weighted images in the brain stem, lentiform nuclei, internal capsule, thalamus, and bilateral frontal lobes.
► On the FLAIR image there is subtle hyperintense signal in several sulci, a nonspecific finding consistent with meningitis, subarachnoid hemorrhage, or elevated CSF protein.
► Postcontrast T1-weighted images show no abnormal enhancement.

Differential Diagnosis

► Vasculitis
► Early cerebritis
► Septic emboli
► Carcinomatous meningitis with infarction

Teaching Points

► Cerebral infarction is a potentially devastating complication of meningitis. The infarcts result from vascular inflammation, vasospasm, and thrombosis.
► Bacterial and tubercular meningitis are the most common causes.
► Small perforating arteries (e.g., lenticulostriates) are most commonly affected and the infarcts most commonly occur at the base of the brain. Larger vessel infarctions are also possible.

Management

► Early recognition of meningitis and antibiotic treatment minimizes the risk of this complication. However, vasculopathy and infarction may occur despite antibiotic treatment.

Further Reading

Kanamalla US, Ibarra RA, Jinkins JR. Imaging of cranial meningitis and ventriculitis. *Neuroimaging Clin North Am.* 2000;10:309-331.

History

▶ 75-year-old woman with progressive dementia

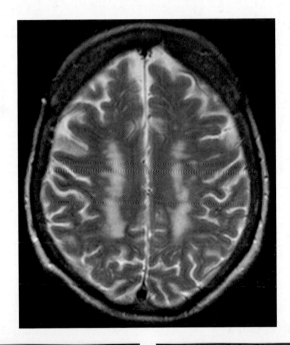

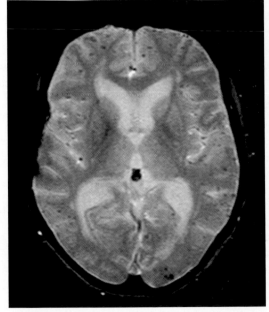

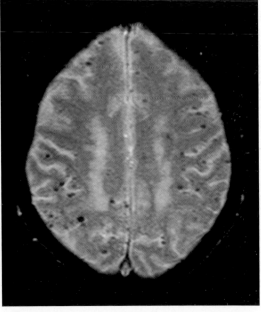

Case 12 Cerebral Amyloid Angiopathy

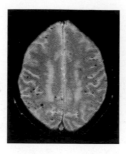

Findings

► There are numerous tiny foci of hypointensity on T2* gradient-echo (GRE) imaging, which are located at the cortical-subcortical regions and consistent with microbleeds.
► Note the sparing of the basal ganglia, thalami, and deep cerebral white matter.

Differential Diagnosis

► Hypertensive microhemorrhages
► Diffuse axonal injury
► Multiple familial cavernous malformations
► Hemorrhagic metastases
► Vasculitis

Teaching Points

► Cerebral amyloid angiopathy (CAA) is a condition characterized by accumulation of beta-amyloid protein in the vessel wall of small to medium arteries supplying the cortical and leptomeningeal regions. These vessels are fragile and prone to microhemorrhage.
► Clinical presentations include acute intracerebral hemorrhage (ICH), transient ischemic symptoms, and dementia. Many patients are asymptomatic.
► CAA represents only 2% of all ICH cases. However, in normotensive patients older than 70, it accounts for 40% to 70% of ICH cases.
► The prevalence of brain microbleeds (BMBs) is approximately 5% in healthy adults, 35% in ischemic stroke patients, and 60% in patients with nontraumatic ICH. BMBs are associated with increasing age, hypertension, and diabetes.
► T2* gradient-echo imaging is highly sensitive for detection of BMBs. In general BMBs are smaller than 5 to 10 mm.
► Imaging findings suggestive of CAA include:
  ▪ Multiple episodes of acute lobar ICH
  ▪ Multifocal BMBs located at the cortical-subcortical region and sparing the deep gray and white matter and brain stem
  ▪ Lacunar infarctions and T2 hyperintensity in the periventricular white matter
► In contrast, BMBs related to hypertension characteristically involve the basal ganglia and thalamus.

Management

► Definitive diagnosis requires biopsy. CAA is considered probable in patients older than 55 who have multiple cortical-subcortical hemorrhages of varying ages and who have no other identifiable cause for bleeding.
► There is no treatment for CAA. However, diagnosis alters the risk–benefit ratio of anticoagulation or thrombolytic therapy. Patients with CAA appear to be at increased risk of warfarin-related ICH.

Further Reading

Chao CP, Kotsenas AL, Broderick DF. Cerebral amyloid angiopathy: CT and MR imaging findings. *Radiographics*. 2006;26:1517-1531.
Cordonnier C, Al Shahi Salman R, Wardlaw J. Spontaneous brain microbleeds: systematic review, subgroup analyses and standards for study design and reporting. *Brain*. 2007;130:1988-2003.

History

▸ 5-year-old with mental status changes

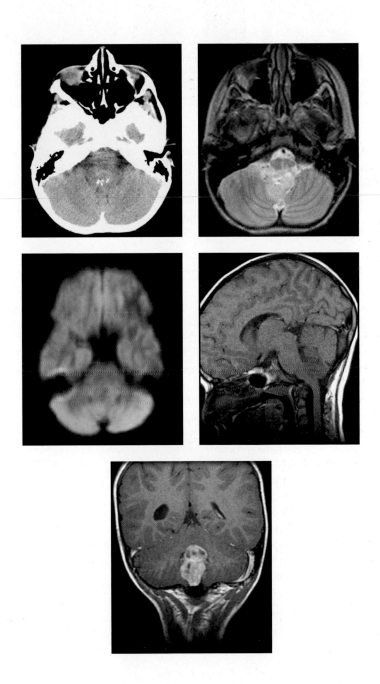

Case 13 Ependymoma

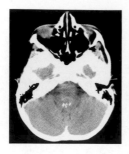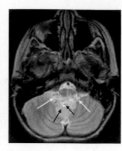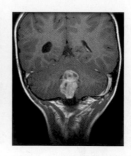

Findings

▶ Noncontrast CT demonstrates a mass in the region of the fourth ventricle. It is iso-attenuating and has coarse internal calcifications.

▶ The mass is hyperintense on T2-weighted images, demonstrates heterogeneous enhancement, and has no restricted diffusion. Punctuate T2 hypointense foci (black arrows) may represent calcification, hemorrhage, or small vessels.

▶ The tumor extends through the foramina of Luschka (white arrows).

Differential Diagnosis

▶ Medulloblastoma
▶ Choroid plexus papilloma
▶ Atypical teratoid/rhabdoid tumor
▶ Cerebellar pilocytic astrocytoma

Teaching Points

▶ Ependymomas are neoplasms that arise from ependymal cells within the ventricles or the central canal of the spinal cord. They account for 10% of all pediatric brain tumors and are the third most common posterior fossa tumor in children (after medulloblastomas and pilocytic astrocytomas).

▶ Approximately 60% of ependymomas arise from the fourth ventricle, usually its floor. In this location, patients often present with obstructive hydrocephalus, at a mean age of 6 years.

▶ Characteristic features on MRI and CT include:
  ▪ A "plastic" growth pattern with extension through the foramina of Luschka and Magendie, into adjacent cisterns, and surrounding vessels and cranial nerves
  ▪ Heterogeneous enhancement, focal calcifications, and hemorrhage

▶ Medulloblastoma is the main differential consideration. Medulloblastoma is less likely to present with calcifications (20%), usually arises near the roof of the fourth ventricle, and often has restricted diffusion.

▶ Supratentorial ependymomas arise from the lateral and third ventricles and occur in older patients (20 years). They are more likely to be extraventricular (70%) and cystic compared to infratentorial ependymomas.

▶ Leptomeningeal spread is less common than with medulloblastoma. It is more often seen in anaplastic and infratentorial ependymomas and younger patients.

Management

▶ Contrast-enhanced MRI of the entire spine should be performed to evaluate for drop metastases.

▶ Primary treatment is surgical resection. The degree of resection correlates with outcome. Residual tumor is treated with radiation therapy.

Further Reading

Koeller KK, Sandburg GD. Cerebral intraventricular neoplasms: radiologic–pathologic correlation. *Radiographics.* 2002;22:1473-1505.

Yuh EL, Barkovich AJ, Gupta N. Imaging of ependymomas: MRI and CT. *Childs Nerv Syst.* 2009;25:1203-1213.

History

▶ 4-year-old boy with seizures

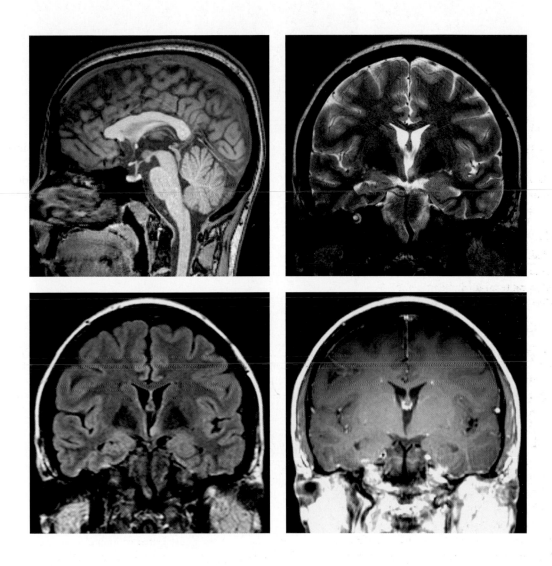

Case 14 Hypothalamic Hamartoma

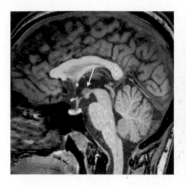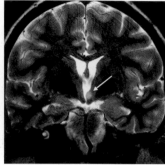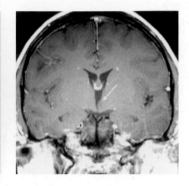

Findings

▶ There is a small round T1 hypointense, T2 hyperintense nodule (arrow) arising from the hypothalamus, adjacent and superior to the left mammillary body.

▶ Postcontrast images demonstrate no enhancement within the lesion.

Differential Diagnosis

▶ Low-grade astrocytoma
▶ Suprasellar germinoma
▶ Langerhans cell histiocytosis
▶ Craniopharyngioma

Teaching Points

▶ Hypothalamic hamartomas (HH) represent a non-neoplastic overgrowth of hypothalamic neurons and glial cells arising from the tuber cinereum (floor of the third ventricle), and are thought to represent a congenital disorder of neuronal migration. They are associated with numerous syndromes, including Pallister-Hall syndrome (HH, polydactyly, craniofacial and renal anomalies).

▶ Patients typically present in early childhood with gelastic seizures (episodes of uncontrollable mechanical laughter), precocious puberty, or both. Seizures may generalize and take on various forms.

▶ HHs are well-defined pedunculated or sessile lesions arising from the tuber cinereum. They usually measure 1 to 3 cm.

▶ On MRI these masses are usually T1 iso- to hypointense, T2 iso- to hyperintense. They lack calcification and contrast enhancement.

▶ The absence of contrast enhancement and long-term stability of size and appearance favor HH over the other differential considerations.

Management

▶ Hormonal suppressive therapy (gonadotropin-releasing hormone agonist therapy) for precocious puberty and antiseizure medications are first-line treatments.

▶ Surgery is performed for failure of medical therapy or rapid growth of the hamartoma. Surgical options include open resection, radiosurgery, and radiofrequency ablation.

Further Reading

Freeman JL, Coleman LT, Wellard RM, et al. MR imaging and spectroscopic study of epileptogenic hypothalamic hamartomas: analysis of 72 cases. *AJNR Am J Neuroradiol*. 2004;25:450-462.

Saleem SN, Said AM, Lee DH. Lesions of the hypothalamus: MR imaging diagnostic features. *Radiographics*. 2007;27:1087-1108.

History

▶ 21-year-old woman presenting to the ED after a generalized tonic-clonic seizure

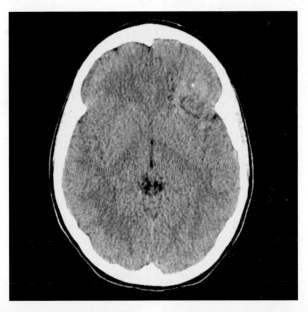

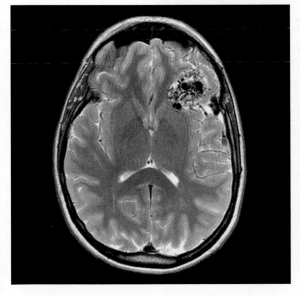

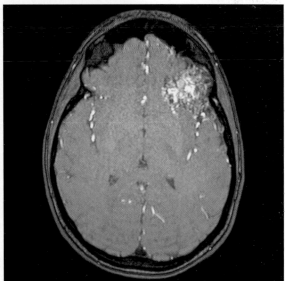

Case 15 Cerebral Arteriovenous Malformation (AVM)

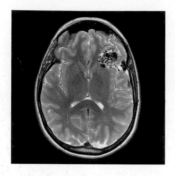 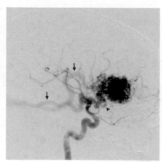

Findings

► The CT shows a heterogeneous mass in the left inferior frontal lobe. Its predominant attenuation is slightly greater than gray matter, and it contains focal calcification.
► The T2-weighted image demonstrates numerous curvilinear flow voids of varying size. There is no edema and little mass effect.
► There is corresponding flow-related enhancement on time-of-flight MRA.
► Injection of the left internal carotid artery shows enlarged MCA branches (arrowhead), a dense vascular nidus, and early draining veins (arrows).

Differential Diagnosis

► With the MRI, the diagnosis of a large AVM is certain, but based on the CT alone the differential includes:
  ▪ Intra-axial neoplasm (e.g., oligodendroglioma)
  ▪ Focal cortical dysplasia

Teaching Points

► AVMs are developmental vascular malformations that have a nidus of small, tortuous, thin-walled, low-resistance vessels that bypass the capillary bed and permit rapid arteriovenous shunting.
► They are usually detected in young or middle-aged adults. Unruptured AVMs may present with headache, seizure, or focal neurologic deficit.
► The estimated risk of rupture is 2% to 4% per year.
► On CT, AVMs typically have the attenuation of the blood in the dural sinuses. Foci of calcification are common.
► MRI demonstrates the enlarged feeding arteries, nidus, and enlarged veins as round or serpiginous flow voids of varying size. The slower-flowing components (usually veins) may enhance after intravenous contrast.
► On MRI, small AVMs may be visible only as an enlarged draining vein. They can be entirely obscured by hemorrhage. When suspicion for AVM is high, catheter cerebral angiography is necessary.
► Angiographic features that should be assessed include the feeding arteries, nidus size and location, the presence of feeding artery or intranidal aneurysms, venous drainage pattern, and the presence of venous stenoses. Feeding artery and intranidal aneurysms and venous stenoses are dangerous features that increase the risk of hemorrhage.
► The Spetzler-Martin classification system uses AVM size, location, and venous drainage pattern to predict the risk of surgical morbidity.

Management

► AVMs may be treated by endovascular embolization with liquid embolics, surgical resection, or radiosurgery. Often, a combination of these techniques is necessary.

Further Reading

Morris P. *Practical Neuroangiography*, 2nd ed. Philadelphia: Lippincott Williams Wilkins; 2007:355-378.

History

▸ 25-year-old man found at home with decreased level of consciousness, aphasia, and spastic quadriparesis

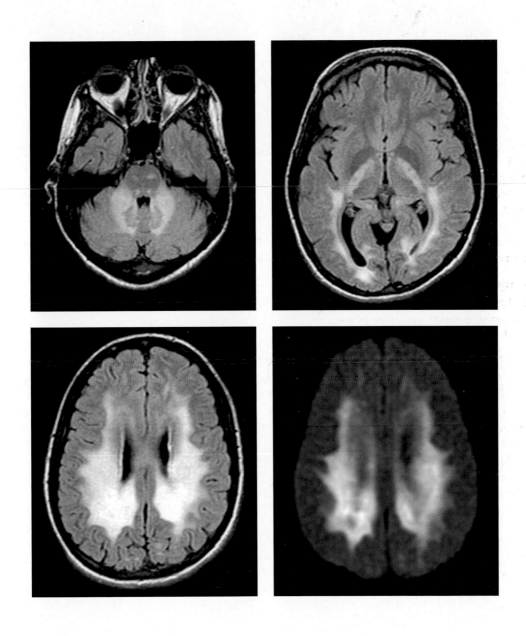

Case 16   Heroin Leukoencephalopathy ("Chasing the Dragon")

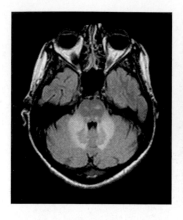 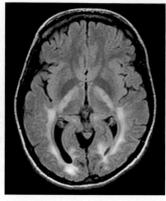 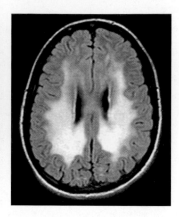

Findings

- There is hyperintense signal FLAIR images throughout the centrum semiovale, posterior limb of the internal capsule, deep cerebellar white matter (sparing the dentate nuclei), and basis pontis.
- DWI shows restricted diffusion in deep white matter.

Differential Diagnosis

- Hypoxic/ischemic encephalopathy
- Other toxic-metabolic leukoencephalopathy

Teaching Points

- "Chasing the dragon" refers to the inhalation of heroin vapors when the freebase form of heroin is heated. Despite the prevalence of heroin inhalation, the leukoencephalopathy resulting from this practice is rare.
- Typically patients present days to months after the toxic exposure and symptoms progress over the course of several weeks. Clinical presentation and progression is highly varied, ranging from mild ataxia and motor restlessness to death.
- MRI findings are specific to this leukoencephalopathy. There is symmetric hyperintense signal on T2-weighted images in the posterior cerebral white matter, splenium of the corpus callosum, posterior limb of the internal capsule, cerebellar peduncles, and cerebellar white matter. There is a predilection for the corticospinal tract and medial lemniscus.
- Gray matter structures are spared.
- When imaging through the posterior fossa, findings can resemble a "bearded man," with the dentate nuclei representing the beard and the corticospinal tracts and medial lemniscus representing the eyes and mouth, respectively.

Management

- Supportive care. Antioxidant therapy has been employed by some but there is no proven specific treatment.

Further Reading

Strang J, Griffiths P, Gossop M. Heroin smoking by "chasing the dragon": origins and history. *Addiction.* 1997;92:673-683.
Wolters EC, van Wijngaarden GK, Stam FC, et al. Leukoencephalopathy after inhaling "heroin" pyrolysate. *Lancet.* 1982;2:1233-1237.

History

► Neonate with poor feeding, hypertonia, posterior arching of the back, and a history of hyperbilirubinemia

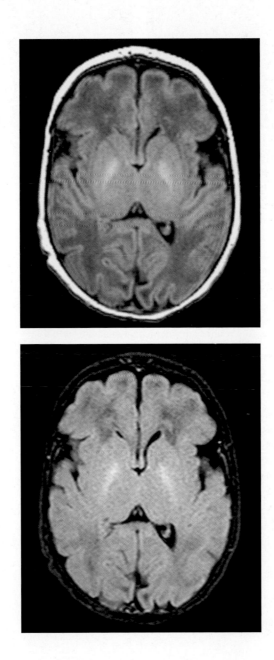

Case 17 Kernicterus

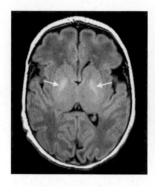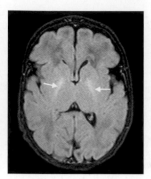

Findings

▶ Axial T1-weighted and FLAIR images show abnormal symmetric hyperintensity in the bilateral globus pallidi (arrows). The thalami and putamina are normal.
▶ The relative hypointensity of the white matter is normal for a neonate with immature myelination.

Differential Diagnosis

▶ Toxic/metabolic: manganese (hyperalimentation), CO poisoning, methylmalonic acidemia
▶ Profound hypoxic-ischemic injury
▶ Hepatic failure

Teaching Points

▶ Kernicterus is a toxic encephalopathy resulting from unconjugated bilirubin injury to the brain in neonates with hyperbilirubinemia.
▶ Serum bilirubin levels do not fully correlate with brain injury, and a multitude of other factors contribute to the disease and its presentation.
▶ History of blood type incompatibility or family history of red blood cell abnormalities is common, but the disorder can be seen in other patients. Initially, patients have nonspecific hypotonia, poor feeding, and decreased alertness, which progresses to hypertonia and posterior arching of the neck and back. Choreoathetoid cerebral palsy, developmental delay, and hearing loss may manifest as the child grows older.
▶ The globus pallidi, subthalamic nuclei, substantia nigra, hippocampi, and dentate nuclei can be involved.
▶ Noncontrast MRI is best imaging tool, but MRI abnormalities may not be present in all patients. Ultrasound occasionally shows subtle globus pallidus hyperechogenicity.
▶ MRI of acutely symptomatic neonates shows symmetric T1 hyperintensity in the globus pallidi and occasionally in the hippocampi, substantia nigra, and dentate nuclei. The diagnosis may be difficult as there is often very subtle T1 hyperintensity in the globus pallidi in normal neonates. Subtle T2 and FLAIR hyperintensity in the globus pallidi may also be present.
▶ In chronic cases, there may be volume loss and T2 hyperintensity of the globus pallidi.

Management

▶ Phototherapy and exchange transfusion are the mainstay of acute-stage treatment.

Further Reading

Coskun A, Yikilmaz A, Kumandas S, et al. Hyperintense globus pallidus on T1-weighted MR imaging in acute kernicterus: is it common or rare? *Eur Radiol.* 2005;15:1263-1267.
Katar S, Akay HO, Taskesen M, et al. Clinical and cranial magnetic resonance imaging (MRI) findings of 21 patients with serious hyperbilirubinemia. *J Child Neurol.* 2008;23:415-417.

History

▶ 27-year-old woman with new-onset seizures

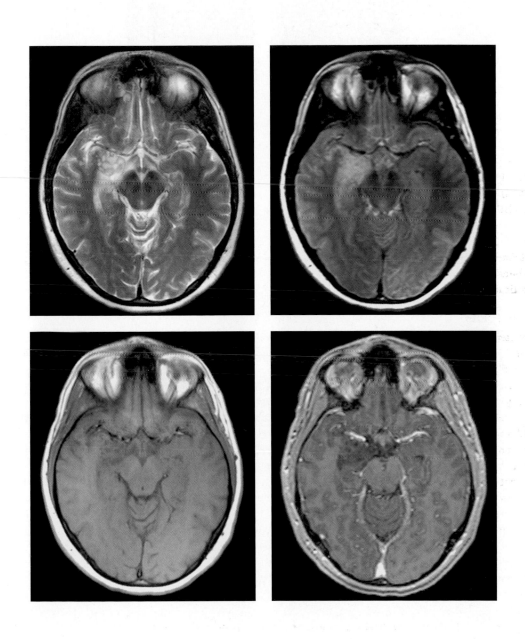

Case 18 Dysembryoplastic Neuroepithelial Tumor (DNET)

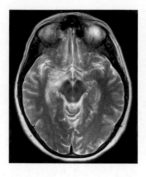 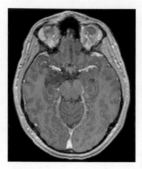

Findings

▶ MRI shows a T2 hyperintense, nonenhancing, cortically based lesion in the right medial temporal lobe with a multicystic ("bubbly") appearance.

▶ There is mild mass effect and little surrounding edema.

Differential Diagnosis

▶ Ganglioglioma
▶ Pleomorphic xanthoastrocytoma
▶ Astrocytoma
▶ Oligodendroglioma
▶ Focal cortical dysplasia

Teaching Points

▶ DNET is a rare benign (WHO grade I) neuroepithelial tumor in children or young adults with a classic clinical history of drug-resistant partial complex seizures.

▶ Histologic criteria include at least one of the following characteristics: a specific glioneuronal element, a nodular component, or an association with cortical dysplasia (more than 50%).

▶ DNETs demonstrate little to no increase in size over time and have an excellent prognosis. Surgical resection is curative in most cases, even if partial.

▶ The temporal lobe is the most common site (approximately 60%); however, these neoplasms may be found in the frontal (31%) and parietal lobes, caudate nucleus, and septum pellucidum.

▶ CT reveals a wedge-shaped, low-attenuation, cortical/subcortical lesion that may be mistaken for an acute infarction. If the tumor is adjacent to the skull, it may remodel the inner table. Calcification is present in one third of cases.

▶ MRI features include:
  ▪ T1 hypointense, T2 hyperintense cortically based lesion, usually without enhancement
  ▪ No peritumoral edema (unless complicated by hemorrhage) or significant mass effect
  ▪ "Bubbly" or multi-septated appearance

▶ These lesions are difficult to distinguish from the other low-grade neoplasms listed in the differential diagnosis on the basis of imaging alone.

Management

▶ Surgical resection

Further Reading

Fernandez C, Girard N, Paz Paredes A, et al. The usefulness of MR imaging in the diagnosis of dysembryoplastic neuroepithelial tumor in children: a study of 14 cases. *AJNR Am J Neuroradiol.* 2003;24:829-834.

Shin JH, Lee HK, Khang SK, et al. Neuronal tumors of the central nervous system: radiologic findings and pathologic correlation. *Radiographics.* 2002;22:1177-1189.

History

► 63-year-old man with left-sided pulsatile tinnitus

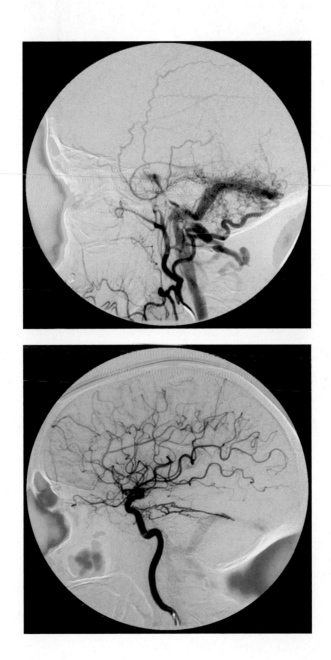

Case 19   Dural Arteriovenous Fistula (DAVF)

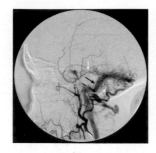 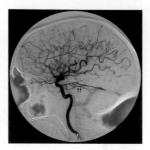

Findings

▶ External carotid artery injection shows a multiple small branches arising from the occipital and middle meningeal arteries (white arrows). There is rapid arteriovenous shunting with early opacification of the transverse and sigmoid sinuses (black arrow).

▶ Internal carotid artery injection shows several dural branches arising from the cavernous internal carotid artery (ICA)supplying the fistula (black double arrow).

▶ There is no cortical venous reflux.

Differential Diagnosis

▶ Arteriovenous malformation (AVM)

▶ Vascular neoplasm (e.g., glomus jugulotympanicum)

Teaching Points

▶ A dural arteriovenous fistula is a vascular malformation of the head or spine that exists within or along the meninges and consists of one or more direct arteriovenous anastomoses. They are distinctly different from brain AVMs in their pathophysiology and evaluation. They are thought to be acquired lesions and may form as a result of trauma or old venous sinus thrombosis.

▶ The most common locations are about the transverse and sigmoid sinuses or cavernous sinus. Common presentations include headache, pulsatile tinnitus, and cranial nerve deficits.

▶ Patients are at risk for intracerebral or subdural hemorrhage when the flow through the fistula is directly into a cortical vein or if it refluxes from a dural sinus into a cortical vein.

▶ While CT and MRI demonstrate cerebral edema or the presence of hemorrhage, the fistula itself is usually difficult to identify. Prominent flow voids may be present on MRI.

▶ MRA may show enlarged arteries and high-velocity flow in cerebral veins or dural sinuses. CTA may show arterial levels of opacification in venous structures or enlarged transosseous channels. Both may show unusual patterns of venous drainage that occur secondary to stenosis or occlusion of primary pathways.

▶ Small AVFs may not be visible on any modality other than high-quality cerebral angiography. Angiographic features that should be specifically assessed include the feeding arteries, venous drainage, and the presence of rapid or retrograde flow in cortical veins.

Management

▶ Treatment is indicated in the setting of cortical venous reflux or intolerable symptoms. The primary treatment modality is endovascular embolization, either transarterial embolization with liquid embolic materials or transvenous occlusion with coils. Surgical occlusion is sometimes necessary.

Further Reading

Cognard C, Januel AC, Silva, NA Jr, et al. Arteriovenous fistulas with cortical venous drainage: new management using Onyx. *AJNR Am J Neuroradiol.* 2008;29:235-241.

Morris P. *Practical Neuroangiography*, 2nd ed. Philadelphia: Lippincott Williams Wilkins; 2007:381-403.

History

► 76-year-old woman with chronic lymphocytic leukemia (CLL), now presenting with several weeks of worsening vision loss, left facial droop, dysarthria, and memory loss

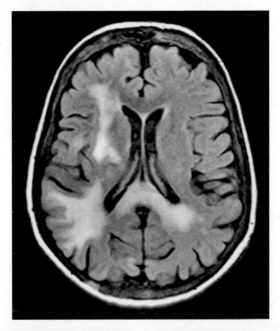

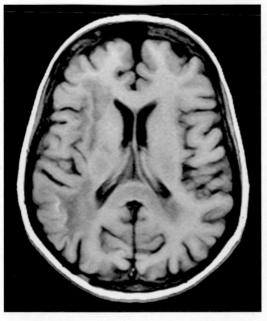

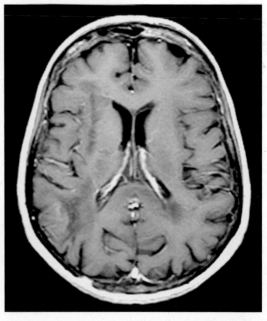

Case 20 Progressive Multifocal Leukoencephalopathy (PML)

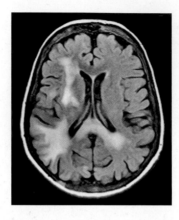

Findings

► FLAIR images show several large areas of hyperintense signal in the white matter of the right cerebral hemisphere and in the splenium of the corpus callosum. Small sites of cortical involvement are present. There is little mass effect.
► There is no abnormal enhancement.

Differential Diagnosis

► HIV encephalitis
► Other viral encephalitis (e.g., cytomegalovirus)
► Acute disseminated encephalomyelitis (ADEM)
► Nonenhancing forms of toxoplasmosis or lymphoma (rare)

Teaching Points

► PML is a demyelinating process caused by the JC polyomavirus. This virus infects or becomes active in patients with severe immunodeficiency, such as AIDS, lymphoproliferative or myeloproliferative disorders, immunosuppressive therapy, or congenital immunodeficiency. Recently cases of PML have occurred in patients with multiple sclerosis undergoing treatment with natalizumab.
► Classic clinical presentation includes focal neurologic deficits, most commonly limb weakness or ataxia. This presentation helps to distinguish PML from HIV encephalitis, which usually presents with global cognitive decline.
► The process predominantly affects white matter, but some involvement of gray matter structures is present in 50% of cases.
► The lesions present on MRI are usually asymmetric and nonenhancing.
► In the setting of recently initiated highly active retroviral therapy (HAART), marginal enhancement is more common. Such patients may experience a marked clinical deterioration, termed "immune reconstitution inflammatory syndrome" (IRIS).

Management

► The diagnosis may be confirmed by the presence of JC viral antigen in the CSF using PCR. The only known effective treatment is reconstitution of the immune system with antiretroviral therapy.

Further Reading

Buckle C, Castillo M. Use of diffusion-weighted imaging to evaluate the initial response for progressive multifocal leukoencephalopathy to highly active antiretroviral therapy: Early experience. *AJNR Am J Neuroradiol.* 2010;31:1031-1035.
Weber T. Progressive multifocal leukoencephalopathy. *Neurol Clin.* 2008;26:833-854.

History

▶ 3-year-old with epilepsy and mild left-sided weakness

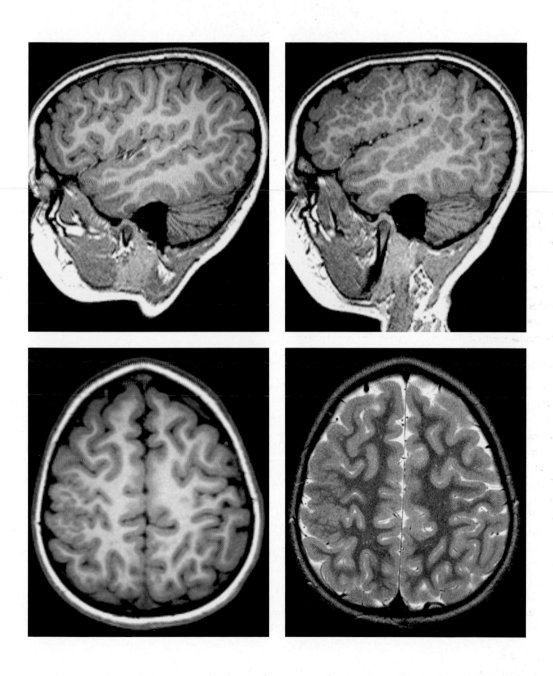

Case 21 Polymicrogyria

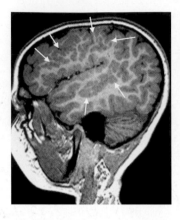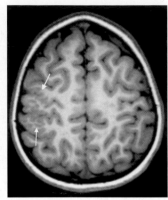

Findings

- ▶ Sagittal T1-weighted images show an area of small, irregular gyri and a serrated appearance to the gray–white junction (arrows) in the perisylvian cortex.
- ▶ Axial T1- and T2-weighted images confirm the abnormal small and irregular gyri. However, there is no signal abnormality in the morphologically abnormal cortex.

Differential Diagnosis

- ▶ Focal cortical dysplasia
- ▶ Pachygyria
- ▶ Schizencephaly

Teaching Points

- ▶ Polymicrogyria is a malformation of abnormal cortical organization. Multiple small irregular gyri are seen.
- ▶ Polymicrogyria may be unilateral or bilateral, focal or diffuse. It may be isolated, sporadic, or syndromic. It may be associated with other brain malformations or seen in conjunction with other findings in diseases such as schizencephaly, congenital cytomegalovirus, or some inborn errors of metabolism.
- ▶ Patients may present at any age. Congenital hemiparesis, seizures, and developmental delay are common symptoms. Symptoms depend on location and extent of involvement and the associated anomalies.
- ▶ High-resolution MR imaging in multiple planes is helpful in establishing the diagnosis. With routine-resolution MRI scans, the cortex may appear thick (pachygyria) or the abnormality may easily be missed.
- ▶ Gray–white junction irregularities and "bumpiness" may be the best clue to the diagnosis. The involved sulci can be shallow or absent. Sometimes there is an abnormal infolding of the brain surface in the areas involved.
- ▶ There is usually no cortical signal abnormality despite the abnormal morphology. The degree of brain myelination may affect the appearance and visualization of the abnormalities.

Management

- ▶ Control of seizures with medication and supportive care remains the mainstay of treatment. Surgery may be performed for accessible lesions in patients with intractable epilepsy.

Further Reading

Barkovich AJ. Current concepts of polymicrogyria. *Neuroradiology.* 2010;52:479-487.
Guerrini R. Genetic malformations of the cerebral cortex and epilepsy. *Epilepsia.* 2005;46 Suppl 1:32-37.

History

▶ Six-week-old infant with new-onset seizures

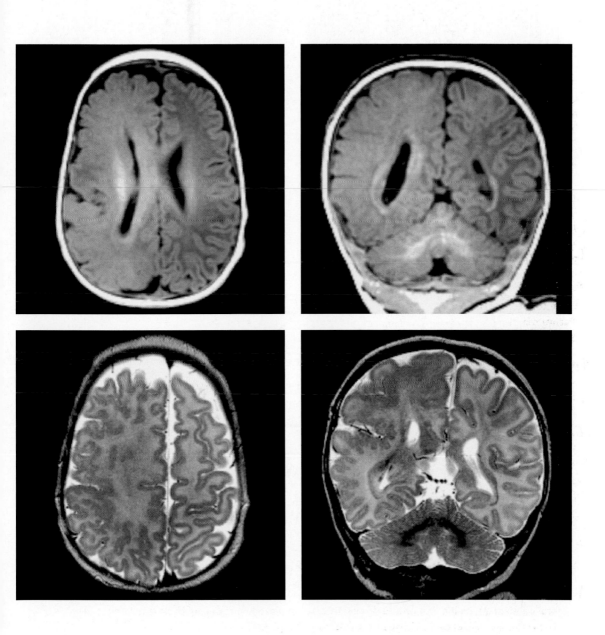

Case 22 Hemimegalencephaly

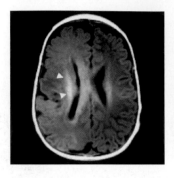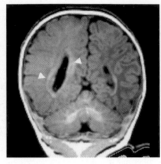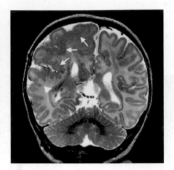

Findings

▸ The right cerebral hemisphere is enlarged.
▸ The right lateral ventricle is slightly larger and abnormally shaped.
▸ In the white matter of the right cerebral hemisphere there is hyperintense signal on T1-weighted images and hypointense signal on T2-weighted images for age. It is both focal (arrowheads) and diffuse, with blurring of gray–white differentiation.
▸ The cortex of the right hemisphere is dysplastic, thick, and polymicrogyric (arrows).

Differential Diagnosis

▸ Gliomatosis cerebri
▸ Hemiatrophy of one hemisphere, such as in Rasmussen encephalitis
▸ Tuberous sclerosis (TS)

Teaching Points

▸ Hemimegalencephaly is a congenital malformation characterized by the abnormal proliferation, migration, and differentiation of neurons. The neurons are giant and decreased in number. There is white matter hypertrophy with increased glial cells and synapses.
▸ The disorder is associated with neurocutaneous and overgrowth syndromes, including tuberous sclerosis, NF-1, and Klippel-Trenaunay-Weber.
▸ Infants present with seizures, psychomotor delay, and contralateral hemiparesis.
▸ The involved hemisphere is asymmetrically enlarged. Unlike acquired cerebral enlargement (e.g., edema, gliomatosis), the ipsilateral ventricle is enlarged as well.
▸ White matter is abnormal with generally advanced myelination and focal heterogeneous signal on T1-weighted images. Neuronal migration abnormalities (e.g., polymicrogyria, pachygyria, heterotopias) may be present. Calcifications may be present.
▸ The disorder may involve only a portion of a hemisphere (focal megalencephaly), often in the occipital lobe.
▸ In later stages there may be secondary brain atrophy later due to prolonged seizures.

Management

▸ In the setting of intractable seizures, hemispherectomy is the treatment of choice.
▸ Careful examination of the contralateral hemisphere is important, as malformations on the other side may preclude hemispherectomy.

Further Reading

Flores-Sarnat L. Hemimegalencephaly: part 1. Genetic, clinical, and imaging aspects. *J Child Neurol.* 2002;17:373-384.
Woo CL, et al. Radiologic–pathologic correlation in focal cortical dysplasia and hemimegalencephaly in 18 children. *Pediatr Neurol.* 2001;25:295-303.

History

▶ Newborn with heart murmur and episodes of desaturation

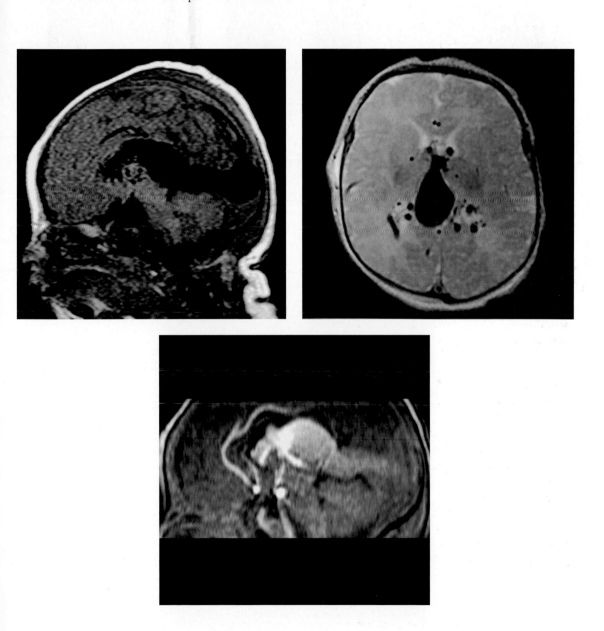

Case 23 Vein of Galen Aneurysmal Malformation (VGAM)

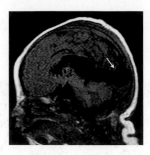

Findings

- Sagittal T1-weighted and axial T2-weighted images show a large flow void along the expected locations of the internal cerebral veins and vein of Galen.
- These aneurysmal veins are continuous with the median vein of the prosencephalon (arrow) and there is no visible straight sinus.
- Sagittal MIP reconstruction from MR angiography shows flow-related enhancement in enlarged arteries and in the aneurysmal vein, consistent with the presence of a high-flow fistula.
- There is no hydrocephalus.

Differential Diagnosis

- Vein of Galen aneurysmal dilatation

Teaching Points

- VGAMs are rare congenital arteriovenous fistulas of the deep venous system. The development of an AV fistula in the embryo at 6 to 11 weeks results in persistence and dilatation of the median vein of the prosencephalon and, usually, hypoplasia of the normal deep venous system.
- VGAMs may be classified into two types:
  - Choroidal VGAMs have a complex network of arteriovenous anastomoses with torrential arteriovenous shunting. Such children usually present shortly after birth with high-output heart failure and hydrocephalus.
  - Mural VGAMs have fewer arteriovenous communications and have lesser degrees of AV shunting. These children present in infancy or early childhood with hydrocephalus or developmental delay.
- Vein of Galen aneurysmal dilatations may appear similar but are really AVMs with drainage into an otherwise normal deep venous system.
- The enlarged vein and presence of hydrocephalus are visible on ultrasound, CT, or MRI. Of these, MRI best demonstrates the arterial and venous anatomy as well as areas of parenchymal damage. MRA shows arterialized flow in the enlarged veins.
- Cerebral angiography is rarely needed until the time of treatment planning.

Management

- Endovascular embolization is the primary treatment modality. In neonates with cardiac failure refractory to medical management, urgent partial embolization decreases the arteriovenous shunting. If possible, treatment is best delayed until 5 to 6 months of age.
- With modern ICU management and endovascular embolization, prognosis has substantially improved and more children now survive without neurologic impairment.

Further Reading

Lasjaunias PL, Chang SM, Sachet M, et al. The management of vein of Galen aneurysmal malformations. *Neurosurgery.* 2006;359: S184-S194.

Morris P. *Practical Neuroangiography*, 2nd ed. Philadelphia: Lippincott Williams Wilkins; 2007:368-373.

History

▶ 3-year-old boy with progressive swelling in the side of the face and periauricular region, not responding to antibiotics

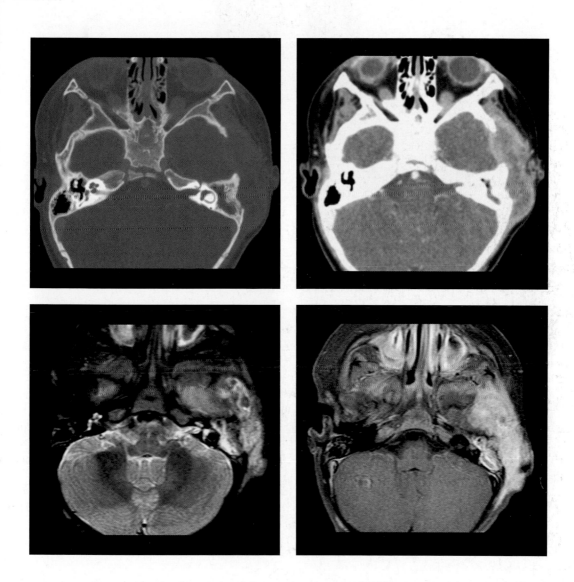

Case 24 Langerhans Cell Histiocytosis

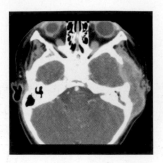

Findings

▶ CT images demonstrate a destructive lesion of the left temporal bone with well-defined bone margins and an associated enhancing soft tissue mass. The left mastoid air cells are opacified.

▶ MR images demonstrate a heterogeneous enhancing mass, mostly hyperintense on T2-weighted images, within and superficial to the left temporal bone.

Differential Diagnosis

▶ Coalescent mastoiditis with extension of infection

▶ Rhabdomyosarcoma

▶ Metastases from neuroblastoma or leukemia

▶ Dermoids or epidermoids

Teaching Points

▶ Langerhans cell histiocytosis (eosinophilic granuloma, histiocytosis X) is a proliferative disease of histiocytes with granuloma formation.

▶ The disease commonly presents in children less than 15 years of age. It may be localized or multifocal. It most commonly occurs in bones but can involve almost any organ. Common areas of involvement are the calvarium, temporal bones, spine (vertebra plana), suprasellar region (thickening of the pituitary infundibulum), extremity bones, thorax, and skin.

▶ Patient symptoms and presentation depend on the area of involvement. Osseous lesions may sometimes be painful. Pituitary stalk lesions present with endocrinopathies and diabetes insipidus. Temporal bone lesions may mimic chronic ear infections.

▶ The bone lesions may be demonstrated on radiographs or CT. They are usually well-defined lytic areas, often with a soft tissue mass.

▶ On bone scans, they may be positive (with a hot peripheral halo), but false-negative rates are high. If lesions are active, they will show increased FDG uptake on PET scans.

▶ On MRI, the lesions are T1-hypointense and T2-hyperintense and enhance avidly. The soft tissue component may appear well defined or infiltrative.

Management

▶ Surgical resection, curettage, steroids, radiation therapy, chemotherapy, and vasopressin supplementation are used in the treatment of this disease. Treatment depends on location and extent of disease and symptoms in each patient.

Further Reading

Kilborn TN, Teh J, Goodman TR. Paediatric manifestations of Langerhans cell histiocytosis: a review of the clinical and radiological findings. *Clin Radiol.* 2003;58:269-278.

Meyer JS, Harty MP, Mahboubi S, et al. Langerhans cell histiocytosis: presentation and evolution of radiologic findings with clinical correlation. *Radiographics.* 1995;15:1135-1146.

History

► 20-month-old with lethargy and vomiting

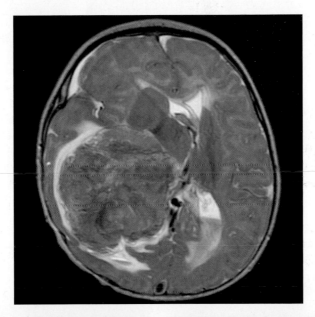

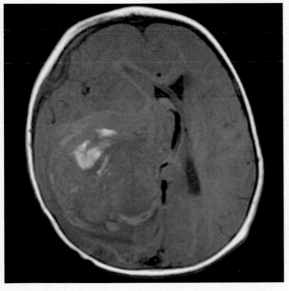

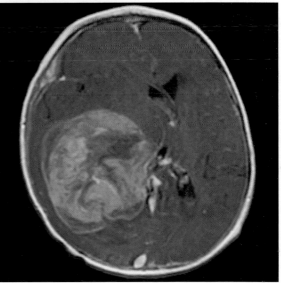

Case 25 Choroid Plexus Carcinoma (CPC)

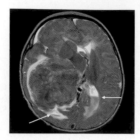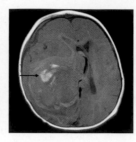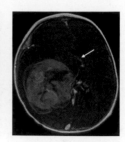

Findings

► MRI shows a large, heterogeneously enhancing mass with lobulated margins, centered within the atrium of the right lateral ventricle.

► There is focal T1 hyperintensity within the tumor (black arrow), likely representing intratumoral hemorrhage. There is a fluid–fluid level within the lateral ventricle due to dependent hemorrhage (white arrows).

► There is T2 hyperintensity and enhancement possibly within the cerebral parenchyma along the tumor margins consistent with parenchymal invasion.

Differential Diagnosis

► Choroid plexus papilloma
► Atypical teratoid-rhabdoid tumor
► Ependymoma
► Subependymal giant cell astrocytoma
► Central neurocytoma
► Metastasis

Teaching Points

► CPC is a malignant choroid plexus tumor arising from the choroid plexus epithelium.
► Choroid plexus tumors are usually found in children under 5 years of age.
► 80% of choroid plexus tumors are papillomas (WHO grade I), which have a 5-year survival rate approaching 100%. The 5-year survival rate of CPC is 25% to 50%.
► Presentation is usually related to hydrocephalus, secondary to increased CSF production.
► Choroid plexus tumors occur more commonly within the lateral ventricles in children, and within the fourth ventricle in adults.
► Contrast-enhanced MRI is the most useful imaging study.
  ▪ CPC is a heterogeneous intraventricular mass with areas of hemorrhage, necrosis, and cystic change. Calcifications are seen in 25%.
  ▪ It is usually T1 isointense with variable T2 signal and prominent enhancement.
  ▪ Choroid plexus tumors have a characteristic finely lobulated appearance along their margins.
► Imaging cannot differentiate between CPC and papilloma, but extraventricular invasion and CSF spread favor CPC.

Management

► Postcontrast imaging of the spine is needed to evaluate for CSF spread.
► Primary treatment is surgical resection with chemotherapy ± radiation therapy.

Further Reading

Koeller KK, Sandberg GD. From the archives of the AFIP: Cerebral intraventricular neoplasms: radiologic–pathologic correlation. *Radiographics.* 2002;22:1473-1505.

Meyers SP, Khademian ZP, Chuang SH, et al. Choroid plexus carcinomas in children: MRI features and patient outcomes. *Neuroradiology.* 2004;46:770-780.

History

▶ 5-month-old presenting with nystagmus and bilaterally abnormal optic discs on eye examination

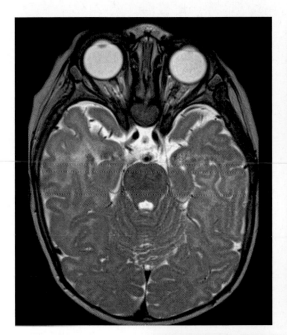
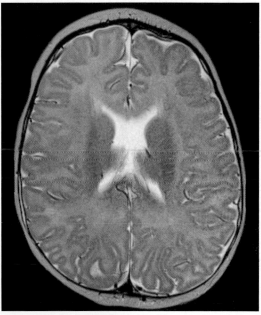
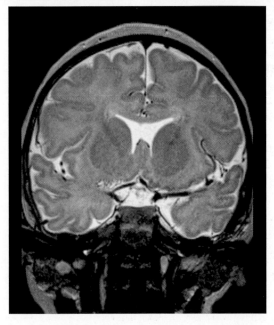

Case 26   Septo-Optic Dysplasia (SOD)

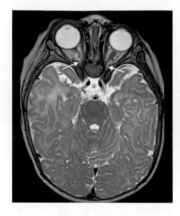 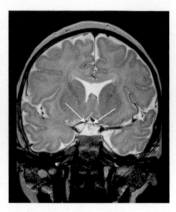

Findings

- ▶ T2-weighted MRI images show abnormally small size of the bilateral optic nerves and the optic chiasm (arrows).
- ▶ The septum pellucidum is absent.

Differential Diagnosis

- ▶ Isolated optic nerve hypoplasia
- ▶ Holoprosencephaly
- ▶ Damage to septum pellucidum in longstanding severe hydrocephalus

Teaching Points

- ▶ Septo-optic dysplasia (SOD, DeMorsier syndrome) is a heterogeneous disorder characterized by hypoplasia of the optic nerves and absence (or partial deficiency) of the septum pellucidum.
- ▶ About two thirds of patients also have disturbances of the hypothalamic–pituitary axis, including an abnormally small pituitary gland or ectopic neurohypophysis.
- ▶ A variety of other malformations can be seen in association with SOD, most commonly schizencephaly (50%). Others include gray matter heterotopia, ventriculomegaly, cortical dysplasia, hippocampal abnormalities, olfactory hypoplasia, and facial abnormalities. In some patients, there is some overlap of findings with lobar holoprosencephaly.
- ▶ The exact etiology is not known and may be multifactorial. A subset of patients have a mutation of the HESX1 gene.
- ▶ Patients may have nystagmus, poor vision, and optic disc hypoplasia on ophthalmologic examination. Those with hypothalamic–pituitary axis disturbance may have a variety of endocrine problems, including growth retardation and hypoglycemia. Epilepsy can be present in patients with associated brain malformations.
- ▶ Coronal MRI provides the best demonstration of the abnormal optic nerves.

Management

- ▶ Therapy includes seizure control in patients with epileptogenic brain malformations and hormonal replacement in those with endocrine abnormalities.

Further Reading

Polizzi A, Pavone P, Ianetti P, et al. Septo-optic dysplasia complex: a heterogeneous malformation syndrome. *Pediatr Neurol.* 2006;34: 66-71.

Riedl S, Vosahlo J, Battelino T, et al. Refining clinical phenotypes in septo-optic dysplasia based on MRI findings. *Eur J Pediatr.* 2008; 167:1269-1276.

History

▶ 67-year-old woman status post evacuation of a subdural hematoma

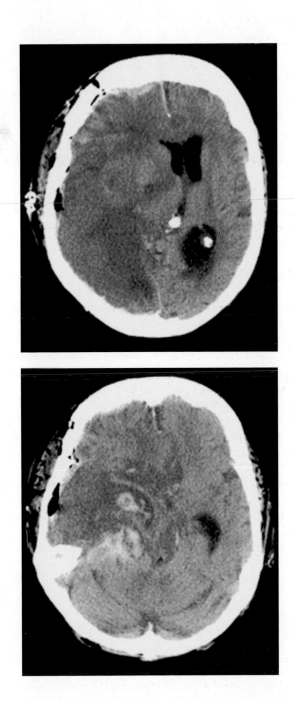

Case 27 Transfalcine, Uncal, and Transtentorial Herniation

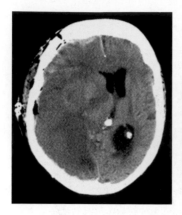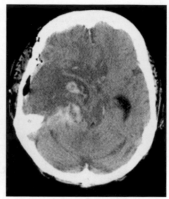

Findings

- ▶ CT after evacuation of the hematoma shows extensive hypoattenuation in the right hemisphere with loss of the gray–white differentiation. There is hemorrhage in the right temporal lobe.
- ▶ The leftward midline shift displaces the medial right frontal and parietal lobes under the falx cerebri, producing transfalcine herniation.
- ▶ The complete effacement of the basilar cisterns and compression of the brain stem are hallmarks of uncal and transtentorial herniation.
- ▶ There is trapping of the left lateral ventricle, resulting in its enlargement.

Teaching Points

- ▶ With increased intracranial pressure resulting from a mass, edema, hemorrhage, or an inflammatory process, the brain can herniate from one compartment into another. Trauma is the most common cause of herniation.
- ▶ It is not uncommon for several different types of herniation to occur concomitantly, as demonstrated here.
- ▶ Subfalcine herniation, with displacement of the cingulate gyrus under the falx, is the most common type of herniation. This type of herniation compresses the ipsilateral ventricle and obstructs the foramen of Monro, resulting in dilatation of the contralateral ventricle. If the anterior cerebral arteries are displaced, they can become occluded, resulting in infarction.
- ▶ The supratentorial brain can herniate downwards and medially in central transtentorial herniation. This results in obliteration of the basilar cisterns and inferior displacement of the third ventricle and brain stem. Complications arising from this include compression of the posterior cerebral (PCA) and basilar arteries (resulting in infarction), Duret hemorrhages in the pons and midbrain, and compression of the oculomotor nerve (resulting in ipsilateral pupillary dilatation).
- ▶ Unilateral downward herniation with medial displacement of the temporal lobe over the incisura is uncal herniation.
- ▶ In the posterior fossa, the cerebellum can herniate downwards through the foramen magnum (tonsillar herniation) or upwards through the incisura, resulting in obliteration of the quadrigeminal cistern. This can obstruct the aqueduct, causing hydrocephalus.
- ▶ Following a craniectomy, the brain can herniate outwards through the skull defect. This known as external herniation.

Management

- ▶ Treatment involves decompression craniectomy and/or removal of the underlying mass or hemorrhage.

Further Reading

Kalita J, Misra UK, Vajpeyee J, et al. Brain herniations in patients with intracerebral hemorrhage. *Acta Neurol Scand.* 2009;199:254-260.

History

▶ 32-year-old woman with altered mental status

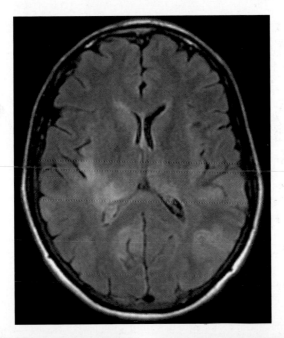

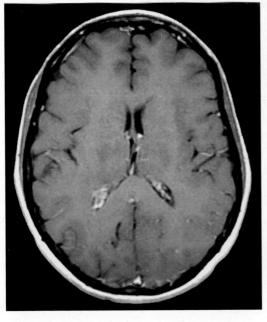

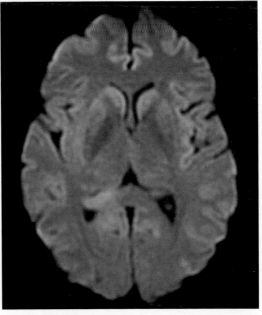

Case 28　Gliomatosis Cerebri

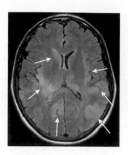

Findings

▶ There are multifocal, ill-defined areas of signal abnormality, hyperintense on FLAIR images and iso-intense on T1-weighted images. They involve the cortex, deep gray nuclei, and white matter of both hemispheres (arrows).
▶ There is mild mass effect with sulcal effacement.
▶ There is no enhancement or restricted diffusion.

Differential Diagnosis

▶ Acute disseminated encephalomyelitis or other demyelinating/dysmyelinating disorder
▶ Viral encephalitis
▶ Vasculitis
▶ Lymphoma (rare, nonenhancing form)
▶ Progressive multifocal leukoencephalopathy

Teaching Points

▶ Gliomatosis cerebri is a rare neoplasm characterized by diffuse infiltration of glial tumor into greater than two cerebral lobes, frequently bilaterally and with relative preservation of the underlying neural structures. It is classified as WHO grade III, but histologic grade and cellular differentiation vary.
▶ Gliomatosis cerebri can be difficult to recognize clinically due to subtle clinical signs. The most common history is indolent personality change and mental status disturbance. Other manifestations include seizures, dementia, and motor or visual deficits.
▶ The imaging findings are often more dramatic than the clinical picture, but they may be subtle. The most commonly affected regions are the hemispheric white matter, followed by the cortical and subcortical gray matter.
▶ The key imaging finding suggestive of gliomatosis is the presence of mass effect, which is often mild. Infectious or inflammatory disease may demonstrate mass effect but may be distinguished clinically.
▶ Most cases demonstrate no or minimal enhancement. Pronounced enhancement or the presence of a focal mass should suggest malignant degeneration into a higher-grade tumor.
▶ MR spectroscopy is nonspecific and demonstrates depressed NAA and elevated choline.
▶ The prognosis is generally poor, with the majority of patients surviving less than 1 year. The functional status at the time of diagnosis determines the length of survival.

Management

▶ MRS and perfusion studies may be used to determine the biopsy site likely to yield highest-grade neoplasm.
▶ Treatment options include corticosteroids, radiation therapy, and chemotherapy, though none has shown much effectiveness for gliomatosis cerebri.

Further Reading

Shin YM, Chang KH, Han MH, et al. Gliomatosis cerebri: comparison of MR and CT features. *AJR Am J Roentgenol.* 1993;161:859-862.
Vates GE, Chang S, Lamborn KR, et al. Gliomatosis cerebri: a review of 22 cases. *Neurosurgery.* 2003;53:261-271.

History

► 67-year-old woman status post cardiac arrest with normal CT at time of admission

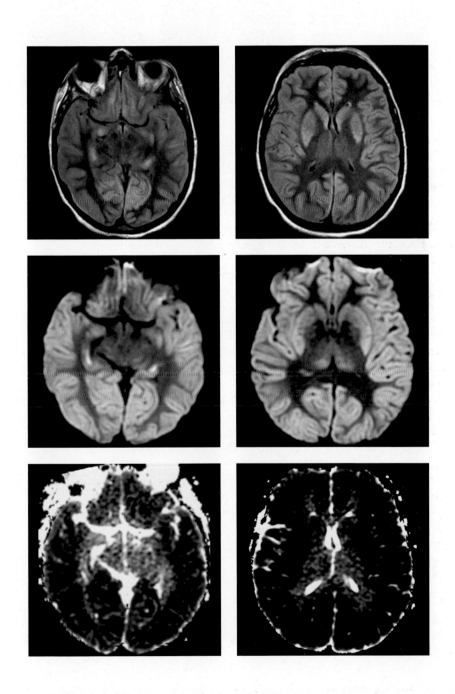

Case 29 Hypoxic-Ischemic Encephalopathy (HIE)

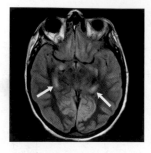 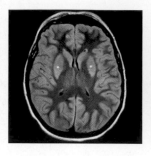 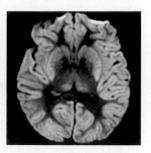

Findings

► There is hyperintense signal on FLAIR and DWI images in bilateral hippocampi (arrows), basal ganglia (asterisks), and the cerebral cortex diffusely.
► ADC maps confirm the presence of restricted diffusion at these sites.
► There is mild cortical swelling and sulcal effacement, consistent with cerebral edema.

Differential Diagnosis

► Creutzfeldt-Jakob disease (CJD)
► Mitochondrial encephalopathy
► Toxic injury

Teaching Points

► HIE results from inadequate delivery of oxygen and nutrients to the cerebrum. Severe global impairment of cerebral blood flow and blood oxygenation may occur in a variety of scenarios (e.g., cardiac arrest, drowning, birth).
► In adults, HIE primarily affects the gray matter structures (areas with excitatory amino acid receptors and high metabolic demand): basal ganglia, thalami, cerebral cortex (particularly sensorimotor and visual cortices), cerebellum, and hippocampi.
► Imaging findings in HIE are variable and dependent on brain maturity (the very young and elderly are most susceptible), severity and duration of insult, and timing of imaging.
► Noncontrast CT is insensitive during the first 24 hours. Findings include diffuse sulcal and ventricular effacement (cerebral edema), diffuse loss of gray–white matter differentiation, and hypoattenuation of the deep gray nuclei.
► MRI is the best imaging modality for the diagnosis of HIE.
  ▪ MR spectroscopy and DWI are the most sensitive sequences for detecting injury within the first few hours.
  ▪ MR spectroscopy reveals elevations in lactate and glutamine-glutamate.
  ▪ DWI shows restricted diffusion. In children, this is often most conspicuous on ADC maps.
  ▪ T2-weighted and FLAIR sequences become abnormal after 12 to 24 hours.
  ▪ Because of delayed apoptotic cell death, a post-anoxic leukoencephalopathy may become visible days to weeks after the initial insult.
► CJD may produce similar changes, but cortical involvement is usually less uniform. It is readily distinguished by history and EEG.

Management

► Treatment is supportive. Neuroprotective strategies, including hypothermia, remain experimental. Extensive HIE, as in this case, carries a poor prognosis.

Further Reading

Huang BY, Castillo M. Hypoxic-ischemic brain injury: imaging findings from birth to adulthood. *Radiographics*. 2008;28:417-439.
Sheerin F, Pretorius P, Briley D, et al. Differential diagnosis of restricted diffusion confined to the cerebral cortex. *Clin Radiol*. 2008;63:1245-1253.

History

► 48-year-old woman with headache

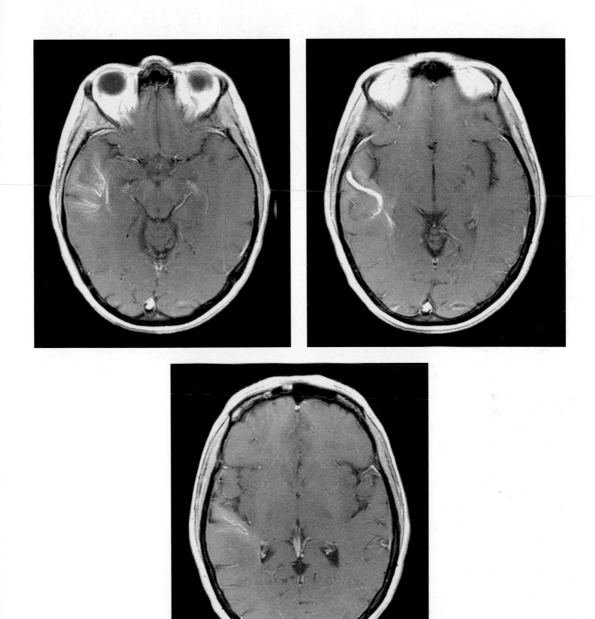

Case 30 Developmental Venous Anomaly

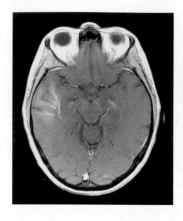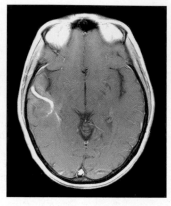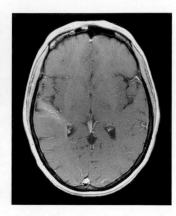

Findings

▶ The postcontrast T1-weighted images show an intracerebral complex of enhancing curvilinear vascular structures in the right temporal lobe.

▶ They coalesce to form a large vein that passes through the cerebral parenchyma to drain superficially.

Differential Diagnosis

▶ Developmental venous anomaly

▶ Arteriovenous malformation (AVM)

Teaching Points

▶ The DVA (formerly known as venous angioma) is a malformation of cerebral venous drainage consisting of an arbor of enlarged medullary veins that drain into a large central trunk that traverses the cerebral parenchyma. The DVA drains normal tissue and does not cause arteriovenous shunting.

▶ DVA represents the most common cerebral vascular malformation and is a frequent incidental finding on MRI studies of the brain.

▶ By itself DVA is usually asymptomatic. Rarely, it may thrombose and produce ischemic or hemorrhagic stroke.

▶ There is a strong association with adjacent cavernous malformation, the incidence of which is about 10%.

▶ Most DVAs are difficult to see on noncontrast CT and MRI. However, the venous channels enhance strikingly on postcontrast imaging. Their unique architecture is described as a caput medusae or hydra.

Management

▶ Angiography is rarely required but is indicated in cases of hemorrhage or when atypical features (e.g., persistence of flow voids on postcontrast T1-weighted images) are present on MRI. The early venous filling and nidus characteristic of AVMs will be absent.

▶ No treatment or follow-up is usually indicated for a DVA. Sudden occlusion of DVAs can have disastrous consequences since they drain normal tissue. For this reason, the identification of any nearby DVA and the preservation of the vein is an important part of surgical treatment of cavernous malformations.

Further Reading

Morris P. *Practical Neuroangiography*, 2nd ed. Philadelphia: Lippincott Williams Wilkins; 2007:353-355.

San Millán Ruíz D, Yilmaz H, Gailloud P. Cerebral developmental venous anomalies: Current concepts. *Ann Neurol.* 2009;66:271-283.

History

▶ 56-year-old man with right face numbness and ophthalmoplegia

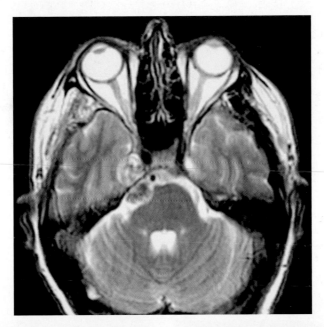

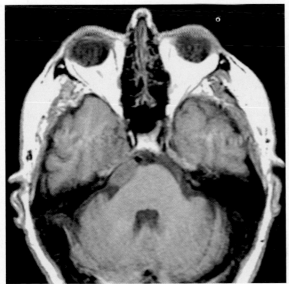

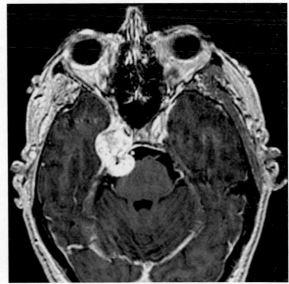

Case 31   Trigeminal Schwannoma

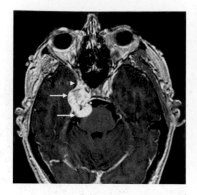 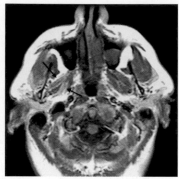

Findings

▸ There is a mass (white arrows) extending along the expected course of the right trigeminal nerve, from the pons to Meckel's cave and the inferior cavernous sinus.

▸ The mass has relatively low signal intensity on T1- and T2-weighted images and shows slightly heterogeneous enhancement.

▸ The mass expands the inferior right cavernous sinus and extends toward the superior orbital fissure (arrowhead).

▸ Note the relative atrophy of the pterygoid muscles on the right (black arrows) compared to the left.

Differential Diagnosis

▸ Trigeminal schwannoma
▸ Meningioma
▸ Metastasis
▸ Perineural tumor spread
▸ Chondrosarcoma

Teaching Points

▸ Cranial neuropathy, including numbness, trigeminal neuralgia, and ophthalmoplegia, are common presenting signs and symptoms.

▸ Trigeminal schwannomas are the second most common intracranial schwannoma. The location of the tumor along the expected course of the trigeminal nerve is the key to suggesting the diagnosis.

▸ 50% of trigeminal schwannomas arise from the segment of the nerve in Meckel's cave, in the medial middle cranial fossa. Approximately 20% remain infratentorial, arising from the trigeminal nerve adjacent to the lateral pons, and 25% extend from the posterior fossa to the middle cranial fossa, as in this case.

▸ It is unusual for intracranial schwannomas to extend extracranially, and vice versa.

Management

▸ Treatment options include stereotactic radiosurgery and operative resection. The surgical approach depends upon tumor location, and a careful assessment of tumor extent is important. Tumor recurs after surgery in up to 25% of patients; recurrence is often related to tumor that couldn't be resected in the cavernous sinus or adjacent to the brain stem.

Further Reading

MacNally SP, Rutherford SA, Ramsden RT, et al. Trigeminal schwannomas. *Br J Neurosurg.* 2008;22:729-738.
Sanders WP, Chundi VV. Extra-axial tumors including pituitary and parasellar. In: Orrison WW. *Neuroimaging.* Philadelphia: Saunders, 2000:643-647.

History

► 61-year-old woman status post trauma

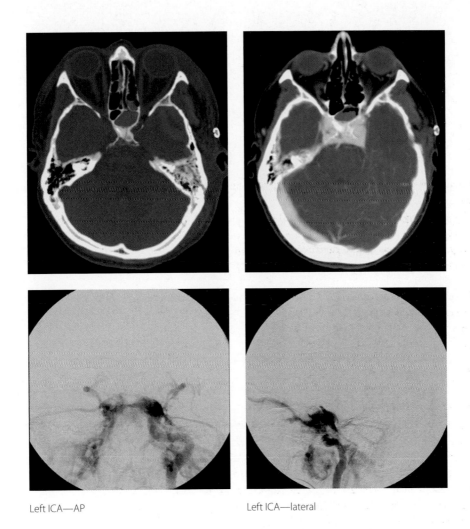

Left ICA—AP

Left ICA—lateral

Case 32 Direct Carotid-Cavernous Fistula (CCF)

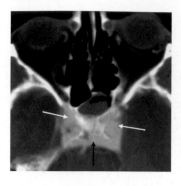 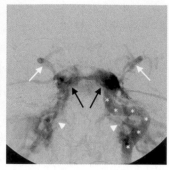 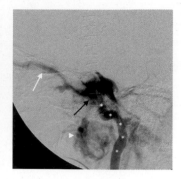

Findings

▶ CT demonstrates fractures of the basisphenoid and the left temporal bone.
▶ On CTA, there is early dense opacification of both cavernous sinuses (white arrows) and the clival venous plexus (black arrow).
▶ Injection of the left internal carotid artery (white asterisks) demonstrates arteriovenous shunting with opacification of both cavernous sinuses (black arrows) in the arterial phase. Venous outflow includes both superior ophthalmic veins (white arrows) and the pterygoid plexus (white arrowheads).

Differential Diagnosis

▶ Clinically, the differential diagnosis includes venous thrombosis and intraorbital hematoma. With these images, however, the diagnosis is clear.

Teaching Points

▶ CCFs are abnormal connections between the carotid arterial system and the cavernous sinus.
▶ There are two main types:
  ▪ Direct communication between the ICA and the cavernous sinus (Barrow type A), which demonstrates high flow and is usually secondary to traumatic laceration of the internal carotid artery (ICA) or rupture of a cavernous ICA aneurysm.
  ▪ Indirect communication between the carotid system and the cavernous sinus via dural branches of the ICA (type B), external carotid artery (ECA) (type C), or both (type D). These lesions, often without clear cause, are better classified as dural arteriovenous fistulas.
▶ Symptoms and signs depend on the magnitude and direction of venous outflow.
  ▪ Anterior drainage through the orbit may produce proptosis, chemosis, and orbital bruit. Prolonged elevation of intraocular pressure may result in permanent vision loss.
  ▪ Posterior drainage into the petrosal sinuses is usually asymptomatic but may produce cranial nerve palsies.
  ▪ Cortical venous drainage will produce venous hypertension and carries the risk of intracerebral hemorrhage.
▶ On CT, proptosis and asymmetric enlargement of the superior ophthalmic vein may be present.
▶ CTA or MRA may demonstrate arterialization of the sinus and draining veins. Time-resolved angiographic techniques are now capable of confirming the diagnosis noninvasively.
▶ Cerebral angiography is necessary to determine the nature of the fistula and fully evaluate the pattern of venous drainage.

Management

▶ Endovascular occlusion of the fistula is the treatment of choice.

Further Reading

Gemmete JJ, Ansari SA, Gandhi D. Endovascular treatment of carotid cavernous fistulas. *Neuroimag Clin North Am.* 2009;19:241-255.
Miller NR. Diagnosis and management of dural carotid-cavernous sinus fistulas. *Neurosurg Focus.* 2007;23:E13.

History

▶ 65-year-old man with 6 months' progressive difficulty sleeping, dizziness, diplopia, slurred speech, memory loss, tremors

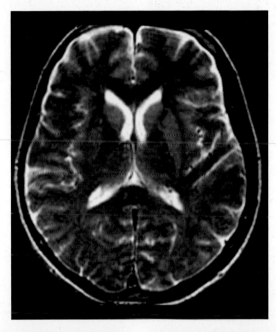

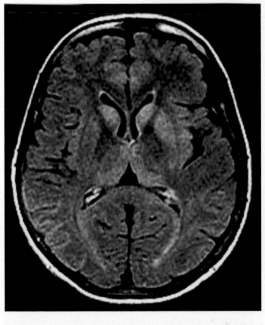

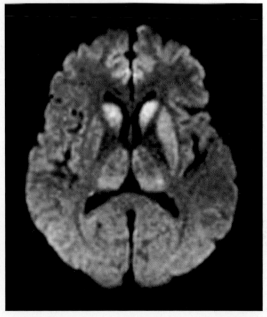

Case 33 Creutzfeldt-Jakob Disease (CJD)

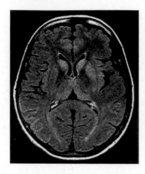 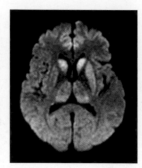

Findings

► The T2-weighted sequence demonstrates subtle hyperintense signal within the caudate head and putamen.
► The FLAIR and DWI sequences demonstrate nearly symmetric hyperintense signal within the caudate head and anterior putamen. There is similar but more subtle abnormality of the thalamus.
► There is similar asymmetric abnormality within the cortical ribbon of the temporal lobes and left insula.

Differential Diagnosis

► Paraneoplastic encephalitis
► Hypoxic-ischemic encephalopathy
► Leigh disease

Teaching Points

► CJD is a rapidly progressive spongiform encephalopathy resulting from prion infection and accumulation of the prion protein in neurons. It is most commonly acquired sporadically (85% of cases) but can be genetically transmitted (familial CJD) or transmitted by ingestion of infected neural tissue (variant CJD) or by iatrogenic contact with contaminated tissues.
► Clinical symptoms include myoclonus, ataxia, and rapidly progressive dementia. The average timefrom diagnosis to death is about 5 months.
► Premortem diagnosis once depended upon the presence of classic clinical symptoms, characteristic epileptiform discharges on EEG, and presence of 14-3-3 protein in the CSF. More recently, MRI has become an important part of the diagnostic evaluation.
► MRI has a high sensitivity and specificity for this disease. There is hyperintense signal in the caudate head, putamen, and thalamus on T2-weighted, FLAIR, and DWI sequences.
► In many patients, similar signal abnormality is present in the large areas of cortical gray matter, typically sparing the sensorimotor cortex.
► The deep gray nuclei most commonly involved are the caudate and anterior putamen. Involvement is usually bilateral and spares the globus pallidus.
► Variant CJD, caused by ingestion of cattle infected by the prion disease known as bovine spongiform encephalopathy, is associated with predominant involvement of the typical signal changes but most marked in the pulvinar of the thalamus.
► In later stages of the disease, the areas involved become atrophic. The signal abnormality on DWI may resolve.

Management

► Autopsy is needed for definitive diagnosis. There is no cure at present for this disease.

Further Reading

Tschampa HJ, Zerr I, Urbach H. Radiological assessment of Creutzfeldt-Jakob disease. *Eur Radiol.* 2007;17:1200-1211.
Young GS, Geschwind MD, Fischbein NJ, et al. Diffusion-weighted and fluid-attenuated inversion recovery imaging in Creutzfeldt-Jakob disease: High sensitivity and specificity for diagnosis. *AJNR Am J Neuroadiol.* 2005;26:1551-1562.

History

▶ 4-year-old with change in mental status, ophthalmoplegia, and dystonia

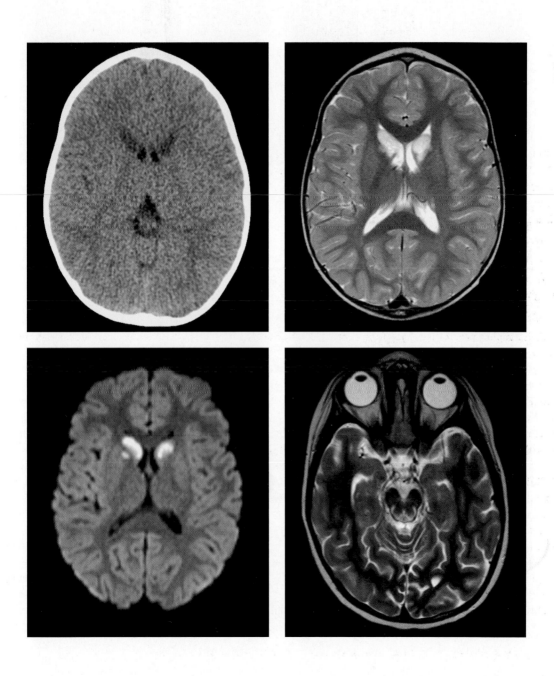

Case 34 Leigh Disease

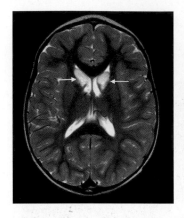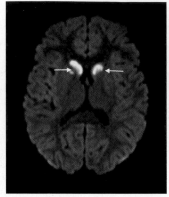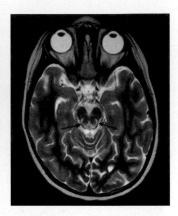

Findings

▶ Axial CT image shows abnormal symmetric hypoattenuation in the head of the caudate nuclei.
▶ Axial T2-weighted and diffusion-weighted images show increased T2 signal and restricted diffusion in the caudate nuclei (white arrows).
▶ An axial T2-weighted image more inferiorly through the level of the midbrain shows symmetric signal abnormality in the dorsal and lateral midbrain (black arrows).

Differential Diagnosis

▶ Hypoxic-ischemic injury

Teaching Points

▶ Leigh disease or syndrome (subacute necrotizing encephalomyelopathy) is a term used to refer to a genetically heterogeneous group of disorders involving energy metabolism, most commonly involving respiratory chain complexes or various parts of the pyruvate dehydrogenase complex.
▶ Patients can present with developmental regression, mental status change, hypotonia, ataxia, dystonia, seizures, swallowing and respiratory problems, and ophthalmoplegia.
▶ On imaging, they are characterized by bilaterally symmetric necrotic and demyelinating lesions involving the basal ganglia, brain stem, cerebellum, and diencephalon. Occasionally the cerebral white matter or spinal cord is also involved.
▶ On CT, the lesions will demonstrate hypoattenuation of the affected areas, though they may occasionally calcify in more chronic stages.
▶ On MRI, they are seen as relatively symmetric areas of hyperintense signal on T2-weighted and FLAIR sequences. Restricted diffusion may be present.
▶ Proton MR spectroscopy may demonstrate increased lactate.

Management

▶ Leigh disease has a poor prognosis, often with death in childhood. There is no cure. Thiamine and dichloroacetate may have benefit. A high-fat, low-carbohydrate diet may be recommended.

Further Reading

Bianchi MC, Sgandurra G, Tosetti M, et al. Brain magnetic resonance in the diagnostic evaluation of mitochondrial encephalopathies. *Biosci Rep.* 2007;27:69-85.
Saneto RP, Friedman SD, Shaw DW. Neuroimaging of mitochondrial disease. *Mitochondrion.* 2008;8:396-413.

History

▶ 43-year-old man presenting with altered mental status

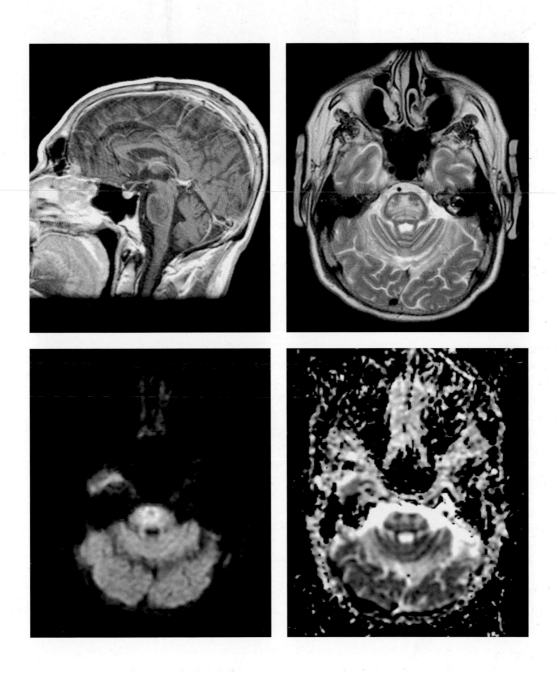

Case 35 Osmotic Demyelination Syndrome (Central Pontine Myelinolysis)

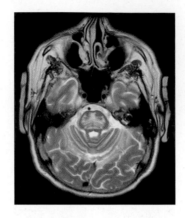

Findings

► There is signal abnormality within the central pons, hyperintense on T2-weighted images and hypointense on T1-weighted images. It spares the periphery and the corticospinal tracts.
► No enhancement or restricted diffusion is present.

Differential Diagnosis

► Brain stem glioma
► Infarction
► Multiple sclerosis
► Toxin exposure
► Hypertensive encephalopathy

Teaching Points

► Osmotic demyelination syndrome encompasses both pontine and extrapontine myelinolysis. It most commonly occurs with rapid iatrogenic correction of severe hyponatremia.
► Oligodendrocytes are very sensitive to osmotic changes, leading to cerebral injury that predominantly affects white matter.
► Patients initially present with symptoms of electrolyte disturbance (seizures, coma). Correction of the electrolytes initially improves symptoms, but then patients develop spastic quadriparesis, pseudobulbar palsy, altered mental status, and coma.
► The pons is the most common site of injury. On MRI there is hyperintense signal on T2-weighted images within the central pons, sparing the periphery and the corticospinal tracts.
► The edema is usually vasogenic, with little restricted diffusion. There is usually no enhancement or mass effect.
► Extrapontine involvement is seen in at least 50% of cases and can occur without significant pontine involvement. Extrapontine sites include the basal ganglia and deep white matter (especially the external capsule). Extrapontine involvement is almost always symmetric.

Management

► Prevention requires slow correction of sodium levels with administration of desmopressin (dDAVP).
► If the patient has been rapidly corrected and develops symptoms, desmopressin can be administered to lower the sodium level.

Further Reading

Howard SA, Barletta JA, Klufas RA, et al. Osmotic demyelination syndrome. *Radiographics*. 2009;29:933-938.

History

▶ 50-year-old man with 2 hours of aphasia and right-sided weakness

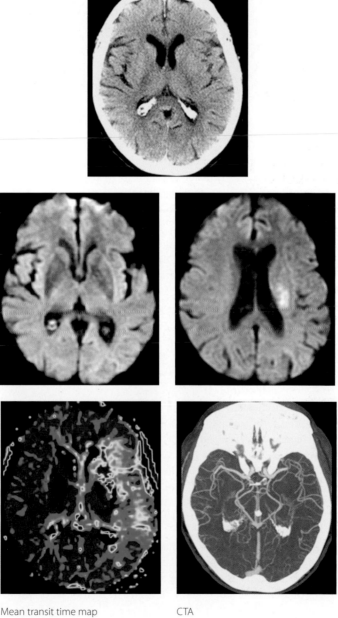

Mean transit time map   CTA

Case 36   Left Middle Cerebral Artery (MCA) Thromboembolism with Perfusion/Diffusion Mismatch

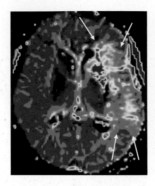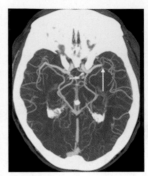

Findings

- Noncontrast CT demonstrates no evidence of infarction, hemorrhage, or mass.
- DWI demonstrates a small area of restricted diffusion in the left corona radiata and putamen.
- Mean transit time (MTT) map obtained using dynamic susceptibility contrast (DSC) perfusion imaging reveals a region of prolonged transit time (white arrows). This area of relative hypoperfusion is much larger than the DWI abnormality.
- CTA reveals a left MCA stem occlusion (white arrow). Note the opacification of the distal left MCA vessels from collateral reconstitution.

Differential Diagnosis

- There is little diagnostic dilemma in this case. Based on the CT alone, however, any of several stroke mimics (e.g., seizure, migraine) also could have been present.

Teaching Points

- Immediate imaging is central to the diagnosis and treatment of acute stroke. It:
  - excludes intracranial hemorrhage or tumor (contraindications to treatment)
  - identifies proximal artery occlusion
  - identifies the irreversibly injured tissue (core infarct)
  - identifies the hypoperfused but viable tissue
- Noncontrast CT is excellent for detecting hemorrhage but insensitive for early ischemic injury.
- CTA or MRA provides evaluation of the patency of proximal cerebral arteries.
- Restricted diffusion on MRI most accurately identifies the core infarct. Alternatively, cerebral blood volume (CBV) on perfusion imaging has been used as a surrogate for infarcted tissue.
- Cerebral blood flow or MTT maps delineate the hypoperfused tissue. The perfusion/diffusion mismatch is taken to represent at-risk penumbral tissue, and at many institutions this is being used for treatment selection outside of the window for intravenous tissue plasminogen activator (IV tPA).

Management

- Acute ischemic stroke is an emergency since tissue viability diminishes rapidly. Current guidelines recommend completion of a CT scan within 25 minutes and interpretation within 45 minutes.
- Approved reperfusion therapies include IV tPA and intra-arterial thrombectomy/aspiration devices (IAT). Treatment is limited by the time from stroke onset: 4.5 hours for IV tPA and 8 hours for IAT.

Further Reading

Latchaw R, Alberts MJ, Lev MH, et al. Recommendations for imaging of acute ischemic stroke: a scientific statement from the AHA. *Stroke.* 2009;40:3646-3678.

Srinivasan A, Goyal M, Al Asri F, et al. State-of-the-art imaging of acute stroke. *Radiographics.* 2006;26:S75–S95.

History

▶ 7-year-old boy with nausea, vomiting, and ataxia

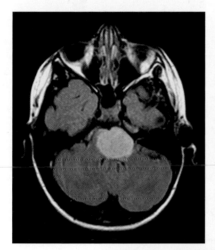 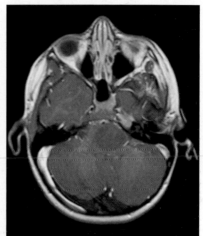

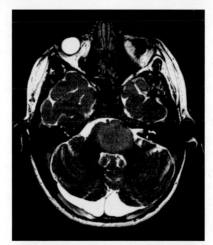

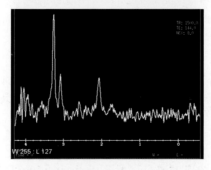

¹H MR spectroscopy

Case 37 Diffuse Pontine Glioma

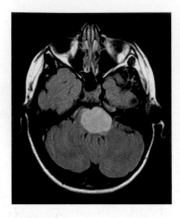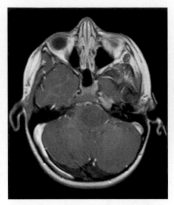

Findings

► There is an expansile, well-demarcated, T2 hyperintense mass centered within the pons. There is no abnormal enhancement.
► MR spectroscopy reveals a choline:creatine ratio greater than 2:1 and marked reduction in NAA:creatine.

Differential Diagnosis

► Brain stem encephalitis
► Demyelinating disease (acute disseminated encephalomyelitis [ADEM], osmotic demyelination)
► Neurofibromatosis type I

Teaching Points

► Brain stem gliomas account for 15% of pediatric brain tumors and 2% of adult tumors. They primarily consist of two types of neoplasm:
  ▪ Diffuse gliomas are typically fibrillary astrocytomas (WHO grade II) that are found in the basis pontis. They carry a poor prognosis: children usually survive only 12 to 15 months, and adults have a median survival of 7 years.
  ▪ Focal gliomas are often pilocytic tumors (WHO grade I) that are located outside of the pons; they have a good prognosis (5-year survival of 95%).
► Diffuse gliomas present with subacute (less than 6 months) onset of multiple cranial nerve palsies, nausea/vomiting, or ataxia.
► Diffuse pontine gliomas are infiltrative and expansile lesions. On CT they are iso- to hypoattenuating.
► On MRI they are hyperintense on T2-weighted images. Enhancement is typically minimal or absent.
► They may engulf the basilar artery and may obstruct (but not invade) the fourth ventricle.
► Proton MR spectroscopy may be helpful for differentiating aggressive neoplastic masses from other possibilities—the neoplasms show markedly elevated choline and decreased NAA.

Management

► Biopsy is generally avoided due to sampling error, risk of morbidity, and limited effect on therapy.
► Radiotherapy is the mainstay of treatment. Other therapies include chemotherapy, and in some cases partial resection depending on patient age and lesion location.

Further Reading

Fisher PG, Breiter SN, Carson BS, et al. A clinicopathologic reappraisal of brain stem tumor classification: Identification of pilocytic astrocytoma and fibrillary astrocytoma as distinct entities. *Cancer.* 2000;89:1569-1576.
Guillamo JS, Monjour A, Taillandier L, et al. Brainstem gliomas in adults: prognostic factors and classification. *Brain.* 2001;124:2528-2539.

History

▶ 60-year-old woman with 4-month history of progressive gait instability, headache, and altered mental status

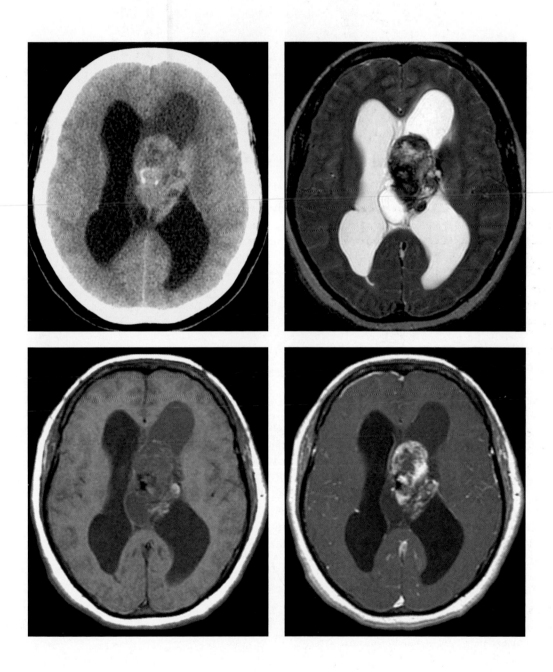

Case 38 Central Neurocytoma

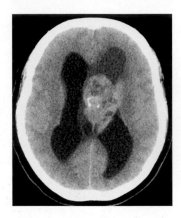

Findings

- A large solid and cystic mass within the body of the left lateral ventricle results in obstructive hydrocephalus.
- On noncontrast CT the mass is heterogeneous with mild general hyperattenuation and foci of coarse calcification
- On MRI, the solid component is T1 iso- to hypointense with mixed T2 hypo- and hyperintensity. The mass demonstrates heterogeneous enhancement.

Differential Diagnosis

- Oligodendroglioma
- Subependymal giant cell astrocytoma (SEGA)
- Ependymoma
- Low-grade or pilocytic astrocytoma
- Choroid plexus papilloma (CPP)
- Meningioma

Teaching Points

- Intraventricular neurocytoma typically occurs in young adults (20 to 40 years of age), has a heterogeneous appearance, and is usually located in the lateral ventricle in the region of the foramen of Monro (resulting in obstructive hydrocephalus), with a broad base of attachment along the septum pellucidum.
- Astrocytoma and ependymoma usually lack cysts and calcification, which are common in neurocytoma.
- SEGA is associated with tuberous sclerosis: look for subcortical and cortical tubers and subependymal nodules.
- CPP most commonly occurs in children and is usually located in the body and trigone of the lateral ventricle. It has characteristic frond-like projections.
- Meningioma typically occurs in the trigone, has a homogeneous appearance, and is found in older patients (over 30 years).
- Oligodendroglioma can be difficult to distinguish from neurocytoma both radiographically and under light microscopy. Diagnosis requires immunohistochemistry or electron microscopy.

Management

- Surgical resection is the treatment of choice. Complete surgical resection is curative due to the benign nature of the tumor.

Further Reading

Chen C, Shen C, Wang J, et al. Central neurocytoma: a clinical, radiological and pathological study of nine cases. *Clin Neurol Neurosurg.* 2008;110:129-136.

Shin JH, Lee HK, Khang SK, et al. Neuronal tumors of the central nervous system: radiologic findings and pathologic correlation. *Radiographics.* 2002;22:1177-1189.

History

▶ Two-year-old boy with three days of intermittent fever, lethargy, nausea, and vomiting. Lumbar puncture revealed CSF leukocytosis

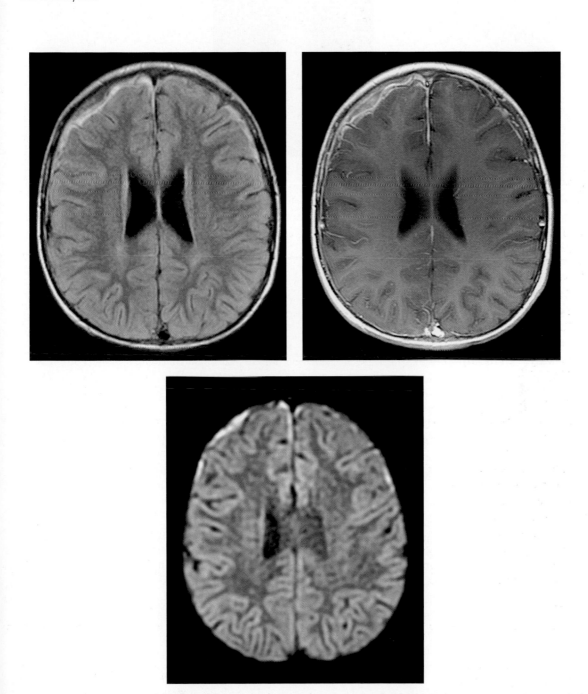

Case 39 Subdural Empyema

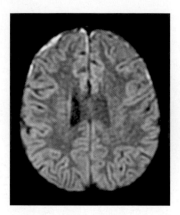

Findings

▸ FLAIR images show hyperintense signal in the subdural spaces along both frontal lobes.
▸ Postcontrast T1-weighted images show a right-sided, rim-enhancing subdural collection.
▸ On DWI, the majority of material in this collection is hyperintense.

Differential Diagnosis

▸ Epidural abscess
▸ Subdural effusion
▸ Subacute or chronic subdural hematoma

Teaching Points

▸ Empyema and epidural abscess are loculated purulent collections in the subdural or epidural space, respectively.
▸ In adults, empyema most commonly results from spread of parameningeal infections (sinusitis, otitis) or as a postsurgical complication. In children, subdural empyema also commonly occurs as a complication of bacterial meningitis.
▸ Presenting symptoms include headache, fever, seizure, confusion, and focal neurologic deficit.
▸ Collections crossing coronal or lambdoid sutures (the right coronal suture in this case) place a collection in the subdural space, distinguishing them from epidural abscess.
▸ The presence of restricted diffusion differentiates subdural empyema from subdural effusion.

Management

▸ The differentiation of subdural empyema and sterile effusion is critical since the former often requires rapid surgical drainage. Conservative therapy with antibiotics alone and close imaging follow-up (preferably MRI) may be used in patients without neurologic deficits.

Further Reading

Kanamalla US, Roldolfo AI, Junkins JR. Imaging of cranial meningitis and ventriculitis. *Neuroimaging Clin North Am.* 2000;10:309-331.
Wong AM, Zimmerman RA, Simon EM, et al. Diffusion-weighted MR imaging of subdural empyemas in children. *AJNR Am J Neuroradiol.* 2004;25:1016-1021.

History

▶ 44-year-old man with slow progressive decline in functional status

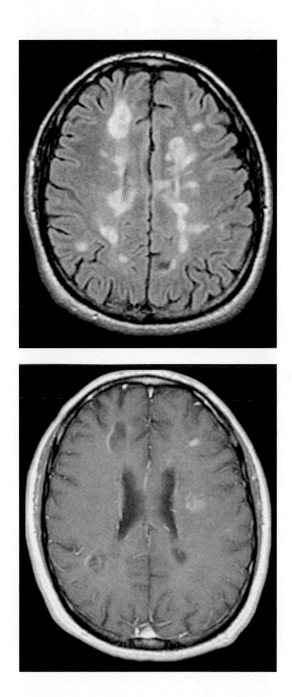

Case 40 Multiple Sclerosis (MS)

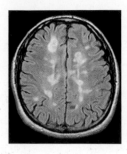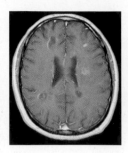

Findings

▶ The FLAIR image shows numerous large hyperintense lesions in the bilateral deep white matter. Many of the lesions have a long axis perpendicular to the surface of the ventricles.

▶ There is little mass effect associated with these lesions.

▶ The postcontrast T1-weighted image shows rim enhancement about some of the lesions.

Differential Diagnosis

▶ Acute disseminated encephalomyelitis (ADEM)

▶ Encephalitis

▶ Cerebral autosomal dominant arteriopathy with subcortical infarcts and leukoencephalopathy (CADASIL)

▶ Vasculitis

Teaching Points

▶ MS is a chronic, persistent inflammatory-demyelinating disease of the CNS. It is characterized by areas of inflammation, demyelination, axonal loss, and gliosis. It has a predilection for the optic nerves, brain stem, spinal cord, and cerebellar and periventricular white matter.

▶ Common signs and symptoms include impaired vision, weakness, numbness, gait disturbance, cranial nerve palsies, and myelopathy. The peak age at diagnosis is 30, with a female predominance.

▶ The white matter lesions are hyperintense on T2-weighted, FLAIR, and proton density images and are variably iso- to hypointense on T1-weighted images.

▶ When demyelination is active, there may be transient enhancement that is typically along the margin of the lesion but may be central. Most enhancement resolves by 6 months.

▶ Large lesions may produce mass effect and simulate CNS neoplasm ("tumefactive MS"). The degree of mass effect is usually less than that from neoplasm and abscess.

▶ Over time cerebral atrophy becomes a prominent feature of the disease.

▶ The criteria for establishing the diagnosis of MS (McDonald criteria) are based on demonstration of lesions disseminated in space (DIS) and disseminated in time (DIT), and exclusion of alternative diagnoses.
  - For DIS, three of four of the following must be present: one enhancing or nine nonenhancing lesions, one juxtacortical lesion, three periventricular lesions, and one infratentorial lesion.
  - For DIT, at least one of the following must be present: enhancing lesion 3 months after clinical onset or new nonenhancing lesion at least 30 days after reference scan.

Management

▶ Corticosteroids are the mainstay of therapy for acute attacks. Numerous other immunomodulating drugs are in use or under investigation.

Further Reading

He J, Grossman RI, Ge Y. Enhancing patterns in multiple sclerosis: evolution and persistence. *AJNR Am J Neuroradiol.* 2001;22:664-669.
Polman CH, Reingold SC, Edan G, et al. Diagnostic criteria for multiple sclerosis:2005 revisions to the "McDonald Criteria." *Ann Neurol.* 2005;58:840-846.

History

▶ 36-year-old man with headache

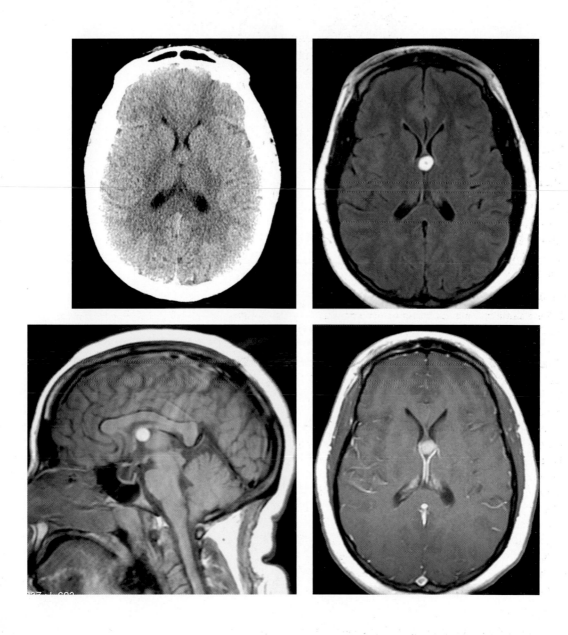

Case 41 Colloid Cyst

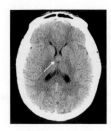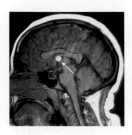

Findings

► CT demonstrates a small mass in the anterior, superior third ventricle (arrow) with attenuation similar to gray matter.
► The lesion is markedly hyperintense on FLAIR and T1-weighted sequences.
► There is no contrast enhancement.

Differential Diagnosis

► A solitary lesion in this location with these characteristics has little else in its differential diagnosis. Based only on the CT image, the differential diagnosis includes:
  ▪ Aneurysm
  ▪ Craniopharyngioma
  ▪ Meningioma
  ▪ Subependymoma
  ▪ Neurocysticercosis
  ▪ Glial or neuronal neoplasm

Teaching Points

► Colloid cyst is a rare nonneoplastic intraventricular lesion that is thought to be endodermal in origin.
► Clinical presentation is variable and nonspecific. The classic history is intermittent headache, which may be positional. Many are discovered incidentally.
► The lesion may cause obstruction of the foramen of Monro and produce acute hydrocephalus. This is a surgical emergency since it may result in brain herniation and sudden death. Ventricular obstruction is not correlated with cyst size.
► The combined CT and MR findings, demonstrating a well-defined, hyperdense, nonenhancing lesion in the anterior-superior third ventricle between the forniceal columns, are virtually pathognomonic for colloid cyst. Peripheral enhancement is rarely seen. MRI signal characteristics are dependent on protein and cholesterol content, and may reveal intracystic fluid levels.
► Other developmental neuroepithelial cysts can occur in this location, but would typically show signal characteristics similar to CSF. Additional cystic lesions should raise the possibility of neurocysticercosis.
► In a clinical (and board examination) setting, the CT image is likely to be encountered first. An appropriately broad differential diagnosis should be offered. It is critical to exclude an aneurysm or other vascular lesion, as an attempted biopsy could prove fatal.

Management

► If the patient is symptomatic or has hydrocephalus, immediate referral to neurosurgery for microsurgical or endoscopic resection is recommended. Resection may also be recommended for symptomatic lesions larger than 1.5 cm. Recurrence is rare after complete resection.

Further Reading

Armao D, Castillo M, Chen H, et al. Colloid cyst of the third ventricle: imaging–pathologic correlation. *AJNR Am J Neuroradiol.* 2000;21:1470-1477.
Jayaraman MV, Boxerman JL. Adult brain tumors. In Atlas SW, ed. *Magnetic Resonance Imaging of the Brain and Spine.* Philadelphia: Lippincott Williams & Wilkins, 2009.

History

▶ 35-year-old woman with headache

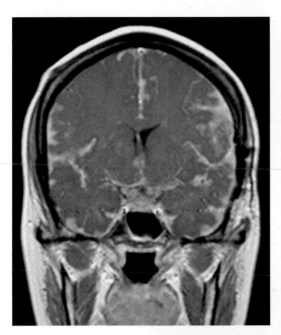
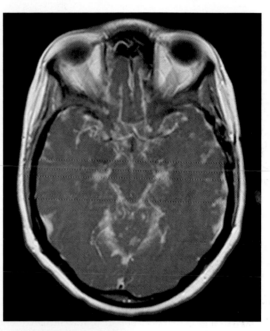
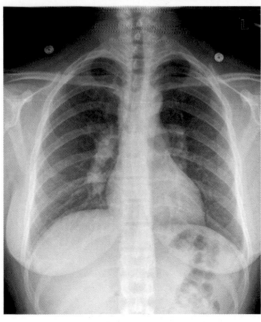

Case 42   Neurosarcoidosis

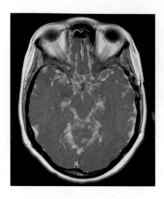

Findings

▶ Postcontrast T1-weighted MRI shows thick, nodular leptomeningeal enhancement, most prominent along the sylvian fissures and basal cisterns.

▶ Bilateral hilar lymphadenopathy is present on the chest x-ray.

Differential Diagnosis

▶ Tuberculosis

▶ Carcinomatous meningitis

▶ Lymphoma

▶ Wegener granulomatosis

▶ Langerhans cell histiocytosis

Teaching Points

▶ Sarcoidosis is a chronic, multisystem inflammatory disorder of unknown cause characterized by noncaseating granulomas.

▶ Most patients present between the ages of 20 and 40. It is most common in African-Americans and there is a slight female predominance.

▶ Neurosarcoidosis occurs in approximately 5% of patients with sarcoidosis. Over 90% of patients with neurosarcoidosis will have an abnormal chest x-ray. Rarely (less than 1% of cases) is neurosarcoidosis the only evidence of disease.

▶ Sarcoidosis can affect any part of the CNS, including the meninges, parenchyma, cranial nerves, spinal cord, and nerve roots. Osseous involvement of the skull and spine also occurs.

▶ Leptomeningeal disease and parenchymal disease are the most common patterns.

  ▪ Leptomeningeal disease may be focal or diffuse. In both forms the enhancement is nodular. Infiltration of the pituitary gland and stalk, hypothalamus, and optic chiasm can be seen.

  ▪ Parenchymal disease is characterized by enhancing periventricular lesions. Vascular involvement may lead to infarcts.

▶ The protean manifestations of neurosarcoidosis make it a "great mimicker." Hilar lymphadenopathy on chest x-ray can be very helpful in suggesting the diagnosis.

Management

▶ Corticosteroids and immunosuppressive drugs are the mainstays of therapy. The disease may be self-limited or progressive.

Further Reading

Shah R, Robertson GH, Curé JK. Correlation of MR imaging findings and clinical manifestations in neurosarcoidosis. *AJNR Am J Neuroradiol.* 2009;30:953-961.

History

▶ Term infant with hypotonia and new-onset seizures (infantile spasms)

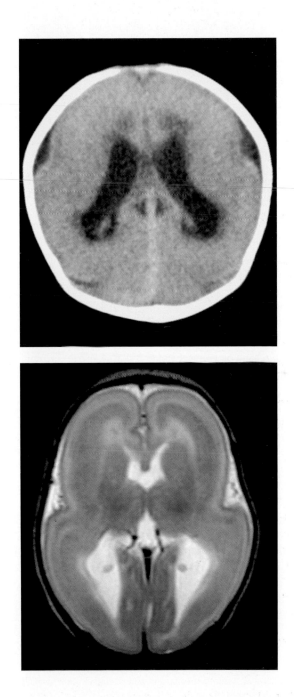

Case 43 Lissencephaly

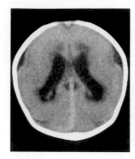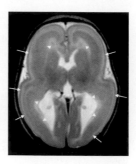

Findings

▶ On noncontrast head CT, the surface of the brain appears abnormally smooth with near-complete absence of normal sulci.
▶ The T2-weighted MR image also shows an abnormally smooth brain surface. There is a thick band of gray matter within the substance of the white matter (arrowheads), which is separated from the cortex by a thin, so-called "cell-sparse" zone of white matter (arrows).
▶ The lateral ventricles are dysmorphic.

Differential Diagnosis

▶ Severe prematurity
▶ Band heterotopia
▶ Congenital cytomegalovirus

Teaching Points

▶ Lissencephaly literally means "smooth brain." The lissencephaly complex is a group of malformations of neuronal migration that is closely related to band heterotopia and agyria-pachygyria (incomplete lissencephaly). In some patients, portions of the brain have a thin smooth surface (agyria) whereas other portions have a thick (pachygyria) or normal-appearing cortex.
▶ Normally cells migrate from the germinal zones near the ventricles to the surface of the brain to form the cortex, and various disorders may result in incomplete migration and cortical formation.
▶ In lissencephaly, there is a thin cell-sparse layer of white matter separating the smooth thin cortex from the thick band of abnormal gray matter deep in the brain.
▶ Lissencephaly may involve only part of the hemisphere.
▶ A number of causative genes and chromosomal abnormalities have been described for these disorders, the best known being the LIS1 and DCX genes.
▶ Patients with lissencephaly present with hypotonia in infancy and early-onset epilepsy and often have significant developmental delay. Prognosis is generally worse than in band heterotopia.
▶ MRI provides the best evaluation of cerebral morphology. The imaging evaluation should always include a search for other malformations, including facial abnormalities (Miller-Dieker syndrome), absence of the corpus callosum, microcephaly, cerebellar hypoplasia, and hippocampal abnormalities.

Management

▶ Management depends on seizure control and management of feeding and airway issues.
▶ Prognosis is generally poor but is related to the extent of malformations in the brain.

Further Reading

Barkovich AJ, Kuzniecki RI, Jackson GD, et al. A developmental and genetic classification for malformations of cortical development. *Neurology.* 2005;65:1873-87.
Dobyns WB. The clinical patterns and molecular genetics of lissencephaly and subcortical band heterotopia. *Epilepsia.* 2010;51 Suppl 1:5-9.

History

▶ 34-year-old woman from Central America, presenting with headache and seizures

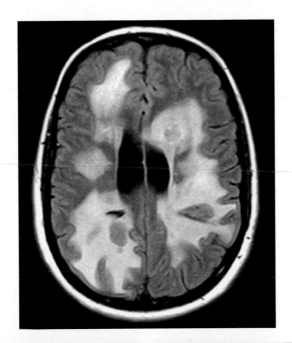

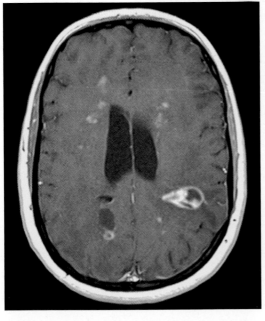

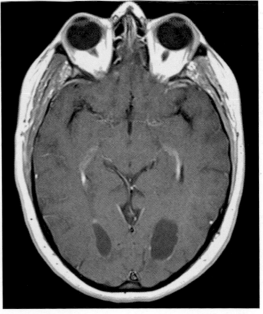

Case 44 Neurocysticercosis

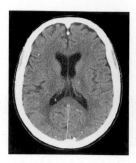

Findings

▶ FLAIR images show extensive hyperintensity, likely vasogenic edema, in the white matter of the cerebral hemispheres.
▶ Postcontrast T1-weighted images show multiple rim-enhancing lesions within the cerebral hemispheres.
▶ Cystic lesions with mural enhancement lie within the occipital horns of the lateral ventricles.
▶ CT from a different patient shows a later form with multiple small cerebral calcifications.

Differential Diagnosis

▶ Septic emboli
▶ Fungal, mycobacterial, or amebic abscess
▶ Metastatic neoplasm
▶ Tumefactive demyelination

Teaching Points

▶ Cysticercosis occurs from the ingestion of eggs of the tapeworm *Taenia solium* with subsequent deposition of the larva in the CNS.
▶ Cysticercosis is one of the leading causes of epilepsy worldwide.
▶ There are four stages of intracerebral larval cyst, with distinct imaging appearances:
  ▪ Vesicular—The viable larva, producing little host response, appears as a nonenhancing cyst with cavity fluid similar to CSF and a small mural nodule (the scolex). This stage will last 2 to 6 years in most cases.
  ▪ Colloidal—With larval death and inflammatory host response, the cysts show alteration of signal within the cyst (usually hyperintense on T1-weighted and T2-weighted imaging), rim enhancement, and edema. It is at this stage that symptoms usually develop.
  ▪ Granular nodular—With gradual resorption of the cyst fluid, a ring-enhancing or nodular lesion remains and there is a gradual decrease in surrounding edema.
  ▪ Calcified—chronic form with small scattered calcific foci, most common at gray–white junctions, best seen on CT
▶ Another common form of CNS infection occurs when the larvae deposit in the subarachnoid or intraventricular spaces, most commonly the fourth ventricle or basal cisterns. The cysts, which often produce CSF obstruction, have variable signal intensity and may or may not demonstrate rim enhancement.

Management

▶ Diagnosis may be based on clinical and radiographic findings. In some cases, biopsy is needed.
▶ Treatment for active intracerebral disease consists of antihelminthic medication (albendazole or praziquantel) and corticosteroids.
▶ Surgery (open or endoscopic) is reserved for patients with cysts that produce symptoms from mass effect or CSF obstruction.

Further Reading

Sumit S, Sharma BS. Neurocysticercosis: a review of current status and management. *J Clin Neurosci.* 2009;16:867-876.
Zee C, Go JL, Kim PE, DiGiorgio CM. Imaging of neurocysticercosis. *Neuroimaging Clin North Am.* 2000;10:391-407.

History

▸ 44-year-old with headache

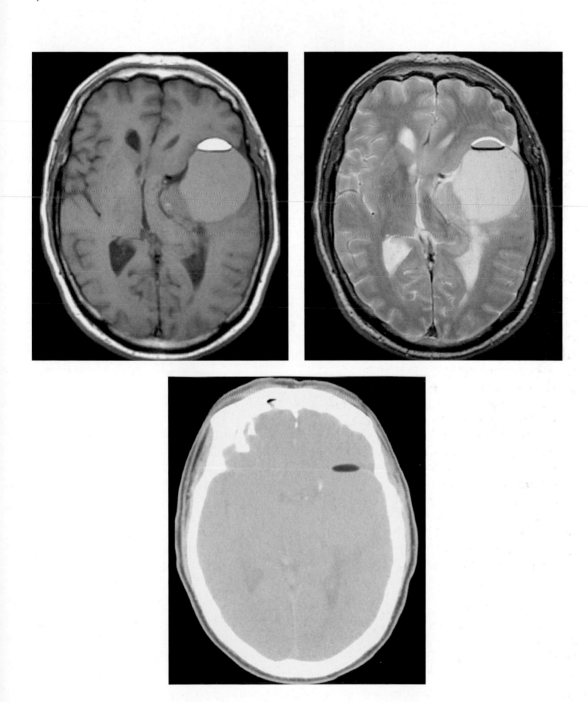

Case 45 Dermoid

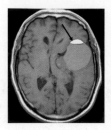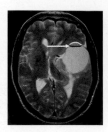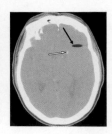

Findings

- There is a large cystic extra-axial mass within the left sylvian fissure.
- Both CT and MR show an air–fluid level with fat layering anteriorly within the cyst (black arrows). Fat demonstrates hyperintense signal on T1-weighted images and low attenuation on CT (–50 to –150 Hounsfield units).
- There is chemical shift artifact at the fat–fluid interface on T2-weighted images in the frequency-encoding direction (white arrow).
- Calcifications are present along the margin of the cyst (bordered white arrow).

Differential Diagnosis

- Teratoma
- Craniopharyngioma
- Lipoma
- Epidermoid cyst

Teaching Points

- Dermoids are rare, congenital, ectodermal inclusion cysts that have dermal elements (hair follicles and sebaceous glands) and contain lipid and cholesterol.
- They usually present with headache or seizure in young adults.
- Dermoids predominantly occur in the midline: sellar/parasellar region > posterior fossa (cerebellar vermis or fourth ventricle).
- Imaging reveals a unilocular cystic mass containing a fat–fluid level. There may be focal rim calcification or rare capsular enhancement.
- Fat-suppressed MRI sequences and CT are useful in definitively demonstrating the fat component.
- Dermoids are prone to rupture. Rupture is more common in large lesions. The cyst contents incite an inflammatory reaction that can cause significant morbidity and mortality. Rupture can be identified on imaging from the presence of subarachnoid or intraventricular fat droplets. Pial enhancement can be seen due to associated chemical meningitis. Hydrocephalus, vasospasm, and infarction may ensue.
- Dermoids may rarely undergo degeneration into squamous cell carcinoma.
- Epidermoid cysts are usually off midline, have signal that matches CSF, and demonstrate restricted diffusion.
- Teratomas contain fat but more commonly occur in the pineal region and are multiloculated, with enhancing nodular components.

Management

- Complete resection is critical: recurrence can occur when residual capsule is present.
- Small lesions or clinically silent ruptures may be followed with imaging to assess for growth and complications.

Further Reading

Osborn AG, Preece MT. Intracranial cysts: radiologic–pathologic correlation and imaging approach. *Radiology.* 2006;27:1211-1216.
Smirniotopoulos JG, Chiechi MV. From the archives of AFIP: Teratomas, dermoids, and epidermoids of the head and neck. *Radiographics.* 1995;15:1437-1455.

History

▶ 53-year-old woman with left-sided sensorineural hearing loss

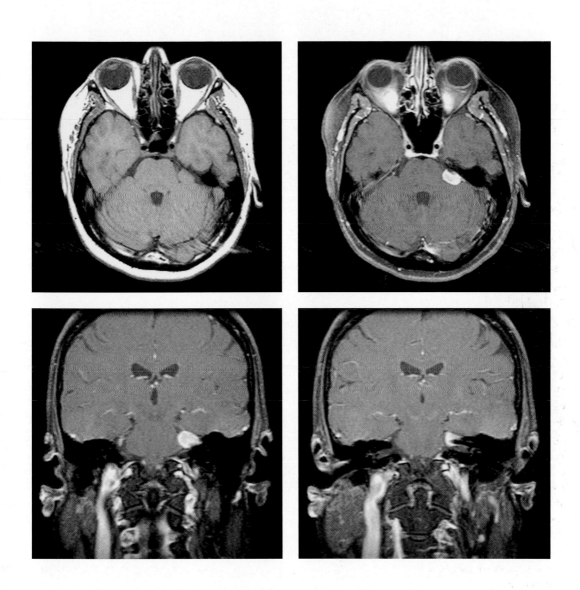

Case 46 Meningioma of Cerebellopontine Angle

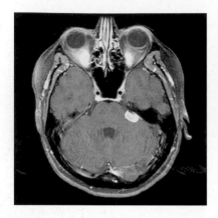 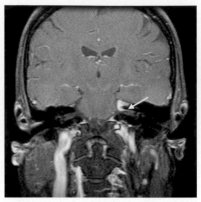

Findings

▶ There is an extra-axial mass in the left cerebellopontine angle, centered above the internal auditory canal (IAC).
▶ The lesion is iso-intense to white matter on precontrast T1-weighted images and enhances uniformly.
▶ There is a tail of dural enhancement that extends into the IAC (arrow).

Differential Diagnosis

▶ Vestibular schwannoma
▶ Metastasis
▶ Lymphoma
▶ Trigeminal schwannoma

Teaching Points

▶ Whereas most vestibular schwannomas are centered in the IAC, meningiomas are generally eccentric. The presence of a "dural tail" may be helpful but is not specific for meningiomas.
▶ Meningiomas are most commonly incidental findings, with cranial nerve findings occurring late—unlike vestibular schwannomas, in which hearing loss is an early clinical symptom.
▶ The presence of calcification or hyperostosis of adjacent bone suggests meningioma.
▶ Widening of the IAC is seen in patients with vestibular schwannomas but is uncommon in meningiomas.

Management

▶ Meningiomas are treated surgically when feasible. As an alternative, or for residual/recurrent disease, radiation therapy can be used.

Further Reading

Glastonbury CM. The vestibulocochlear nerve, with an emphasis on the normal and diseased internal auditory canal and cerebellopontine angle. In: Swartz JD, Loevner LA. *Imaging of the Temporal Bone*, 4th ed. New York: Thieme, 2009:510-513.
Swartz JD. Lesions of the cerebellopontine angle and internal auditory canal: diagnosis and differential diagnosis. *Semin Ultrasound CT.* 2004;25:332-352.

History

► 31-year-old man with systemic lupus erythematosus admitted with visual auras, fevers, and positive blood cultures

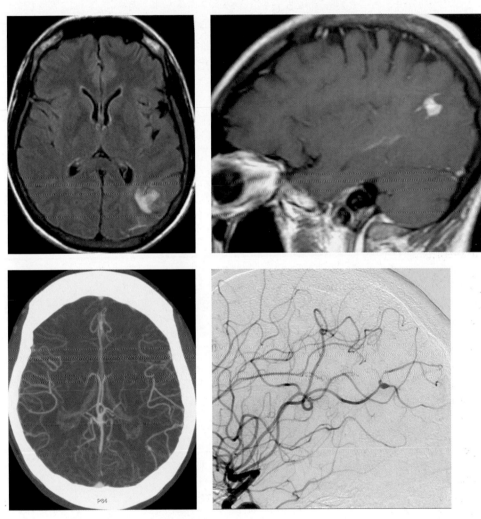

Left common carotid artery

Case 47 Mycotic Aneurysm

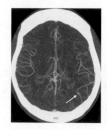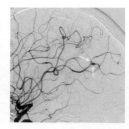

Findings

- On MRI, there is a focal subcortical lesion in the left parietal lobe with heterogeneous hyperintense signal on FLAIR and postcontrast T1-weighted images. There is mild mass effect.
- The CT angiogram shows a small site of aneurysmal dilatation in a distal left MCA branch (arrow, left).
- The catheter angiogram shows a focal fusiform aneurysm (arrows, right) in a distal branch of the MCA. There is irregular narrowing in the parent vessel at this site.

Differential Diagnosis

- Vasculitis/vasculopathy
- Dissecting aneurysm
- Intravascular lymphoma (rare)

Teaching Points

- Mycotic or infectious aneurysms result from septic embolization to the arterial vasa vasorum with spread of infection through the intima, leading to destruction of the vessel wall and resultant aneurysmal dilatation.
- They are rare compared to saccular (berry) aneurysms and account for only 2% to 4% of total aneurysm cases.
- Mycotic aneurysms may be secondary to bacterial, fungal, or viral infections. They usually occur in the setting of bacterial endocarditis (in up to 10% of infective endocarditis cases).
- The most common presentation is intracranial hemorrhage. Like other pseudoaneurysms, mycotic aneurysms have an higher risk of rupture than saccular aneurysms.
- CT or MR imaging may reveal subarachnoid or intraparenchymal hemorrhage, infarction, or edema. Regional enhancement may occur secondary to cerebritis.
- Cerebral angiography is the gold standard for any patient with clinical suspicion for mycotic aneurysm. Angiographic features of mycotic aneurysm include:
  - Peripheral location
  - Fusiform or irregular morphology
  - Adjacent arterial irregularity, stenosis, or occlusion
  - Changing morphology on repeat imaging

Management

- All cases are treated emergently with antibiotics for 4 to 6 weeks.
- Ruptured aneurysms are treated with immediate closure of the aneurysm (surgical or endovascular).
- For medically managed aneurysms, serial angiography is valuable since response of the vessel injury is variable. Aneurysms may regress, enlarge, or remain unchanged.

Further Reading

Colen TW, Gunn M, Cook E, et al. Radiologic manifestations of extra-cardiac complications of infective endocarditis. *Eur Radiol.* 2008;18:2433-2445.

Kannoth S, Thomas SV. Intracranial microbial aneurysm (infectious aneurysm): current options for diagnosis and management. *Neurocrit Care.* 2009;11:120-129.

History

▸ Neonate with facial anomalies, hypotonia, and microcephaly

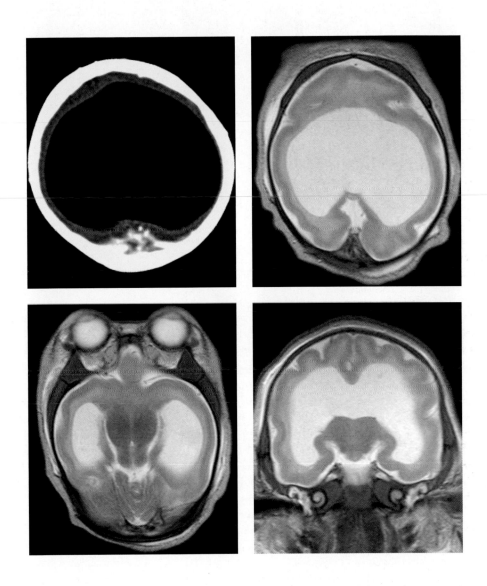

Case 48   Holoprosencephaly (Alobar)

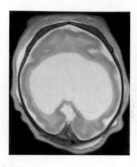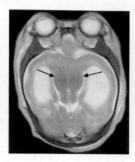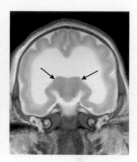

Findings

▶ Axial CT image shows a large rounded ventricle. There is a fully circumferential rind of brain tissue around the ventricle.

▶ Axial and coronal T2-weighted MR images show absence of the septum pellucidum with a large single monoventricle.

▶ There is fusion of the frontal lobes anteriorly, and fusion of the thalami in the midline (arrows).

Differential Diagnosis

▶ Severe hydrocephalus with ruptured septum pellucidum

▶ Hydranencephaly

▶ Large bilateral open lip schizencephaly

▶ Agenesis of the corpus callosum with large interhemispheric cyst

Teaching Points

▶ Holoprosencephaly (HPE) is a spectrum of malformations characterized by incomplete separation of the cerebral hemispheres and lack of cleavage of midline structures. The septum pellucidum and anterior midline falx are absent and there is usually a single azygous anterior cerebral artery. Patients have varying degrees of fusion of the hemispheres, basal ganglia, hypothalami, and thalami.

  ▪ In the alobar form, there is very little separation of the hemispheres, with a single monoventricle, absence of a distinct third ventricle, agenesis of the corpus callosum, and fused thalami and basal ganglia.

  ▪ In the semilobar form, there is more separation of the hemispheres posteriorly, with a partially formed third ventricle, and fusion of the basal ganglia and ventral thalami. The splenium of the corpus callosum is present, but the anterior corpus callosum and frontal horns are not developed.

  ▪ In the lobar form, which may be quite subtle, the hemispheres are separated but there is poor formation of the anterior corpus callosum and fusion of small parts of the adjacent frontal lobes.

▶ In some patients, there is a dorsal cyst, sometimes in communication with the ventricles.

▶ There are a range of associated facial malformations, including midline facial clefts, hypotelorism, cyclopia, single midline maxillary incisor tooth, and single nares.

▶ Clinical signs and symptoms include microcephaly, facial anomalies, developmental delay, seizures, hypothalamic dysfunction, and pituitary hormonal deficiencies.

Management

▶ Treatment is mainly supportive, along with treatment of endocrine dysfunction and seizures.

Further Reading

Hahn JS, Barnes PD. Neuroimaging advances in holoprosencephaly: Refining the spectrum of the midline malformation. *Am J Med Genet C Semin Med Genet.* 2010;154C:120–132.

Hahn JS, Pinter JD. Holoprosencephaly: genetic, neuroradiological, and clinical advances. *Semin Pediatr Neurol.* 2002;9:309–319.

History

▶ 3-year-old with developmental delay and seizures since infancy

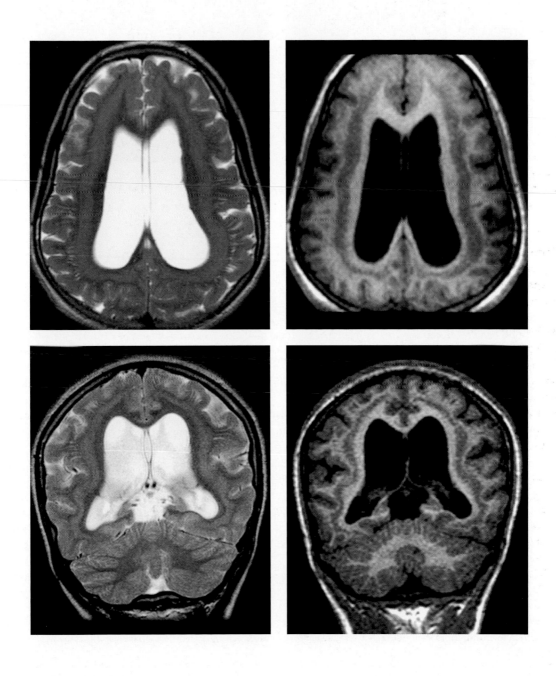

Case 49   Band Heterotopia

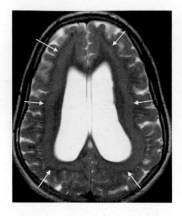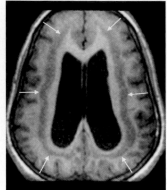

Findings

► There is a smooth band-like layer of abnormal tissue running parallel to the cortex deep within the substance of the white matter. It follows the T1 and T2 signal intensity of gray matter on all sequences (arrows).

Differential Diagnosis

► Lissencephaly
► Zellweger syndrome (peroxisomal disorder)

Teaching Points

► Subcortical band heterotopia is a malformation of neuronal migration that is closely related to and in the same spectrum as lissencephaly and so-called agyria-pachyria. DCX (doublecortin) and LIS1 gene mutations are involved.
► In band heterotopia, in contrast to lissencephaly, the convolutions of the overlying cortex are relatively preserved, though they are often not completely normal. Just as in lissencephaly, band heterotopia may not involve the entire hemisphere.
► Over 90% of the patients are female. Patients with band heterotopia present with early-onset epilepsy and often have significant developmental delay. Swallowing problems and aspiration pneumonia are common.
► A smooth layer of gray matter deep to the cortex will give the appearance of a "double cortex."
► If band heterotopia is thin or incomplete, it may be difficult to diagnose. Coronal imaging and MRI sequences with good gray–white discrimination will help identify the abnormalities.
► Band heterotopia is genetically distinct from other forms of gray matter heterotopia. Other heterotopias include nodular subependymal (most common) and nodular subcortical. MRI is much more sensitive than CT in detecting these abnormalities.

Management

► Management depends on seizure control and management of swallowing and airway issues. Prognosis is related to the extent of malformations in the brain.

Further Reading

Barkovich AJ, Kuzniecki RI, Jackson GD, et al. A developmental and genetic classification for malformations of cortical development. *Neurology.* 2005;65:1873-1887.
Dobyns WB. The clinical patterns and molecular genetics of lissencephaly and subcortical band heterotopia. *Epilepsia.* 2010;51(Suppl 1):5-9.

History

▶ 13-year-old with headache

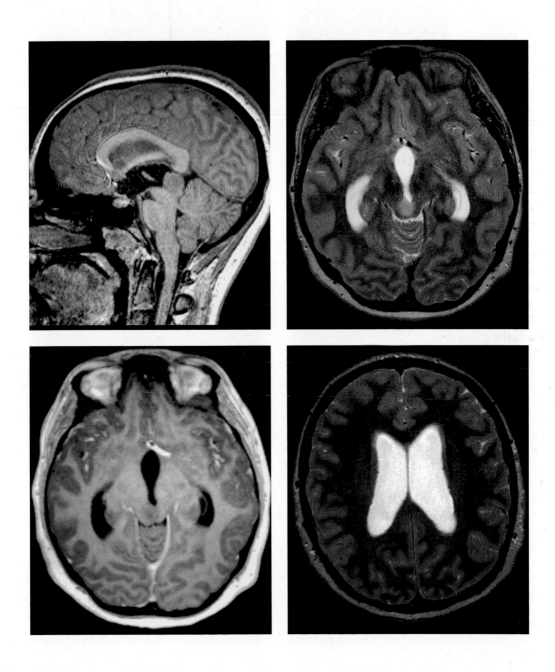

Case 50   Tectal Glioma

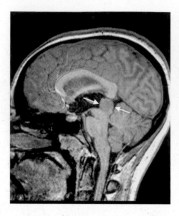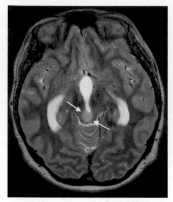

Findings

- ▶ The sagittal T1-weighted image shows abnormal expansion of the tectal plate by a rounded mass (arrows).
- ▶ Axial T2-weighted and post-contrast T1-weighted images show the lesion to be T2-hyperintense and non-enhancing.
- ▶ There is hydrocephalus with enlargement of the third and lateral ventricles due to the obstruction caused by stenosis of the cerebral aqueduct.

Differential Diagnosis

- ▶ Aqueductal stenosis (non-neoplastic)
- ▶ Metastasis
- ▶ Pineal tumor

Teaching Points

- ▶ The majority of tectal gliomas are low-grade astrocytomas that arise in the tectal plate (quadrigeminal plate) and near the aqueduct of Sylvius. They are uncommon tumors and are more commonly seen in children and young adults.
- ▶ The mass effect from the lesion (even if the tumor is small) can cause narrowing or obstruction of the aqueduct, producing hydrocephalus in the third and lateral ventricles.
- ▶ Patients most commonly present with symptoms of hydrocephalus, including headache, vomiting, and change in mental status. Some may present with gaze palsies.
- ▶ On CT, diagnosis can be difficult or sometimes impossible on routine CT, and only hydrocephalus may be seen.
- ▶ On MRI, there is tectal thickening or a frank mass in the tectum. The masses are hyperintense on T2-weighted and FLAIR sequences. Only a minority enhance with contrast.

Management

- ▶ Most lesions grow very slowly or remain stable. Initial management is CSF shunting/diversion to treat hydrocephalus.
- ▶ Periodic MR imaging is recommended. If the tumor progresses, radiotherapy, chemotherapy, or occasionally debulking surgery is performed.

Further Reading

Bowers DC, Georgiades C, Aronson LJ, et al. Tectal gliomas: natural history of an indolent lesion in pediatric patients. *Pediatr Neurosurg.* 2000;32:24-29.

Dağlioğlu E, Cataltepe O, Akalan N. Tectal gliomas in children: the implications for natural history and management strategy. *Pediatr Neurosurg.* 2003;38:223-231.

History

▶ 3-year-old boy with behavioral change and progressive difficulty walking

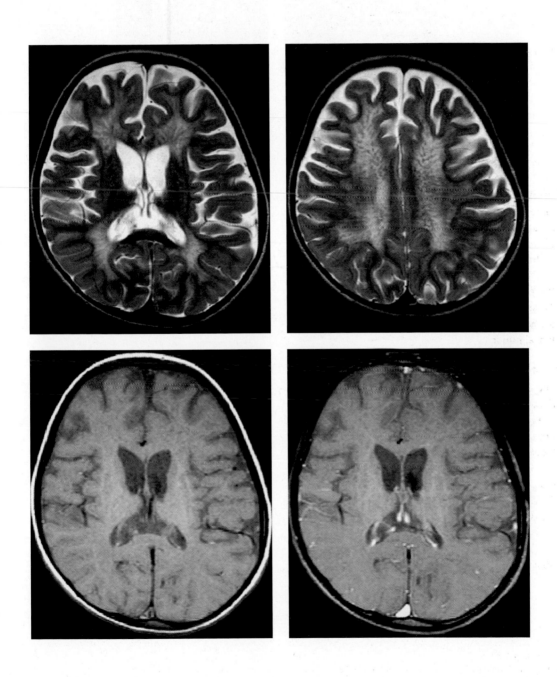

Case 51 Metachromatic Leukodystrophy

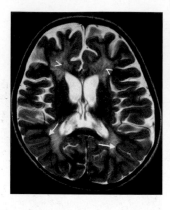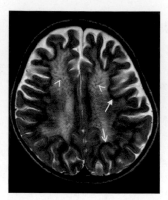

Findings

▸ Axial T2-weighted images show abnormal confluent hyperintensity in the white matter of the centrum semiovale and corona radiata, in a "butterfly-like" configuration. There are multiple linear "tigroid" stripes in the white matter (arrowheads). The subcortical white matter U-fibers remain relatively spared in most areas (arrows). There is mild cerebral volume loss.

▸ Pre- and post-contrast T1-weighted images show no contrast enhancement in the areas of white matter abnormality.

Differential Diagnosis

▸ Periventricular leukomalacia (PVL)
▸ TORCH infections
▸ Krabbe's disease

Teaching Points

▸ Metachromatic leukodystrophy (MLD) is a lysosomal storage disease due to deficiency of arylsulfatase A, resulting in defective catabolism of sulfatides, one of many components of myelin. It has autosomal dominant inheritance and has late-infantile, juvenile, and adult forms.

▸ Infants present with hypotonia and weakness. In older children and adults, gait abnormalities, stiffness, vision problems, bulbar symptoms, and intellectual impairment are common.

▸ On CT there are areas of decreased attenuation in the white matter, typically without calcification or enhancement.

▸ On MRI, there is often confluent hemispheric white matter T2 hyperintensity involving both the anterior and posterior white matter, in a butterfly configuration. In the early stages, the subcortical U-fibers are spared and remain relatively hypointense. There is no contrast enhancement.

▸ The perivenular regions in the white matter are initially spared, resulting in linear tigroid stripes in the white matter. These tiger stripes are common in but not specific to MLD.

▸ As the disease progresses, the subcortical U-fibers become involved and there is brain atrophy.

Management

▸ The disease is fatal and death often occurs within a few years. Treatment is symptomatic and supportive. Bone marrow transplantation may delay progression in some patients.

Further Reading

Cheon JE, Kim IO, Hwang YS, et al. Leukodystrophy in children: a pictorial review of MR imaging features. *Radiographics.* 2002;22: 461-476.

Faerber EN, Melvin J, Smergel EM. MRI appearances of metachromatic leukodystrophy. *Pediatr Radiol.* 1999;29:669-672.

History

▶ 48-year-old man with HIV and one week of frontal headache. He presents to the ER with left-sided weakness

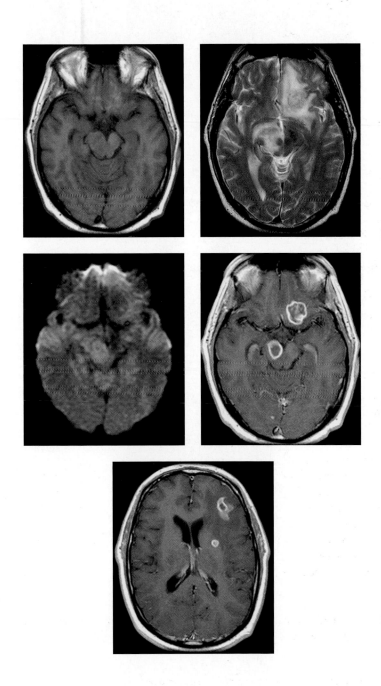

Case 52 CNS Toxoplasmosis

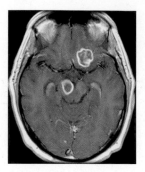

Findings

▶ Postcontrast T1-weighted images show several large rim-enhancing lesions in the cerebral hemispheres and midbrain. They are present in both basal ganglia and subcortical white matter.
▶ T2-weighted images show surrounding edema and heterogeneous internal signal
▶ The lesions are iso-intense on DWI.

Differential Diagnosis

▶ In the setting of HIV or other immunocompromised states, the most likely possibilities are:
  ▪ Lymphoma
  ▪ Mycobacterial, fungal, or pyogenic abscesses
  ▪ Metastatic neoplasm

Teaching Points

▶ Toxoplasmosis is an intracellular parasite found throughout the world and acquired through ingestion of undercooked meat or exposure to cat feces.
▶ In immunocompetent humans, the infection produces few if any symptoms. However, it is a major source of encephalitis in AIDS patients.
▶ Unlike congenital toxoplasmosis, calcification is uncommon.
▶ MRI is the imaging modality of choice for evaluation of patients with HIV and focal neurologic deficits or global cognitive impairment.
▶ On MRI, toxoplasmosis most commonly produces ring-enhancing masses, hyperintense on T2-weighted images. There is usually substantial surrounding edema.
▶ Toxoplasmosis and lymphoma are the two most common causes of ring-enhancing masses in the HIV or immunocompromised populations. Both have a predilection for the basal ganglia and often produce multiple lesions.
▶ When compared to CNS lymphoma, toxoplasmosis is more likely to have thin uniform walls, multiple lesions, and subcortical lesions. Lymphoma is more likely to involve the ependyma and leptomeninges.
▶ Advanced imaging studies such as PET, thallium-201 SPECT, MR spectroscopy, DWI, and MR perfusion have shown promise in the discrimination of toxoplasmosis and lymphoma.
▶ Unlike pyogenic abscesses, toxoplasmosis rarely produces restricted diffusion within the abscess cavity.

Management

▶ When both toxoplasmosis and lymphoma remain considerations in an immunocompromised patient, presumptive treatment with pyrimethamine or sulfadiazine is begun.
▶ If this therapy fails to provide clinical or imaging improvement within two weeks, brain biopsy is indicated.

Further Reading

Kornbluth CM, Destain S. Imaging of rickettsial, spirochetal, and parasitic infections. *Neuroimaging Clin North Am.* 2000;10:375-390.

History

▶ 9-year-old with headaches and seizures

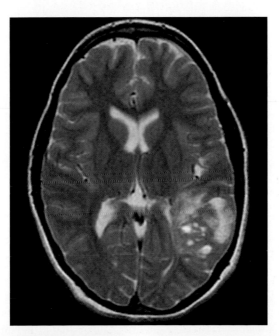

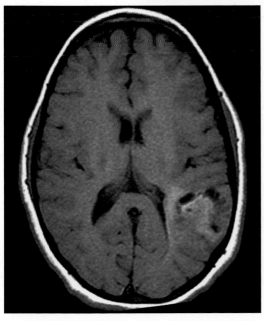

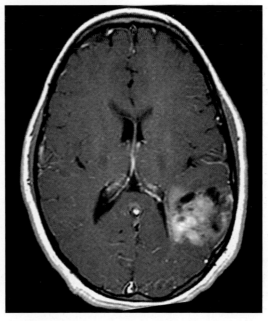

Case 53 Pleomorphic Xanthoastrocytoma (PXA)

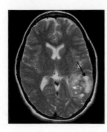 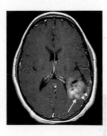

Findings

- ► There is a left parietal lobe mass extending from the cortex to the periventricular white matter.
- ► It has heterogeneous signal characteristics, predominantly hyperintense on the T2-weighted image. There are cystic (black arrow) and nodular enhancing (white arrow) components.
- ► It has relatively mild mass effect for its size and minimal surrounding edema.
- ► Note the linear dural enhancement adjacent to the mass (arrowheads).

Differential Diagnosis

- ► Ganglioglioma
- ► Pilocytic astrocytoma
- ► Dysembryoplastic neuroepithelial tumor
- ► Oligodendroglioma

Teaching Points

- ► PXA is a cortically based astrocytic neoplasm. It usually demonstrates benign behavior (WHO grade II), with a 10-year survival rate of 70%. However, aggressive variants exist and there is malignant transformation in up to 20% of cases.
- ► PXA usually occurs in children and adolescents, presenting as a supratentorial mass. Seizure is the most common clinical symptom.
- ► On CT, the tumor is typically iso-attenuating to gray matter and noncalcified.
- ► MRI features that suggest this mass include:
  - ▪ Cortical involvement with the mass abutting the pial surface
  - ▪ T1 iso-intense and mildly T2 hyperintense to gray matter with minimal peritumoral edema
  - ▪ Heterogeneous enhancement that includes a dural component
  - ▪ Presence of cystic areas (in 50%)
- ► Gangliogliomas are cortically based masses that can have solid and cystic components, but they often have calcification and do not involve the meninges.
- ► Pilocytic astrocytomas often have solid and cystic components, but these tumors usually involve the posterior fossa, hypothalamus, or optic chiasm.
- ► Dysembryoplastic neuroepithelial tumors are peripheral tumors with a "soap bubble" appearance at the cortical margin. The majority demonstrate minimal to no enhancement.
- ► Oligodendrogliomas often have heterogeneous calcifications.

Management

- ► Surgical resection is the primary treatment. Extent of resection influences rate of recurrence and outcomes.
- ► Chemotherapy and radiation therapy do not typically alter patient outcomes, but radiation therapy is occasionally used in patients with recurrent tumors.

Further Reading

Fouladi M, Jenkins J, Burger P, et al. Pleomorphic xanthoastrocytoma: favorable outcome after complete surgical resection. *Neuro Oncol.* 2001;3:184-192.

Koeller KK, Henry JM. From the archives of the AFIP: Superficial gliomas: radiologic-pathologic correlation. *Radiographics.* 2001;21:1533-1556.

History

▶ 57-year-old woman with decreased vision in one eye

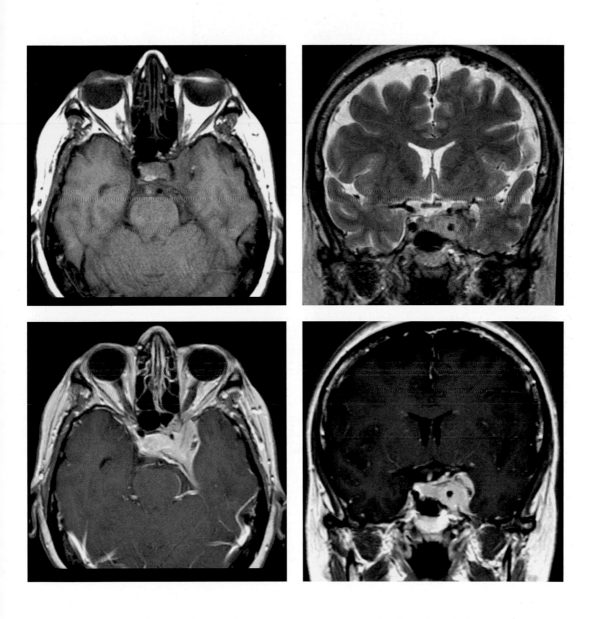

Case 54 Cavernous Sinus Meningioma

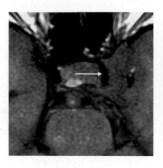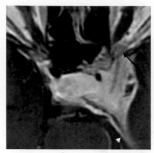

Findings

- There is abnormal material within an expanded left cavernous sinus.
- It is iso-intense on T1-weighted images and mildly hyperintense on T2-weighted images, and enhances homogeneously.
- The mass encases and mildly narrows the left cavernous internal carotid artery (white arrow).
- There is an enhancing dural tail along the petrous apex (white arrowhead).
- The mass extends into the left orbital apex (black arrow), where it exerts mass effect on the optic nerve.

Differential Diagnosis

- Nerve sheath tumor
- Pituitary adenoma
- Chordoma/chondrosarcoma
- Metastasis
- Sarcoidosis or other granulomatous process
- Tolosa-Hunt syndrome

Teaching Points

- Meningioma is the most common tumor of the cavernous sinus.
- Because the cavernous sinus contains numerous cranial nerves and is adjacent to the orbit and sella, cavernous sinus lesions are usually symptomatic. Clinical presentations include ophthalmoplegia, facial pain, and visual loss.
- MRI is the best way to evaluate the full extent of cavernous sinus lesions and to assess relationships with important neurovascular structures.
- Characteristic imaging findings of meningioma include:
  - Encasement with narrowing of the internal carotid artery (ICA)
  - Tumoral calcification or hyperostosis (best seen on CT)
  - Presence of an enhancing dural tail (up to 60%)
- Among cavernous sinus masses, it is important to consider ICA aneurysm, which may demonstrate heterogeneous signal due to thrombosis.

Management

- Asymptomatic cavernous sinus meningiomas are managed conservatively.
- In the presence of symptoms or significant tumor growth, radiosurgery or combined partial resection and radiosurgery provides good tumor control with low morbidity.

Further Reading

Tang Y, Booth T, Steward M, et al. The imaging of conditions affecting the cavernous sinus. *Clin Radiol.* 2010;65:937-945.
Walsh MT, Couldwell WT. Management options for cavernous sinus meningiomas. *J Neurooncol.* 2009;92:307-316.

History

► 4-month-old with large head size

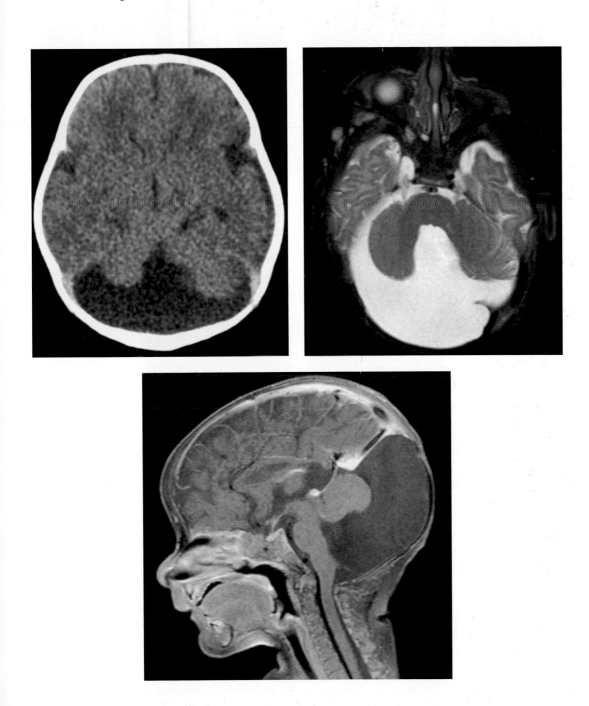

Case 55 Dandy-Walker Malformation

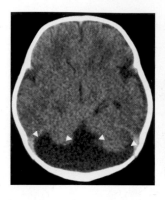 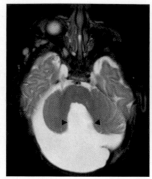 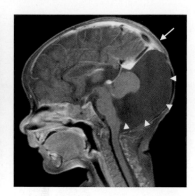

Findings

- ▶ Both CT and MRI show an enlarged fourth ventricle and cystic dilatation of the posterior fossa (arrowheads).
- ▶ The torcula is located much more superiorly than normal (arrow).
- ▶ The cerebellar vermis is severely hypoplastic, the cerebellum is rotated upwards, and the cerebellar hemispheres are slightly small.

Differential Diagnosis

- ▶ Hypoplastic vermis with rotation (formerly Dandy-Walker variant)
- ▶ Mega cisterna magna
- ▶ Retrocerebellar arachnoid cyst
- ▶ Cerebellar hypoplasia

Teaching Points

- ▶ Dandy-Walker malformation (DWM) is characterized by an enlarged cystic posterior fossa and superiorly positioned torcula. There is lambdoid–torcula inversion (torcular confluence of venous sinuses located above lambdoid sutures). The fourth ventricle is large and the vermis is hypoplastic with upward rotation. There are variable degrees of hypoplasia of the cerebellar hemispheres and compression of the brain stem.
- ▶ Dandy-Walker spectrum of posterior fossa anomalies, listed from the most severe form to least severe:
  - ▪ DWM
  - ▪ Hypoplastic vermis with rotation—here there is variable hypoplasia of the vermis and mild upward vermian rotation but a normal-sized posterior fossa with normal position of the torcula.
  - ▪ Mega cistern magna—a common entity, considered a normal variant, in which the vermis and fourth ventricle are normal and the cistern is often crossed by leaflets of falx cerebelli and small veins
- ▶ In DWM, infants present with large head size and bulging fontanel. Hydrocephalus is also common. Prognosis depends on other associated brain malformations and the degree of cerebellar hypoplasia.

Management

- ▶ Ventriculoperitoneal shunting (if there is hydrocephalus), with or without shunting of the posterior fossa cyst, remains the mainstay of treatment.

Further Reading

Patel S, Barkovich AJ. Analysis and classification of cerebellar malformations. *Am J Neuroradiol.* 2002;23:1074-1087.
Ten Donkelaar HJ, Lammens M. Development of the human cerebellum and its disorders. *Clin Perinatol.* 2009;36:513-530.

History

▶ 58-year-old man with ataxia, slurred speech, difficulty swallowing, involuntary laughing, rigidity, and bradykinesia

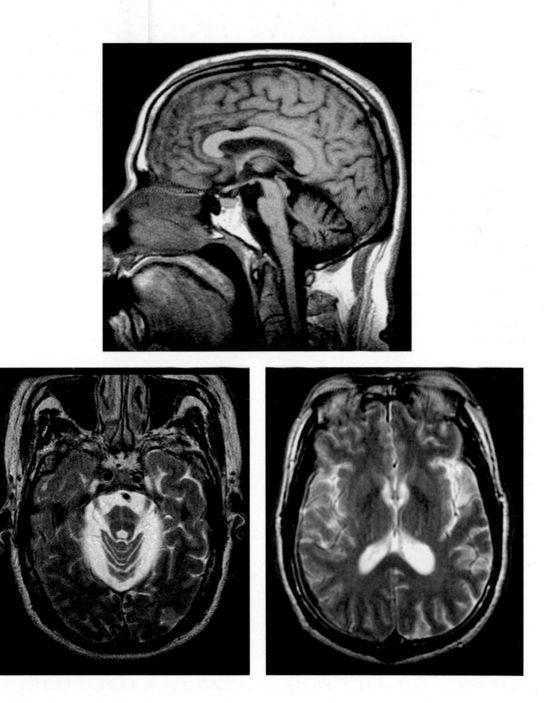

Case 56 Multiple System Atrophy

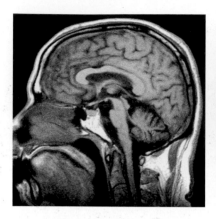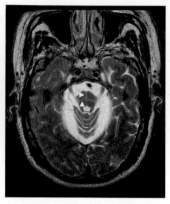

Findings

▶ Sagittal T1-weighted images show marked atrophy of the pons and cerebellum.
▶ T2-weighted images show coronally and sagittally oriented bands of hyperintense signal in the pons (arrowheads). There is subtle hyperintense signal along the lateral margin of the putamen.

Differential Diagnosis

▶ Olivopontocerebellar degeneration
▶ Spinocerebellar ataxia

Teaching Points

▶ Multiple system atrophy (MSA) is a progressive neurodegenerative disorder characterized by parkinsonism mixed with varying degrees of cerebellar ataxia, and autonomic dysfunction. Earlier names for forms of this disease include Shy-Drager syndrome, striatonigral degeneration, and olivopontocerebellar atrophy.
▶ Definitive diagnosis requires pathologic demonstration of striatonigral and olivopontocerebellar degeneration and presence of α-synuclein-positive cytoplasmic inclusions.
▶ Early diagnosis, particularly differentiation from Parkinson's disease, is difficult.
▶ Features on MRI include:
  ▪ Atrophy of the cerebellum, pons, and middle cerebellar peduncles
  ▪ Putaminal atrophy and development of curvilinear T2-hyperintense signal along the lateral margin of the putamen
  ▪ Hyperintense signal on T2-weighted images in the pons along the transverse pontocerebellar fibers ("hot cross bun" sign)
▶ [18]FDG PET may demonstrate hypometabolism in the brain stem, striatum, or cerebellum.

Management

▶ There is no cure for MSA. Anti-parkinsonian medications are relatively ineffective. Treatment is focused on ameliorating orthostatic hypertension and other symptoms.

Further Reading

Gilman S, Wenning GK, Low PA, et al. Second consensus statement on the diagnosis of multiple system atrophy. *Neurology.* 2008;71: 670-676.
Seppi K, Schocke MFH, Wenning GK, et al. How to diagnose MSA early: the role of magnetic resonance imaging. *J Neural Transm.* 2005;112:1625-1634.

History

▶ 46-year-old woman with altered mental status 9 days after coil occlusion of a ruptured cerebral aneurysm

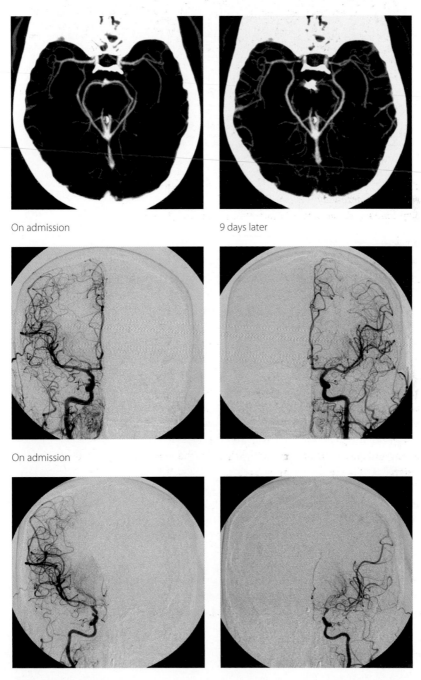

On admission

9 days later

On admission

Day 9 angiogram

Case 57   Cerebral Vasospasm

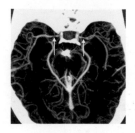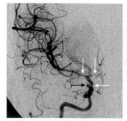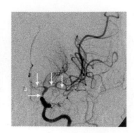

Findings

- ▸ MIP image from the Day 9 CT angiogram demonstrates multiple areas of narrowing in the proximal middle cerebral arteries bilaterally (white arrows).
- ▸ AP projection cerebral angiograms reveal multiple areas of moderate and severe narrowing, involving the intracranial internal carotid and the proximal anterior and middle cerebral arteries (white arrows).
- ▸ The stenoses have smooth margins and occur over relatively long segments of the vessels.
- ▸ There is an incidental (unruptured) right internal carotid artery (ICA) aneurysm (black arrow).

Differential Diagnosis

- ▸ Intracranial atherosclerosis
- ▸ CNS vasculitis/vasculopathy

Teaching Points

- ▸ Vasospasm is the delayed, subacute narrowing of the intracranial vasculature following subarachnoid hemorrhage (SAH), usually secondary to aneurysm rupture.
- ▸ Angiographically evident vasospasm occurs in 60% of patients with aneurysmal SAH and produces clinical symptoms (termed "delayed ischemic neurologic deficits") or infarction in 30%. It causes half of the deaths in patients surviving to aneurysm treatment.
- ▸ Vasospasm risk is related to the amount of subarachnoid and intraventricular hemorrhage, features stratified in the Fisher grading scale for CT scans.
- ▸ It typically occurs 4 to 20 days after SAH and is usually most severe at 7 to 10 days. It may involve either proximal or distal intracerebral arteries.
- ▸ Symptoms depend on the territory affected and range from global cognitive impairment to focal deficits.
- ▸ Transcranial Doppler ultrasound detects elevated blood velocities due to vasospasm and is used to screen patients in the intensive care setting. Drawbacks include operator dependence and limited evaluation of the anterior cerebral arteries and posterior circulation.
- ▸ CT angiography may be used to confirm equivocal cases but may overestimate the degree of vessel narrowing. The role of CT or MR perfusion-weighted imaging is under investigation.
- ▸ Catheter angiography is the gold standard method for evaluating the severity of vessel narrowing. The stenoses are typically smoothly marginated and may occur over long segments of the vessels.

Management

- ▸ The calcium channel antagonist nimodipine is given prophylactically to reduce vasospasm-related morbidity.
- ▸ Induced hypervolemia and hypertension are used to maintain cerebral perfusion in the setting of documented vasospasm.
- ▸ When medical therapy fails, endovascular techniques (intra-arterial vasodilators and balloon angioplasty) are performed.

Further Reading

Bederson JB, Connolly Jr ES, Batjer HH, et al. Guidelines for the management of aneurysmal subarachnoid hemorrhage. *Stroke.* 2009;40: 994-1025.

Keyrouz SG, Diringer MN. Clinical review: Prevention and therapy of vasospasm in subarachnoid hemorrhage. *Critical Care.* 2007;11:220.

History

▶ 46-year-old woman with one-day history of headache, found unconscious the next day. In the emergency room, she is afebrile, normotensive, and unresponsive

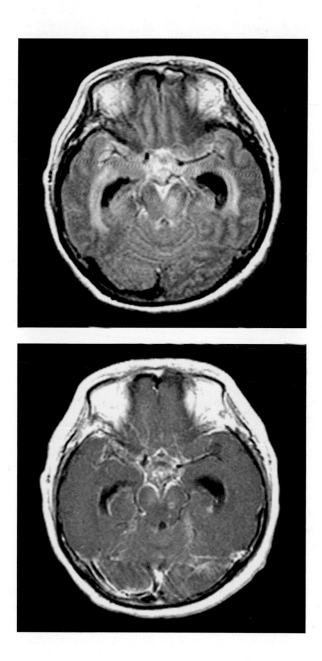

Case 58 Bacterial Meningitis and Ventriculitis (*S. Pneumoniae*)

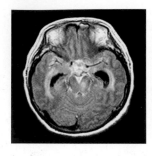 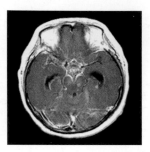

Findings

- There is hyperintense signal in the sulci and basal cisterns on the FLAIR sequence and thin abnormal enhancement in the suprasellar cistern and along the surface of the midbrain. On postcontrast T1-weighted images, there is subtle enhancement in the sulci about the inferior frontal lobes.
- There is moderate ventriculomegaly (enlargement of the temporal horns).
- There is hyperintense signal in periventricular white matter on FLAIR imaging and subependymal enhancement.
- There is signal abnormality and abnormal enhancement in the left cerebral peduncle, consistent with subacute infarction or abscess.

Differential Diagnosis

- Carcinomatous meningitis
- Lymphoma
- Leptomeningeal dissemination of primary CNS neoplasm
- Sarcoidosis
- Langerhans cell histiocytosis
- Chemical meningitis (e.g., ruptured dermoid, intrathecal medication)

Teaching Points

- Pyogenic meningitis is infection of the CSF and leptomeninges, usually by bacteria.
- The most common organisms in pyogenic meningitis vary with patient demographic. In neonate, *E. coli* and group B streptococcus predominate. In older children and adults, *S. pneumoniae*, *N. meningitidis*, and *L. monocytogenes* are most common. In postoperative patients, staphylococcal species are usually responsible.
- Lumbar puncture is the test of choice for diagnosis of meningitis. The role of advanced imaging is to establish the absence of contraindication to lumbar puncture and to detect the complications of meningitis.
- The earliest imaging sign of meningitis is hyperintense signal in the subarachnoid space on FLAIR imaging.
- Thin leptomeningeal enhancement along the basal cisterns and sulci may be present.
- Complications of pyogenic meningitis include hydrocephalus (communicating or obstructive), ventriculitis, venous thrombosis, arterial infarction (usually perforating arteries), subdural/epidural empyema, cerebritis, and cerebral abscess.

Management

- Bacterial meningitis can progress rapidly and when this disease is suspected, antibiotic therapy should be instituted prior to diagnostic procedures. CSF sampling is needed to establish the diagnosis and choose optimal antibiotic therapy.
- Complications of meningitis (e.g., hydrocephalus, ventriculitis, empyema, and cerebral abscess) may require surgical intervention.

Further Reading

Ferreira N, Otta G, Amaral L, da Rocha A. Imaging aspects of pyogenic infections of the central nervous system. *Topics Magn Reson Imaging.* 2005;16:145-154.

Kanamalla US, Roldolfo AI, Junkins JR. Imaging of cranial meningitis and ventriculitis. *Neuroimaging Clin North Am.* 2000;10:309-331.

History

▶ 30-year-old man with headaches and psychosis

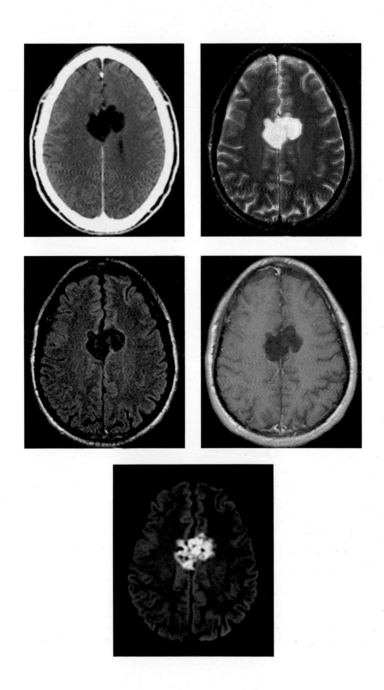

Case 59 Epidermoid Cyst

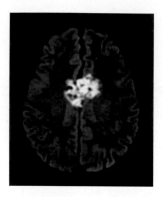

Findings

▶ There is a mass within the interhemispheric fissure with undulating borders that scallop the bilateral medial frontal lobes.

▶ The lesion is nonenhancing and has signal characteristics similar to CSF on CT as well as T1-weighted and T2-weighted MRI.

▶ However, it demonstrates mildly heterogeneous signal on FLAIR and hyperintense signal on DWI.

Differential Diagnosis

▶ Arachnoid cyst

▶ Abscess

▶ Dermoid cyst

Teaching Points

▶ Epidermoid cysts are benign congenital ectodermal inclusion cysts arising from an anomaly of neural tube closure early in embryogenesis.

▶ Lesions grow slowly and can remain clinically silent for years. They most often present in adults, usually with headache. They can produce compressive symptoms (e.g., cranial nerve palsy) when present at the skull base.

▶ The cysts are most commonly located off midline within the cerebellopontine angle cistern (40% to 50%), followed by the fourth ventricle (20%) and parasellar region (20%).

▶ Cyst contents include debris, keratin, and cholesterol laid down in a lamellar fashion.

▶ Epidermoids are extra-axial, infiltrative, lobulated masses. They may engulf neural and vascular structures.

▶ On CT they have uniform attenuation consistent with fluid.

▶ On T1- and T2-weighted MRI, signal in the mass matches that of CSF.

▶ The key imaging findings are the incomplete nulling of signal on the FLAIR sequence and the presence of marked hyperintensity on DWI.

Management

▶ Primary treatment is microsurgical resection. This is often complicated by encased neurovascular structures.

▶ Recurrence is common if the lesion is incompletely resected. Subarachnoid seeding also may occur. Follow-up imaging is important to assess for these sequelae.

Further Reading

Chen CY, et al. Intracranial epidermoid cyst with hemorrhage: MR imaging findings. *Am J Neuroradiol.* 2006;27:427-429.
Osborn AG, Preece MT. Intracranial cysts: radiologic-pathologic correlation and imaging approach. *Radiology.* 2006;239:650-664.

History

▶ 21-year-old man status post motor vehicle collision

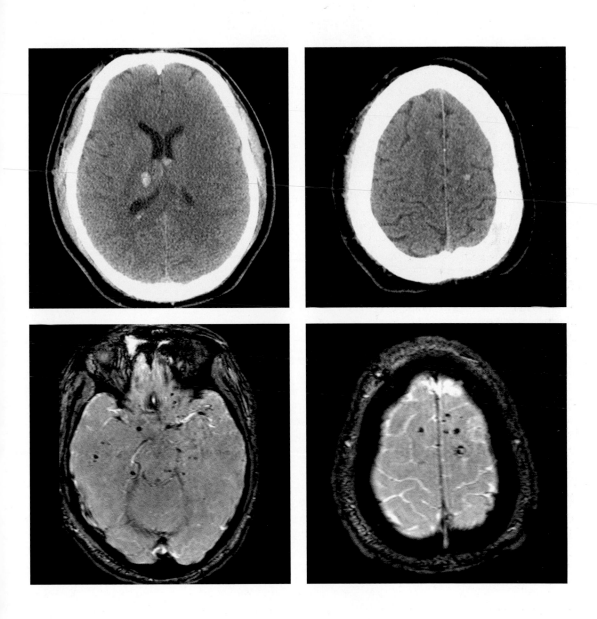

Case 60   Diffuse Axonal Injury

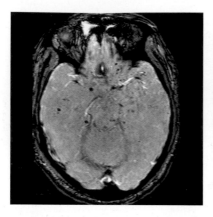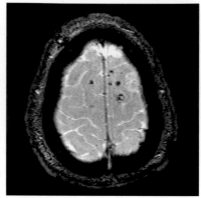

Findings

- ► CT images show multiple small hemorrhagic foci at the cortical gray–white matter junctions and in right thalamus.
- ► On the MRI, the susceptibility-weighted imaging (SWI) sequence shows many more sites of hemorrhage, visible as small foci of signal loss.

Differential Diagnosis

- ► Cerebral amyloid angiopathy
- ► Multiple cavernous malformations

Teaching Points

- ► Diffuse axonal injury (DAI) is a result of traumatic axonal stretching seen in the setting of deceleration injuries, most commonly high-speed motor vehicle accidents.
- ► The injury occurs where brain tissues of different densities intersect; this is why injuries most commonly involve the gray–white matter junctions. In more severe injuries the corpus callosum and dorsolateral brain stem are involved.
- ► The clinical presentation is variable depending on the severity of the injury. In mild cases transient loss of consciousness and retrograde amnesia is typical. Severe cases result in coma.
- ► CT demonstrates punctate foci of hemorrhage that result from shearing of small vessels. It usually underestimates the extent of injury.
- ► MRI, particularly heavily T2*-weighted or SWI sequences, provides more sensitive detection of microhemorrhage.
- ► MRI may also show non-hemorrhagic shear injury as foci of edema and restricted diffusion.
- ► When present, DAI lesions are focal and multiple with an ovoid shape parallel to the long axis on the involved axon. Autopsy series show that the extent of axonal injury is underestimated by imaging, even with current modalities.

Management

- ► Supportive therapy

Further Reading

Ezaki Y, Tsutsumi K, Morikawa M, Nagata I. Role of diffusion-weighted magnetic resonance imaging in diffuse axonal injury. *Acta Radiol.* 2006;47:733-740.

Gentry L, Knopp E. Head trauma. In: Atlas S, ed. Magnetic Resonance Imaging of the Brain and Spine, 4th ed. Philadelphia: Lippincott Williams, 2008:908-911.

History

▶ 45-year-old woman with history of stage IV gastroesophageal junction adenocarcinoma, now with slurred speech and ataxia

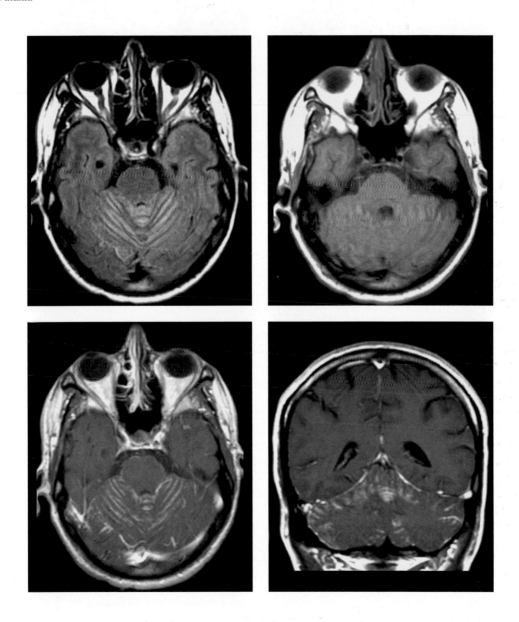

Case 61 Leptomeningeal Carcinomatosis

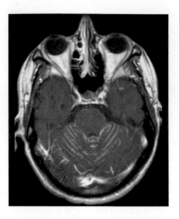

Findings

▸ On the FLAIR sequence, there is curvilinear hyperintense signal outlining the cerebellar folia.
▸ Postcontrast T1-weighted images show linear and nodular enhancement coating the surfaces of the cerebellum and pons.

Differential Diagnosis

▸ Sarcoidosis
▸ Infectious meningitis
▸ Wegener's granulomatosis and other inflammatory disorders

Teaching Points

▸ Leptomeningeal carcinomatosis represents infiltration of the leptomeninges by malignant cells metastasizing from systemic neoplasia. It occurs most commonly via hematogenous seeding with subsequent CSF spread.
▸ It tends to involve the basal cisterns and posterior fossa, theoretically due to slow CSF flow and gravity.
▸ Clinical presentations include headache, meningitis-like symptoms, and multifocal neurologic dysfunction, including cranial nerve palsies.
▸ Both CSF cytology and MR imaging play important roles in the diagnosis. MRI with postcontrast imaging has a sensitivity of 70%. With a series of three lumbar punctures, CSF sampling has a sensitivity of about 90%. MRI detects disease in up to 50% of patients with a negative CSF cytology.
▸ MRI characteristics cannot readily differentiate between the diagnostic possibilities, and diagnosis largely hinges on known history of malignancy and CSF findings.

Management

▸ Treatment options include radiation and intrathecal chemotherapy.

Further Reading

Collie DA, Brush JP, Lammie GA, et al. Imaging features of leptomeningeal metastases. *Clin Radiol*. 1999;54:765-771.
Kesari S, Batchelor TT. Leptomeningeal metastases. *Neurol Clin North Am*. 2003;21:25-66.
Maroldi R, Ambrosi C, Farina D. Metastatic disease of the brain: extra-axial metastases (skull, dura, leptomeningeal) and tumour spread. *Eur Radiol*. 2005;15:617-626.

History

▶ 13-year-old girl with short stature and frequent headaches

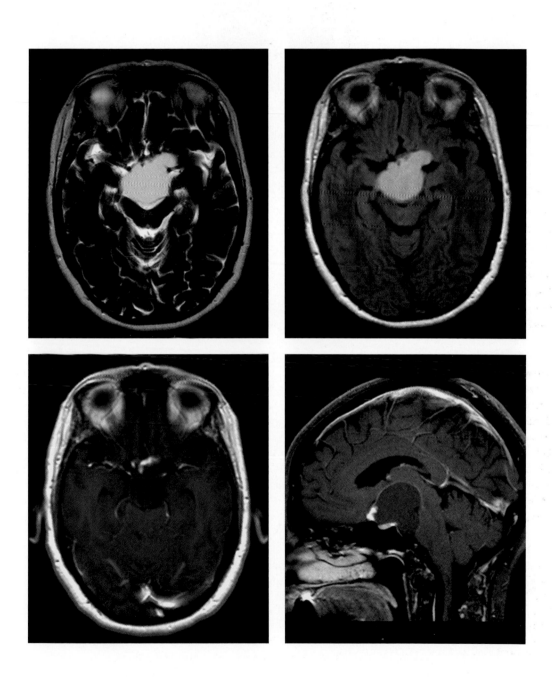

Case 62   Craniopharyngioma

Different patient

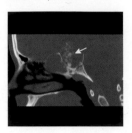

Different patient

Findings

▶ There is a large cystic, sellar and suprasellar mass with nodular mural enhancement.
▶ The cyst is hyperintense on the FLAIR sequence, consistent with proteinaceous contents.
▶ It deforms the sella and compresses the pituitary, third ventricle, and brain stem.
▶ On a CT from another patient (this page), coarse calcifications (arrow) are identified within a sellar and suprasellar mass.

Differential Diagnosis

▶ Rathke cleft cyst
▶ Dermoid/epidermoid cyst
▶ Germinoma
▶ Cystic pituitary adenoma
▶ Hypothalamic-chiasmatic glioma
▶ Partially thrombosed aneurysm

Teaching Points

▶ Craniopharyngioma is a benign epithelial neoplasm that is thought to arise from adenohypophyseal metaplasia or ectopic remnants of Rathke's pouch.
▶ It accounts for 5% to 10% of pediatric intracranial tumors and is the most common pediatric suprasellar tumor (~50%).
▶ There are two histologic types.
  ▪ The adamantinomatous type is more common in children and is usually cystic, calcified, and enhancing.
  ▪ The papillary type typically occurs in adults (>50 years) as a solid, enhancing tumor.
▶ Clinical presentation is related to mass effect on the optic chiasm (visual disturbance), pituitary gland (growth hormone deficiency in children, hypogonadism in adults), and ventricles (headaches and nausea/vomiting).
▶ Craniopharyngiomas are usually centered in the suprasellar (>90%) region with variable intra- and parasellar extension. They can extend into all cranial fossae, the ventricles, and the retroclival region.
▶ CT scan is useful to identify calcification. Cysts demonstrate variable density due to proteinaceous or hemorrhagic contents.
▶ MRI provides a better assessment of tumor extent. The cyst contents have variable signal on T1- and T2-weighted sequences due to differences in protein, cholesterol, and blood content.
▶ Significant enhancement should not be seen in Rathke cleft cysts, arachnoid cysts, or dermoids/epidermoids.
▶ Germinomas and gliomas with cystic/necrotic components may appear similar to craniopharyngioma, but calcification is uncommon.

Management

▶ These neoplasms may be treated with surgical resection but the extent of resection is often limited by proximity or adherence to vital structures. Residual neoplasm is usually treated with radiation therapy.

Further Reading

Karavitaki N, Cudlip S, Adams C, et al. Craniopharyngiomas. *Endocrinol Metab Clin North Am.* 2008;37:173-193.
Tsuda M, Takahashi S, Higano S, et al. CT and MR imaging of craniopharyngioma. *Eur Radiol.* 1997;7:464-469.

History

▶ 8-year-old boy with new onset of epilepsy

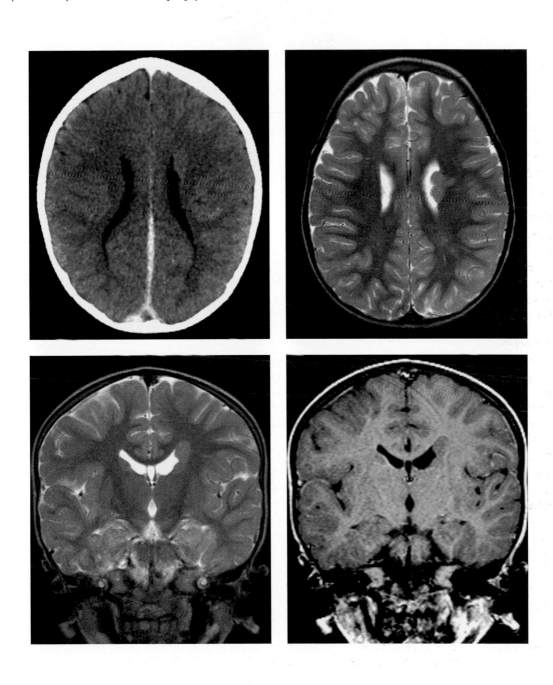

Case 63 Gray Matter Heterotopia

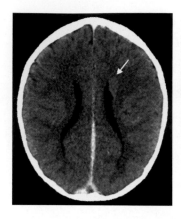 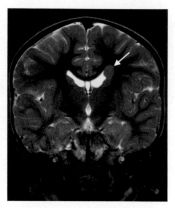

Findings

▶ Contrast-enhanced CT shows a noncalcified nodular mass in the subependymal region of the left lateral ventricle (arrow).
▶ On T2-weighted and postcontrast T1-weighted MRI sequences the lesion (arrow) follows the signal of gray matter. It does not enhance.

Differential Diagnosis

▶ Subependymal nodules of tuberous sclerosis
▶ Normal body and tail of caudate nucleus

Teaching Points

▶ Gray matter heterotopia is a disorder of cortical development in which collections of nerve cells are seen in abnormal locations due to arrested neuronal migration.
▶ Gray matter heterotopias may appear band-like, nodular subependymal (most common), or nodular subcortical. Subependymal nodular heterotopias as in these case are adjacent to and often indent the margin of the lateral ventricle.
▶ Seizures and developmental delay are the most common clinical symptoms. Small heterotopias may be asymptomatic.
▶ Heterotopias may be seen in isolation or in association with a variety of brain malformations such as Chiari II, cephaloceles, or agenesis of the corpus callosum. Some cases are familial.
▶ Heterotopias follow the attenuation and signal intensity of gray matter on CT and all MRI pulse sequences, respectively. MRI is much more sensitive than CT in detecting these lesions. They do not enhance and generally do not calcify.

Management

▶ Antiepileptic medication is used for patients with seizures. Surgery is reserved for patients with medically refractory epilepsy and small accessible lesions. For extensive lesions, corpus callosotomy is occasionally performed.

Further Reading

Barkovich AJ, Kuzniecki RI, Jackson GD, et al. A developmental and genetic classification for malformations of cortical development. *Neurology.* 2005;65:1873-1887.
Spalice A, Parisi P, Nicita F, et al. Neuronal migration disorders: clinical, neuroradiologic and genetics aspects. *Acta Paediatr.* 2009;98: 421-433.

History

▶ Routine second-trimester prenatal ultrasonography in a mother with diabetes

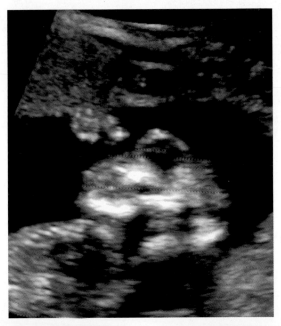

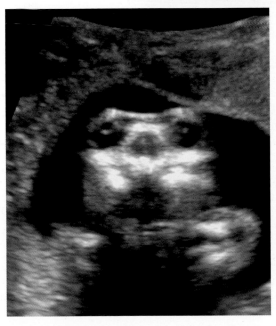

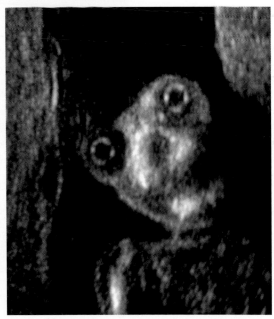

Case 64 Anencephaly

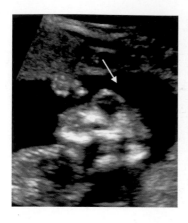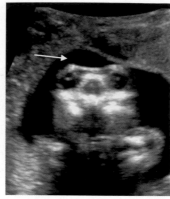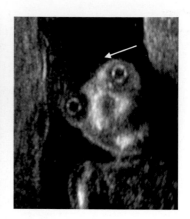

Findings

▶ Ultrasound images of the fetal head demonstrate absence of the cranial vault and supratentorial brain structures above the orbit (arrows).

Differential Diagnosis

▶ Acrania
▶ Large encephalocele or meningocele
▶ Severe microcephaly
▶ Amniotic band syndrome

Teaching Points

▶ Anencephaly is a neural tube defect in which large portions of the skull, scalp, and brain fail to form. The forebrain is absent or severely hypoplastic and the remaining brain structures and brain stem are exposed and often dysfunctional.
▶ There is a higher risk in mothers with insulin-dependent diabetes mellitus, folic acid deficiency, and use of medications with folic acid antagonist properties.
▶ On ultrasound, a small crown–rump length can be an early finding and clue. There is no calvarium and brain tissue is absent above the orbits during second-trimester imaging. Diagnosis can often be confidently made on ultrasound. Fetal MRI may confirm an equivocal ultrasound but usually is not needed.
▶ Polyhydramnios is common secondary to impaired swallowing function because of the brain abnormality. The eyes often appear protuberant secondary to shallow orbits. There is a high incidence of associated cervical or lumbar neural tube defects. Genitourinary defects and cleft lip or palate are also seen with higher frequency.

Management

▶ Anencephaly is a lethal malformation and most newborns die within hours to a few days.

Further Reading

Aubry MC, Aubry JP, Dommergues M. Sonographic prenatal diagnosis of central nervous system abnormalities. *Childs Nerv Syst.* 2003;19:391-402.
Dias MS, Partington M. Embryology of myelomeningocele and anencephaly. *Neurosurg Focus.* 2004;16:1-16.

History

▸ 6-year-old boy with headache and fever

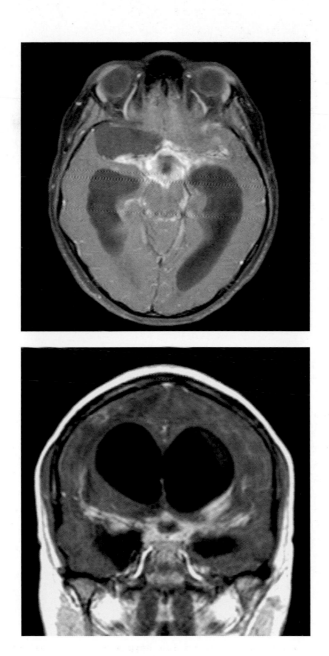

Case 65 Tuberculous Meningitis

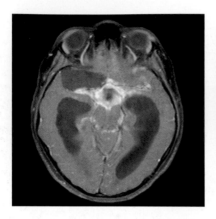 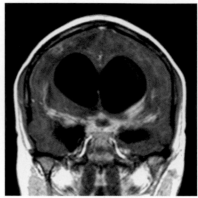

Findings

▸ The postcontrast T1-weighted MRI studies show thick leptomeningeal enhancement along the basal cisterns and sylvian fissures and thinner leptomeningeal enhancement along the brain surface. There is intracerebral extension to the inferior left frontal lobe.

▸ There is marked ventriculomegaly. An arachnoid cyst is present in the right middle cranial fossa, and it may be incidental or a result of the inflammatory exudate.

Differential Diagnosis

▸ Pyogenic meningitis
▸ Fungal or amebic meningitis
▸ Lymphoma
▸ Leptomeningeal carcinomatosis
▸ Sarcoidosis

Teaching Points

▸ Tuberculous meningitis, unlike pyogenic meningitis, usually results from hematogenous seeding of the brain and subsequent rupture of intracerebral infection into the subarachnoid space.

▸ Patients present with fever, headache, nausea, meningismus, and cranial nerve palsies. CSF analysis shows lymphocytosis and decreased glucose.

▸ The MRI or CT demonstrates thick abnormal leptomeningeal enhancement, typically along the basal cisterns.

▸ Hydrocephalus, usually communicating, is common and results from thick gelatinous inflammatory exudate impairing CSF resorption.

▸ Inflammatory vasculopathy is another common complication, usually manifest as infarcts in the distribution of the small perforating arteries.

▸ The other common form of tuberculous CNS infection is intracerebral granuloma, identified on imaging as multiple ring-enhancing and nodular-enhancing foci.

Management

▸ The diagnosis is confirmed by CSF sampling with direct identification of the mycobacteria or their growth on culture. Negative AFB staining should not preclude treatment when suspicion is high.

▸ Treatment consists of combination therapy with antituberculous drugs and, when needed, CSF shunting.

Further Reading

Shah GV. Central nervous system tuberculosis: Imaging manifestations. *Am J Neuroradiol.* 2000;10:355-374.

History

▶ 3-year-old boy presenting with seizures. There is a birthmark on the left side of the upper face

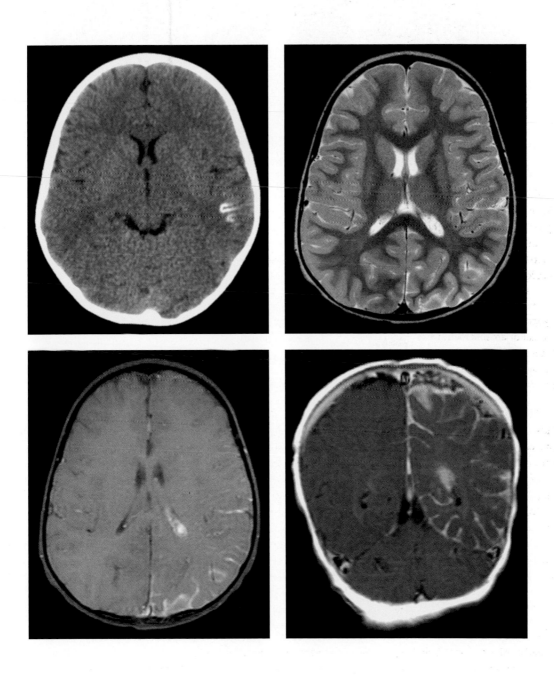

Case 66 Sturge-Weber Syndrome (Encephalotrigeminal Angiomatosis)

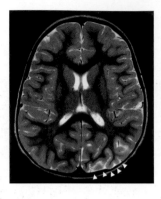 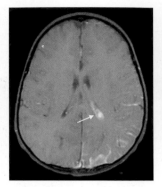 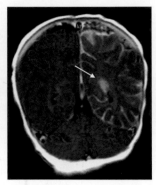

Findings

▶ Axial noncontrast CT demonstrates curvilinear and gyriform calcification in the left cerebral hemisphere.

▶ Axial T2-weighted MRI shows subtle focal volume loss in the left occipitoparietal region (arrowheads).

▶ Postcontrast axial and coronal T1-weighted images show intense leptomeningeal enhancement along with asymmetric enlargement and enhancement of the left choroid plexus (arrows).

Differential Diagnosis

▶ Meningitis

▶ Leptomeningeal metastases

▶ Other vascular malformations

▶ Subacute infarcts with enhancement

Teaching Points

▶ Sturge-Weber syndrome, or encephalotrigeminal angiomatosis, is a sporadic congenital syndrome consisting of facial nevus flammeus (port wine stain) in the distribution of the trigeminal nerve, choroidal angiomas in the eye, and pial angiomatosis in the brain (ipsilateral to the facial abnormalities). The cerebral angiomatous component is thought to be due to a malformation in the development of cortical veins.

▶ Patients often have seizures or glaucoma in infancy and may develop progressive hemiparesis and developmental delay.

▶ In 20% of patients, the brain manifestations are bilateral. Rarely, there is no facial nevus flammeus.

▶ Radiographs may show curvilinear calcifications along the surface of the brain ("tram-track" calcifications). CT is more sensitive and the calcifications are typically gyriform. CT may initially be normal.

▶ MRI with contrast is much more sensitive in detecting the pial angiomatosis changes. The ipsilateral choroid plexus is almost always enlarged and may be the only early manifestation of disease.

▶ Over time the extent of demonstrable brain abnormality in the affected hemisphere may increase. The extent and degree of enhancement and calcification increases and eventually leads to progressive atrophy and gliosis of the involved portions of the brain due to chronic venous ischemia.

Management

▶ Seizure control is the mainstay of treatment. It may require resection of the involved lobes or hemisphere.

Further Reading

Adams ME, et al. A spectrum of unusual neuroimaging findings in patients with suspected Sturge-Weber syndrome. *Am J Neuroradiol.* 2009;30:276-281.

Smirniotopoulos JG. Neuroimaging of phakomatoses: Sturge-Weber syndrome, tuberous sclerosis, von Hippel-Lindau syndrome. *Neuroimaging Clin North Am.* 2004;14:171-183.

History

▶ 59-year-old with seizures and lethargy

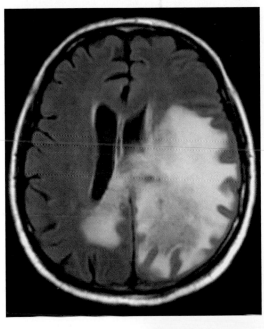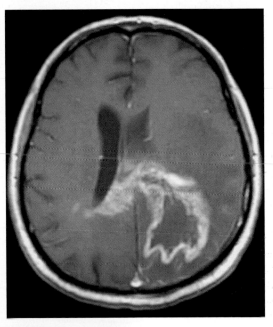

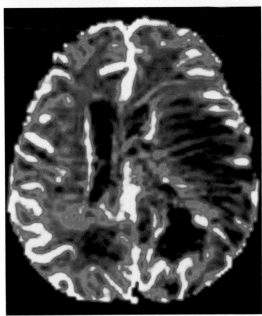

CBV map

Case 67   Glioblastoma Multiforme (GBM)

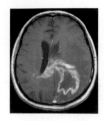 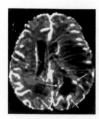

Findings

- There is a large, peripherally enhancing mass expanding the left cerebral hemisphere. There is extensive surrounding hyperintense signal on FLAIR imaging.
- The signal abnormality and enhancement cross the corpus callosum to involve the right parietal lobe.
- Areas of elevated cerebral blood volume, CBV (arrows) are present within the enhancing tissue.

Differential Diagnosis

- Abscess
- Metastases
- Tumefactive demyelination
- Lymphoma
- Radiation necrosis

Teaching Points

- GBM is a high-grade (WHO grade IV) astrocytic tumor with poor prognosis. Despite best current therapy, average survival is 14 months.
- GBM is most common in adults and is usually supratentorial.
- The usual appearance is an irregularly enhancing mass containing cystic/necrotic components and hemorrhagic foci. Often there is an extensive surrounding area of T2 prolongation and expansion. This nonenhancing component consists of both interstitial edema and cancer cells.
- Within the solid and enhancing components of GBM:
  - MR spectroscopy demonstrates elevated choline:creatine ratio and depressed N-acetylaspartate.
  - MR perfusion imaging reveals elevated CBV.
- Abscesses have a central area of restricted diffusion and a thin peripheral T2-hypointense rim.
- Metastases are often multiple and round and occur at the gray–white matter junction.
- Tumefactive demyelination may involve the corpus callosum and can appear identical to GBM. However, it often has less mass effect and an incomplete peripheral rim of enhancement.
- Lymphoma typically enhances homogeneously, except in the setting of AIDS, where it may be necrotic. Lymphomas can cross the corpus callosum and often demonstrate restricted diffusion and relatively hypointense signal on T2-weighted images.
- Radiation necrosis may be difficult to differentiate from recurrent GBM. Clinical history and advanced imaging techniques are needed.

Management

- Biopsy and resection are performed to confirm the diagnosis and debulk the neoplasm. Followed by postoperative chemotherapy and radiation. Salvage chemotherapy and anti-angiogenic treatment for recurrence.

Further Reading

Brandes AA, Tosoni A, Franceschi E, et al. Glioblastoma in adults. *Crit Rev Oncol Hematol.* 2008;67:139-152.

Law M, Cha S, Knopp EA, et al. High-grade gliomas and solitary metastases: differentiation by using perfusion and proton spectroscopic MR imaging. *Radiology.* 2002;222:715-721.

History

▶ 60-year-old man with depression

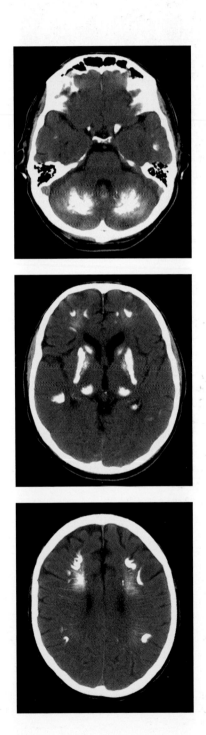

Case 68   Fahr Disease

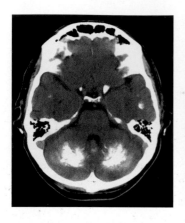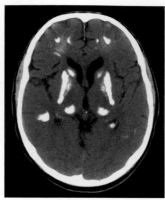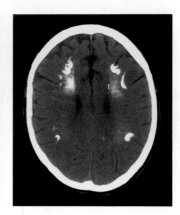

Findings

▶ There are symmetric areas of calcification centered in the dentate nuclei, lentiform nuclei, thalami, and subcortical white matter.

Differential Diagnosis

▶ While there are many causes of bilateral basal ganglia calcifications, this pattern of symmetric striopallidodentate calcinosis in an adult has a limited differential diagnosis:
  ▪ Hypoparathyroidism
  ▪ Pseudohypoparathyroidism
  ▪ Hyperparathyroidism

Teaching Points

▶ Fahr disease is a group of disorders of uncertain etiology marked by deposition of calcium and other minerals in the basal ganglia, dentate nucleus, other deep gray nuclei, and cerebral white matter.
▶ Patients may present with movement disorders, cognitive impairment, or cerebellar dysfunction. About one third of patients are asymptomatic.
▶ There are both sporadic and inherited forms of this phenomenon.
▶ The calcifications are readily demonstrated on CT but may be difficult to identify on MRI.

Management

▶ Evaluation for disorders of calcium metabolism is necessary. In the absence of such metabolic diseases, there is no known treatment.

Further Reading

Manyam BV. What is and what is not "Fahr's disease." *Parkinsonism Relat Disord.* 2005;11:73-80.

History

▶ 16-year-old girl with headaches

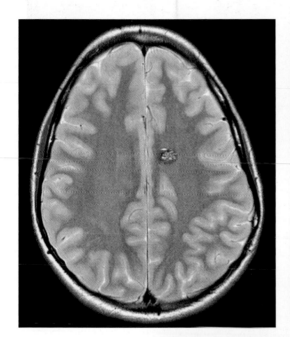 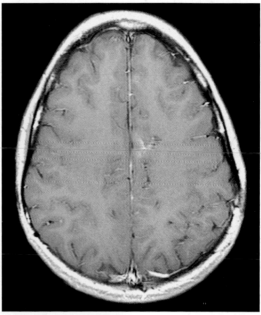

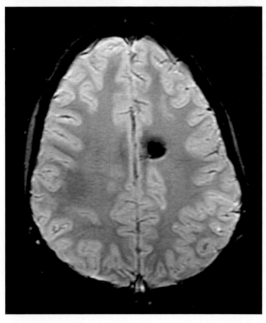

Case 69 Cavernous Malformation (CM)

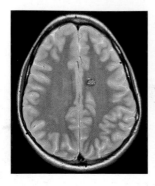 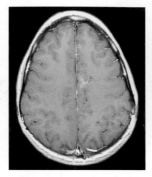 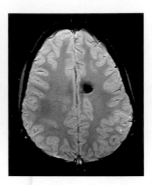

Findings

▶ There is a well-circumscribed ovoid lesion in the left centrum semiovale.
▶ On T2-weighted images it has a rim of markedly hypointense signal and a central multiseptate area of hyperintense signal.
▶ There is curvilinear enhancement adjacent to the lesion, possibly a small developmental venous anomaly (DVA).
▶ Susceptibility-weighted imaging shows "blooming" of the signal loss associated with the lesion, corroborating the presence of blood products.

Differential Diagnosis

▶ Hemorrhagic metastasis
▶ Intracerebral hemorrhage of other etiology (e.g., arteriovenous malformation, amyloid angiopathy, diffuse axonal injury)

Teaching Points

▶ CMs are developmental vascular malformations consisting of a circumscribed collection of thin-walled vessels. Even asymptomatic lesions almost always show evidence of prior microhemorrhage with formation of a border of gliosis and old blood products about the abnormal vessels. Unlike AVMs, there is no arteriovenous shunting.
▶ They commonly present with seizures or with hemorrhage and resultant focal neurologic deficits.
▶ Lesions with prior symptomatic hemorrhage have a 4.5% annual risk of rebleeding. Lesions without prior hemorrhage have an annual hemorrhage risk of less than 1%.
▶ While many CMs are sporadic, there are inherited forms. Familial CMs are often multiple.
▶ On CT, CMs are visible as partially calcified masses. Small or noncalcified cavernous malformations are difficult to detect.
▶ MRI is both sensitive and specific. T2-weighted images will demonstrate the central area of abnormal vessels as a "bubbly" area of hyperintensity. This area is surrounded by a complete rim of hypointense signal that represents old blood products.
▶ Small CMs may be visible only on T2*-weighted images as foci of susceptibility-related signal loss.
▶ While hemorrhagic metastasis may mimic a CM, it is rare for a metastasis to have a complete ring of blood products about its margin.
▶ There is an association between CMs and DVAs, and they are often found in close proximity. Detection of DVAs is important since care is taken to avoid them during surgery.

Management

▶ CMs that have bled and are in relatively safe locations are surgically resected. Asymptomatic lesions and those in areas with substantial surgical morbidity (e.g., brain stem) may be followed.

Further Reading

Morris P. *Practical Neuroangiography*, 2nd ed. Philadelphia: Lippincott Williams Wilkins, 2007:348-351.
Tung GA, Blitstein MK. MRI of cerebral microhemorrhages. *AJR Am J Roentgenol.* 189:720-725.

History

▶ 4-year-old with seizures and developmental delay and white patches on the skin

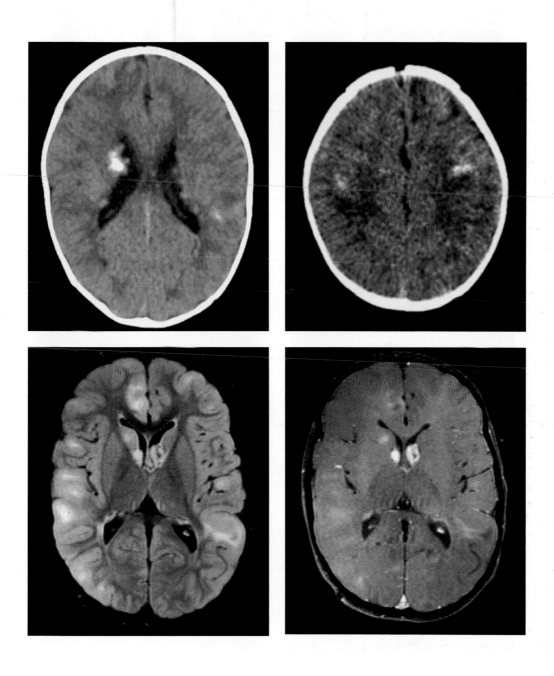

Case 70 Tuberous Sclerosis

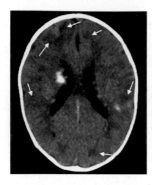 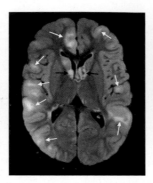 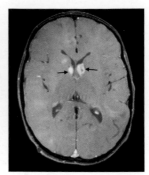

Findings

► Axial noncontrast CT images demonstrate multiple foci of subcortical and cortical hypoattenuation in the brain bilaterally (white arrows).
► In some areas, there are foci of subcortical calcification. There are multiple densely or partially calcified nodules along the ependymal surface of the lateral ventricles.
► The FLAIR sequence shows numerous areas of cortical and subcortical high signal intensity (white arrows).
► There are enhancing nodular masses near the foramina of Munro bilaterally (black arrows).

Differential Diagnosis

► Congenital infections (TORCH)
► Multiple subependymal gray matter heterotopias (do not calcify)

Teaching Points

► Tuberous sclerosis (epiloia or Bourneville disease) is a phakomatosis with autosomal dominant inheritance, though many cases are *de novo* mutations.
► Patients often present with seizures, developmental delay, and skin lesions.
► There are several cerebral manifestations of tuberous sclerosis.
  ▪ Multiple cortical/subcortical tubers, which appear as areas of gyral thickening, subcortical and cortical signal abnormality (hyperintense on T2-weighted mages, iso- or hypointense on T1-weighted images). They may show radiating signal abnormality from the cortex towards the ventricles. Some have subcortical calcification.
  ▪ Subependymal nodules (hamartomas) along the lateral ventricles. They are often calcified, especially in older children. They may or may not enhance with contrast.
  ▪ Subependymal giant cell astrocytomas (SEGAs) are slow-growing grade I tumors that arise near the foramina of Munro and are distinguished from the other subependymal nodules by demonstration of growth and larger size.
► Skin lesions of tuberous sclerosis include facial angiofibromas, hypomelanotic macules (ash leaf spots), and periungual fibromas. Other manifestations include cardiac rhabdomyomas, renal or other organ angiomyolipomas, lung disease similar to lymphangioleiomyomatosis, retinal hamartomas, and cysts in the kidneys, pancreas, or bone.

Management

► Antiepileptic medication for seizures is the mainstay of treatment. SEGAs that grow are surgically resected. Tubers that are thought to be responsible for seizures may occasionally be resected.

Further Reading

Kalantari BN, Salamon N. Neuroimaging of tuberous sclerosis: spectrum of pathologic findings and frontiers in imaging. *AJR Am J Roentgenol.* 2008;190:W304-309.
Lin DD, Barker PB. Neuroimaging of phakomatoses. *Semin Pediatr Neurol.* 2006;13:48-62.

History

▶ 48-year-old man with history of right insular glioblastoma multiforme status post resection, chemotherapy, and involved-field radiation therapy

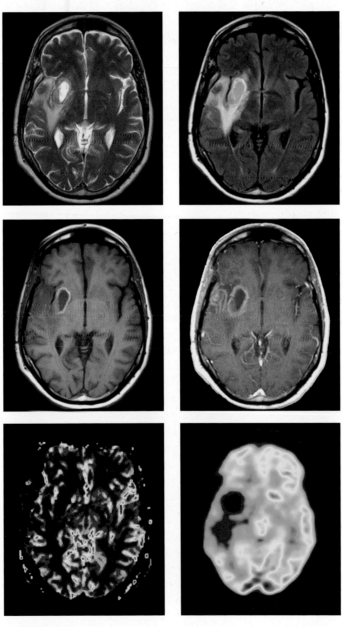

Cerebral blood volume   PET

Case 71 Radiation Necrosis

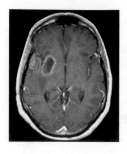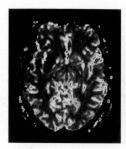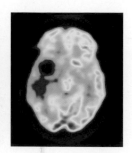

Findings

► There is T2 hyperintensity and mild expansion in the right anterior temporal lobe and subinsular region with irregular enhancement. The resection cavity has a T1- and T2-hyperintense rim, consistent with the presence of blood products.
► MR perfusion-weighted imaging (PWI) demonstrates corresponding decreased cerebral blood volume (CBV).
► FDG PET reveals corresponding hypometabolism.

Differential Diagnosis

► Recurrent neoplasm
► Abscess
► Foreign body reaction
► Subacute infarction

Teaching Points

► Radiation necrosis represents ischemic injury to the cerebral parenchyma. It usually occurs 6 months to 2 years after radiation therapy.
► The challenge is to distinguish radiation necrosis from recurrent neoplasm. Standard morphologic imaging is unreliable. Functional imaging techniques are helpful in making this distinction.
  ▪ MR PWI usually reveals increased CBV in recurrent tumor versus decreased CBV in radiation necrosis.
  ▪ MR spectroscopy (not shown) in recurrent tumor demonstrates decreased NAA and increased choline/creatine ratio. Radiation necrosis usually demonstrates marked reduction in all metabolites.
  ▪ DWI demonstrates higher levels of diffusivity in radiation necrosis than in recurrent neoplasm.
  ▪ FDG PET tends to have increased metabolism in recurrent tumor versus decreased metabolism in radiation necrosis.
► Radiation injury has a broad spectrum of imaging findings in addition to necrosis:
  ▪ Focal or confluent areas of abnormal signal intensity in the white matter (leukoencephalopathy)
  ▪ Mineralizing microangiopathy (subcortical and basal ganglia calcifications)
  ▪ Necrotizing leukoencephalopathy
  ▪ Radiation-induced cavernous malformations or capillary telangiectasias
► Foreign body reaction may be indistinguishable from recurrent tumor or radiation necrosis on imaging, and diagnosis is largely based on history.

Management

► Stereotactic biopsy remains the gold standard for differentiating radiation necrosis from recurrent tumor. The condition may be treated conservatively, but when it is symptomatic, treatment with surgical resection, bevacizumab, hyperbaric oxygen, or corticosteroids may be beneficial.

Further Reading

Alexiou GA, Tsiouris S, Kyritsis AP, et al. Glioma recurrence versus radiation necrosis: accuracy of current imaging modalities. *J Neurooncol.* 2009;95:1-11.
Barajas RF, Chang JS, Segal MR, et al. Differentiation of recurrent glioblastoma multiforme from radiation necrosis after external beam radiation therapy with dynamic susceptibility-weighted contrast-enhanced perfusion MR imaging. *Radiology.* 2009;253:486-496.

History

▶ 58-year-old woman with ataxia

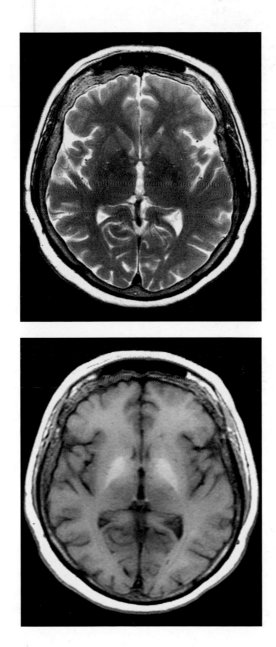

Case 72 Chronic Liver Disease

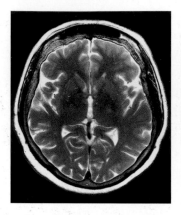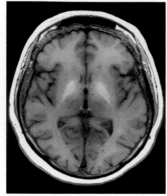

Findings

▶ The T2-weighted image appears normal.
▶ The T1-weighted image shows symmetric, abnormal, relatively uniform, hyperintense signal within the globus pallidus.

Differential Diagnosis

▶ Total parenteral nutrition
▶ Manganese (Mn) toxicity
▶ Radiation and chemotherapy for CNS neoplasm
▶ Neurofibromatosis I

Teaching Points

▶ Mn accumulation is thought to be the mechanism by which chronic liver dysfunction produces symmetric pallidal T1 shortening.
▶ There is poor correlation between this finding and neurologic status. The finding is commonly present in patients without clinical abnormalities.
▶ CT is usually normal.
▶ T1-weighted MR images show hyperintense signal in the globus pallidus. The other deep gray nuclei may show similar changes.
▶ Clinically evident hepatic encephalopathy is associated with the development of signal changes in the corticospinal tracts: hyperintense signal on FLAIR images and increased diffusion.

Management

▶ The various causes of this pallidal signal abnormality (listed above) produce similar imaging findings. The diagnosis is usually apparent from clinical history. Reversal of the inciting pathology often leads to resolution of the imaging findings.

Further Reading

Morgan MY. Cerebral magnetic resonance imaging in patients with chronic liver disease. *Metab Brain Dis*. 1998;13:273-290.
Rovira A, Alonso J, Cordoba J. MR imaging findings in hepatic encephalopathy. *Am J Neuroradiol*. 2008;29:1612-1621.

History

▶ 3-year-old girl with upper respiratory infection one week ago, now presents with profound lethargy

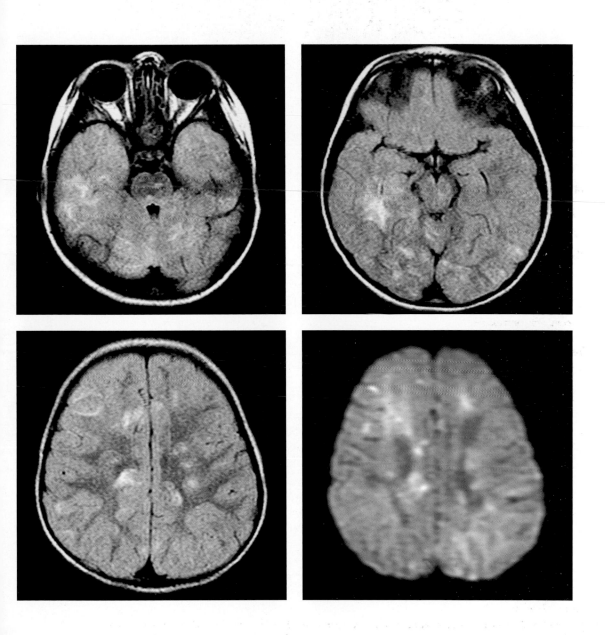

Case 73 Acute Disseminated Encephalomyelitis (ADEM)

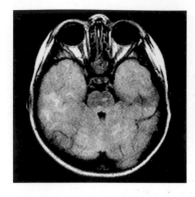 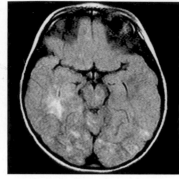 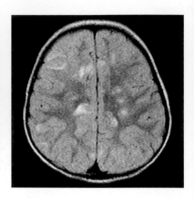

Findings

▶ FLAIR images show numerous asymmetric hyperintense lesions in the white matter of the cerebral hemispheres, cerebellum, and brain stem.

▶ Many of the lesions are hyperintense on DWI.

Differential Diagnosis

▶ Multiple sclerosis (MS)

▶ Encephalitis

▶ Vasculitis

Teaching Points

▶ ADEM is an immune-mediated, monophasic, demyelinating disorder of the CNS. The disease has a predilection for children and is usually precipitated by a viral infection or vaccination (Epstein-Barr, influenza A, mumps, measles, chickenpox).

▶ The presenting features include an acute encephalopathy with multifocal neurologic signs and deficits. These include headaches, drowsiness, cranial nerve palsies, ataxia, seizures, and coma. Patients present 1 to 2 weeks after the viral illness/immunization. Most patients completely recover, but there is a 10% to 20% mortality rate. Spinal involvement is seen in 30% of cases.

▶ A rare variant of ADEM with hemorrhage (acute hemorrhagic leukoencephalopathy) has a rapid course with poor prognosis.

▶ Imaging findings are similar to MS with multifocal T2-hyperintense white matter lesions. The lesions in ADEM are more likely to involve gray matter and usually do not involve the callosal/septal interface.

▶ Monophasic course also helps distinguish ADEM from MS. The lesions may be large, but show mild mass effect. Enhancement may be present, similar to findings in MS.

Management

▶ Corticosteroids are the mainstay of therapy, with plasmapheresis used for more severe cases.

Further Reading

Rossi A. Imaging of acute disseminated encephalomyelitis. *Neuroimaging Clin North Am.* 2008;18:149-161.
Tenenbaum S, Chitnis T, Ness J, et al. Acute disseminated encephalomyelitis. *Neurology.* 2007;68:S23-36.

History

► 35-year-old man with new-onset seizures

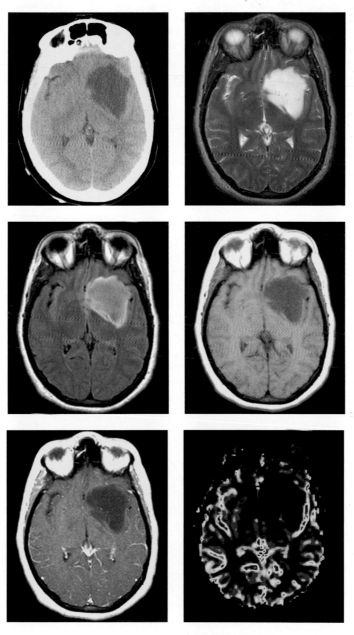

Cerebral blood volume

Case 74 Low-grade Fibrillary Astrocytoma

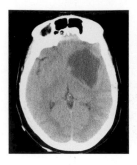 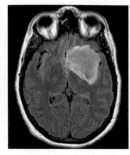 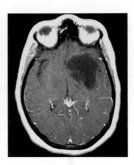

Findings

- ▶ Noncontrast CT demonstrates a hypoattenuating mass involving the left frontal and subinsular white matter and the left basal ganglia. There is mild local mass effect.
- ▶ The mass is homogeneously T1-hypointense and T2-hyperintense with no significant enhancement on post-gadolinium images. The mass is hyperintense on the FLAIR sequence. There is little surrounding edema.
- ▶ Perfusion imaging demonstrates decreased cerebral blood volume relative to normal brain.

Differential Diagnosis

- ▶ Anaplastic astrocytoma
- ▶ Oligodendroglioma
- ▶ Subacute infarction
- ▶ Encephalitis

Teaching Points

- ▶ Fibrillary astrocytoma (FA) is the most common type of low-grade astrocytoma and most frequently presents in young adults, with a mean age of 35 years.
- ▶ Seizure is the most common presenting symptom and is seen in approximately 75% of cases.
- ▶ Survival is variable and determined largely by whether there is malignant progression to a higher-grade astrocytoma (anaplastic astrocytoma or glioblastoma multiforme). Median survival may be up to 10 years.
- ▶ The majority are located in the supratentorial brain. They can be focal or diffuse, but there is usually infiltration beyond the margins demonstrated on imaging.
- ▶ On CT, cysts and calcification are rare.
- ▶ On MR imaging, low-grade astrocytomas typically demonstrate T1 hypointensity, T2 hyperintensity, and no significant enhancement. There may be significant overlap between the appearance of FA, anaplastic astrocytoma, and oligodendroglioma.
- ▶ Low relative cerebral blood volume on perfusion-weighted imaging may help differentiate low-grade astrocytoma from other neoplasms.
- ▶ If enhancement of the mass develops as the lesion is being followed, it suggests progression to a higher-grade neoplasm.

Management

- ▶ Patients with few symptoms and lesions in eloquent areas may be followed.
- ▶ When necessary, the primary treatment is surgical resection with or without radiation therapy.

Further Reading

Cha S. Update on brain tumor imaging: from anatomy to physiology. *Am J Neuroradiol.* 2006;27:475-487.

Wessels PH, Weber WE, Raven G, et al. Supratentorial grade II astrocytoma: biological features and clinical course. *Lancet Neurol.* 2003;2:395-403.

History

▶ 68-year-old man with memory loss

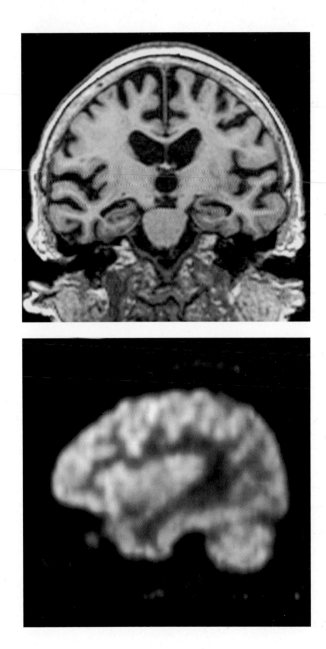

Case 75 Alzheimer's Disease

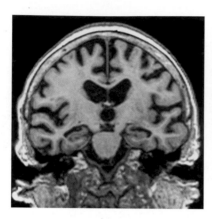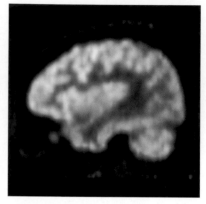

Findings

► Coronal thin-section T1-weighted images show bilateral hippocampal atrophy, proportionately greater than the diffuse cerebral atrophy present.
► [18]FDG-PET shows relative hypometabolism in the posterior parietal and temporal lobes.

Differential Diagnosis

These imaging findings strongly suggest the presence of Alzheimer's disease (AD). The primary clinical problems are early recognition and differentiation from other causes of dementia (i.e., vascular dementia, frontotemporal dementia, and dementia with Lewy bodies).

Teaching Points

► AD is a progressive neurodegenerative disorder characterized by deposition of β-amyloid plaques and neurofibrillary tangles in the brain. There is also loss of the neurotransmitter acetylcholine in affected regions.
► Patients present with a slowly progressive dementia in which consciousness is preserved but memory and cognitive functions are impaired.
► Currently, premortem diagnosis is established by clinical examination and neuropsychological testing, but definitive diagnosis relies upon histopathology.
► Imaging of the brain is recommended to exclude nondegenerative causes of dementia.
► There is substantial support for the use of advanced imaging in distinguishing AD patients from normal and from patients with other dementias. Further, these tests may allow diagnosis of AD prior to the presence of clinically evident disease.
  ▪ MRI performed with thin coronal sections is reliably able to detect tissue loss in the hippocampus and entorhinal cortex early in the course of the disease.
  ▪ [18]FDG PET shows decreased metabolic activity in the parietal and temporal lobes.
  ▪ Direct imaging of β-amyloid with novel radiopharmaceuticals and PET or SPECT shows early promise.

Management

► There is no cure for AD. There is modest and temporary improvement with oral cholinesterase inhibitors.

Further Reading

Fennema-Notestine C, McEvoy LK, Hagler DJ, et al. Structural neuroimaging in the detection and prognosis of pre-clinical and early AD. *Behav Neurol.* 2009;21:3-12.
O'Brien JT. Role of imaging techniques in the diagnosis of dementia. *Br J Radiol.* 2007;80:S71-S77.

History

▶ 27-year-old patient with a history of epistaxis, dyspnea, prior transient ischemic attacks, and headaches

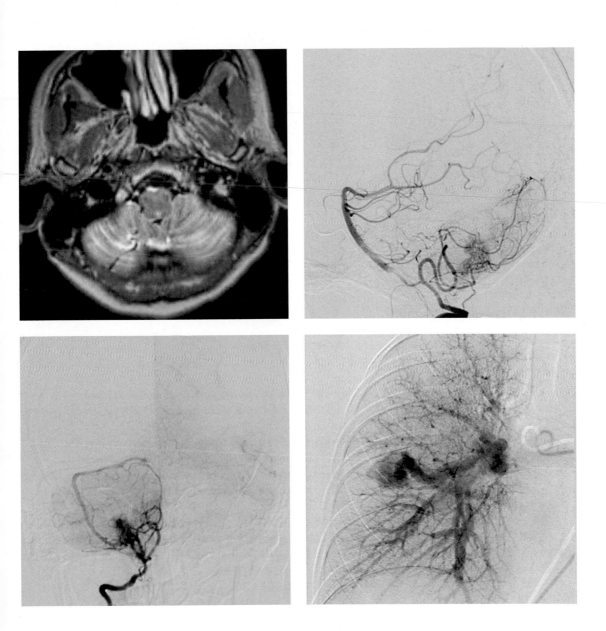

Case 76   Osler-Weber-Rendu Syndrome (Hereditary Hemorrhagic Telangiectasia [HHT])

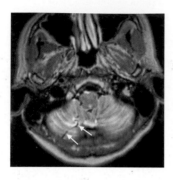 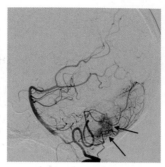 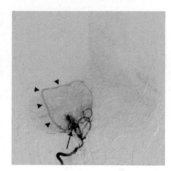

Findings

- ▶ Axial T2-weighted MRI shows an abnormally prominent vascular flow void coursing within the right cerebellar hemisphere (white arrows).
- ▶ Catheter angiogram of the vertebral artery shows an abnormal tangle of vessels (black arrows) with an early-phase draining vein (arrowheads), consistent with an arteriovenous malformation.
- ▶ Pulmonary arteriogram shows abnormally dilated vessels and early filling of enlarged venous channels (arrows), consistent with a pulmonary arteriovenous malformation (pAVM).

Differential Diagnosis

- ▶ Multiple intracranial malformations without HHT
- ▶ Multiple intracranial developmental venous anomalies (venous angiomas)

Teaching Points

- ▶ Osler-Weber-Rendu syndrome (HHT) is an autosomal dominant vascular phakomatosis characterized by mucocutaneous and visceral telangiectasias and multiple arteriovenous malformations of the lungs, brain, liver, spine, and gastrointestinal tract.
- ▶ The vascular malformations in HHT can lead to hemorrhage. Epistaxis is the most common symptom. The risk of bleeding in cerebral AVMs in HHT is lower than it is in those without HHT, but hemorrhage can occur.
- ▶ Pulmonary AVMs can cause right-to-left shunting with dyspnea, cyanosis, polycythemia, and heart failure. Bland and septic emboli to the brain via the pulmonary shunt may cause stroke or cerebral abscesses.
- ▶ CT and MRI can show the cerebral AVMs or cerebral abscesses.
- ▶ T2-weighted MR imaging may show abnormal flow voids in the AVMs. Susceptibility imaging may show microhemorrhages or telangiectasias. Time-of-flight MRA may not demonstrate the smaller AVMs. Contrast-enhanced MRI is more sensitive in demonstrating the vascular abnormalities, both the telangiectasias and the AVMs. Catheter cerebral angiography is most sensitive in demonstrating the cerebral AVMs.

Management

- ▶ Brain and spine AVMs in HTT can be treated by surgery, endovascular methods, and stereotactic radiosurgery. Pulmonary AVMs are embolized to prevent right-to-left shunt complications and to prevent cerebral embolism.

Further Reading

Carette MF, Nedelcu C, Tassart M, et al. Imaging of hereditary hemorrhagic telangiectasia. *Cardiovasc Intervent Radiol.* 2009;32:745-757.
Fulbright RK, Chaloupka JC, Putman CM, et al. MR of hereditary hemorrhagic telangiectasia: prevalence and spectrum of cerebrovascular malformations. *Am J Neuroradiol.* 1998;19:477-484.

History

▶ 76-year-old man with new headache and speech difficulty

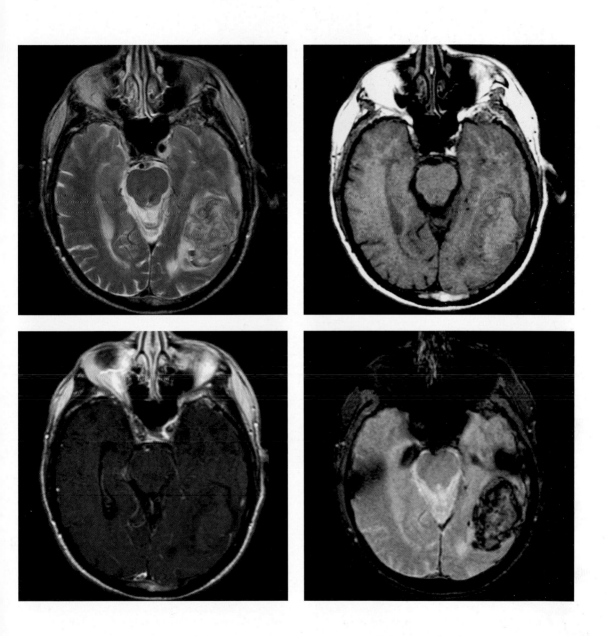

Case 77 Intracerebral Hemorrhage (Hyperacute)

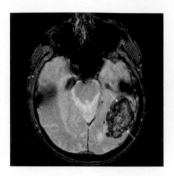

Findings

▶ There is a 3-cm lesion in the left posterior temporal lobe with moderate mass effect.

▶ It is T1 iso-intense and T2 hyperintense to the adjacent brain parenchyma, without enhancement.

▶ On the gradient-echo (or T2*-weighted) sequence it has a peripheral hypointense rim (arrows) surrounding a partially isointense center.

Differential Diagnosis

▶ Primary intracerebral hemorrhage (e.g., hypertensive bleed, cerebral amyloid angiopathy)

▶ Hemorrhagic neoplasm

▶ Vascular malformation (e.g., arteriovenous malformation, cavernous malformation)

▶ Venous sinus thrombosis

▶ Vasculopathy (e.g., vasculitis, mycotic or pseudoaneurysm)

▶ Coagulopathy

▶ Trauma

Teaching Points

▶ MR signal characteristics of intracranial hemorrhage are determined by the paramagnetic effects of the hemoglobin breakdown products, the magnetic field strength, and the pulse sequence used.

▶ Stages of intracerebral hemorrhage

Stage	Time course	CT	T1	T2	GRE	Mass effect	Components
Hyperacute	<12 hours	Hyperdense	Iso-intense	High intensity	Central iso-intensity, peripheral low intensity	+++	Central oxyhemoglobin, peripheral deoxyhemoglobin
Acute	12 hours to 2 days	Hyperdense	Iso-intense	Low intensity	Diffuse low intensity	+++	Deoxyhemoglobin
Early subacute	2 to 7 days	Hyperdense	High intensity	Low intensity	Diffuse low intensity	+++/++	Intracellular methemoglobin
Late subacute	1 to 4 weeks	Isodense	High intensity	High intensity	Iso-intense	+/-	Extracellular methemoglobin
Chronic	>1 month	Hypodense	Low intensity	Low intensity	Low intensity	-	Hemosiderin

Management

- ▶ Additional imaging is performed to help differentiate among the possible etiologies.
  - ▪ Noncontrast CT will identify the calcifications that may be present with some neoplasms, vascular malformations, and aneurysms.
  - ▪ Postcontrast MRI sequences are helpful in identifying underlying neoplasm.
  - ▪ Gradient-echo sequences may reveal multiple microhemorrhages to suggest amyloid angiopathy or multiple cavernous malformations.
  - ▪ Noninvasive vascular imaging (CTA, MRA) is more sensitive for detecting aneurysm and vascular malformation.
- ▶ Close interval follow-up imaging is performed to assess for hematoma growth and increased mass effect. If mass effect becomes severe enough to produce clinical deterioration, operative decompression may be necessary.
- ▶ If no source of hemorrhage is identified from clinical and imaging investigation, delayed vascular imaging and repeat MRI are often obtained.

Further Reading

Anzalone N, Scott R, Riva R. Neuroradiologic differential diagnosis of cerebral intraparenchymal hemorrhage. *Neurol Sci.* 2004;25 Suppl 1:S3-5.

Kidwell CS, Wintermark M. Imaging of intracranial hemorrhage. *Lancet Neurol.* 2008;7:256-267.

History

▶ 50-year-old woman with "worst headache of life"

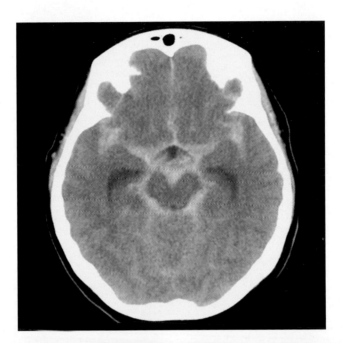

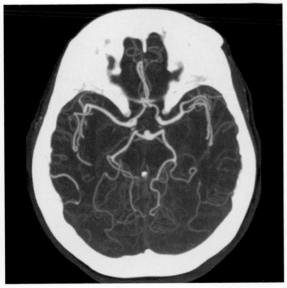

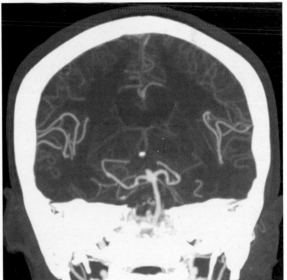

Case 78 Nontraumatic Subarachnoid Hemorrhage (Ruptured Basilar Tip Aneurysm)

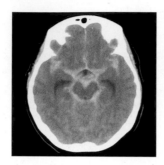 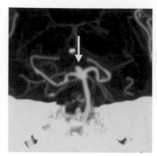

Findings

▶ Noncontrast CT scan demonstrates high-attenuation material within the suprasellar, interpeduncular, and ambient cisterns as well as the sylvian and interhemispheric fissures, consistent with subarachnoid hemorrhage (SAH).

▶ There is dilatation of the temporal horns due to hydrocephalus.

▶ Coronal maximum intensity projection (MIP) images demonstrate a superiorly directed outpouching arising from the basilar artery terminus (arrow), consistent with basilar tip aneurysm.

Differential Diagnosis

▶ Non-aneurysmal perimesencephalic SAH

▶ Traumatic SAH

Teaching Points

▶ Nontraumatic SAH accounts for up to 5% of all new strokes. 80% are related to rupture of a cerebral aneurysm.

▶ Aneurysmal SAH (aSAH) is a neurologic emergency, with a case fatality rate of approximately 50%. Survivors are functionally dependent in one third of cases.

▶ Patients often present with the "worst headache of life." Prognosis is related to the patient's level of consciousness, age, and amount of SAH.

▶ Noncontrast CT is the best test for detecting SAH. If negative and clinical suspicion remains high, a lumbar puncture is performed. If SAH is present, vascular imaging with CT or catheter angiography is mandatory to identify any cerebral aneurysm or vascular malformation.

▶ The sensitivities of both CT and lumbar puncture diminish rapidly over a few days. In cases of subacute presentation, MRI with FLAIR imaging may detect occult SAH as the presence of hyperintense signal in the subarachnoid space.

▶ Saccular or "berry" aneurysms typically arise from the arteries of the circle of Willis at bifurcations. The most common locations include the anterior and posterior communicating arteries, internal carotid artery, middle cerebral artery bifurcations, and basilar artery terminus.

Management

▶ Ruptured aneurysms must be treated urgently with endovascular coiling or open surgical clipping to prevent early rebleeding.

▶ Continuous monitoring in the neurointensive care setting is required for detection and management of SAH-related vasospasm or hydrocephalus.

Further Reading

Suarez JI, Tarr RW, Selman WR. Aneurysmal subarachnoid hemorrhage. *N Engl J Med*. 2006;35:387-396.

Velthuis BK, Rinkel GJ, Ramos RM, et al. Subarachnoid hemorrhage: aneurysm detection and preoperative evaluation with CT angiography. *Radiology*. 1998;208:423-430.

History

▶ Neurologically devastated child with large head, paralysis and hyperreflexia

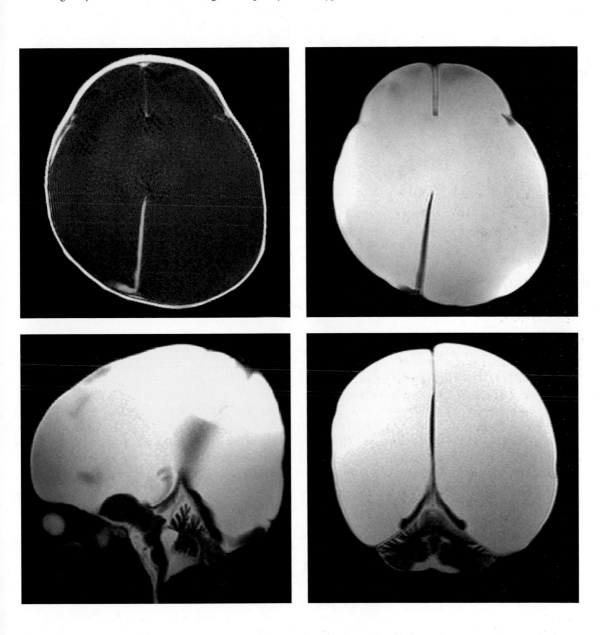

Case 79 Hydranencephaly

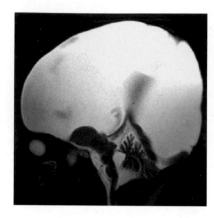 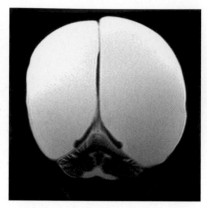

Findings

▶ Axial T1-weighted and triplanar T2-weighted images show absence of nearly all supratentorial brain tissue, with an enlarged cranial vault filled with CSF. The brain stem, parts of the diencephalon, and cerebellum are present. There is only a minimal rind of residual tissue in the occipital regions.

Differential Diagnosis

▶ Alobar holoprosencephaly
▶ Maximal hydrocephalus
▶ Large bilateral open-lip schizencephaly

Teaching Points

▶ Hydranencephaly is thought to be caused by prenatal bilateral internal carotid artery vascular occlusion leading to destruction and liquefaction of the supratentorial brain.
▶ Patients may be macrocephalic, normocephalic, or microcephalic depending on degree of CSF secretion and absorption. There is severe developmental failure and hyperreflexia. Only brain-stem function is present.
▶ Cerebral falx is often fully or mostly intact. Posterior fossa structures and brain stem are relatively spared. Basal ganglia remain separate if present. Often residual small peripheral islands of hemispheric brain tissue will be seen.
▶ In alobar holoprosencephaly, there is a large monoventricle, but there is fusion of midline structures and the falx is often absent.
▶ In maximal hydrocephalus, there is a thin rim of brain tissue left along the cranial vault and falx (though it might be quite difficult to see on CT).
▶ In large bilateral open-lip schizencephaly there are large bilateral middle cerebral artery distribution defects, with the margins of the defect lined by gray matter. The pathophysiology is thought to be similar to hydranencephaly.

Management

▶ CSF diversion by a shunt will treat the progressive macrocephaly but will not affect the severe underlying deficits. Prognosis is generally very poor, but with extensive medical support, survival of up to several years has been reported.

Further Reading

McAbee GN, Chan A, Erde EL. Prolonged survival with hydranencephaly: report of two patients and literature review. *Pediatr Neurol.* 2000;23:80-84.
Sutton LN, Bruce DA, Schut L. Hydranencephaly versus maximal hydrocephalus: an important clinical distinction. *Neurosurgery.* 1980;6:34-38.

History

► Newborn with an abnormality detected on cranial ultrasound

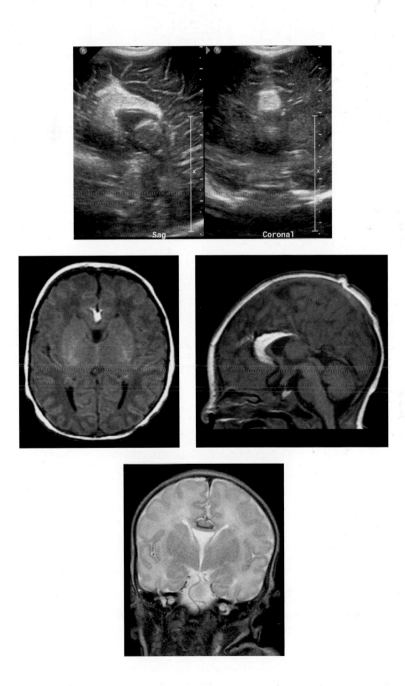

Case 80 Dysgenesis of Corpus Callosum with Lipoma

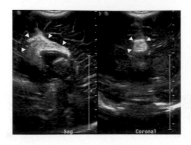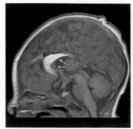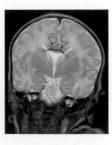

Findings

▶ Ultrasound demonstrates a hyperechoic midline mass along the anterior corpus callosum and interhemispheric fissure (arrowheads).

▶ T1-weighted sagittal MRI shows a hyperintense mass adjacent to the anterior aspect of corpus callosum. The anterior body and genu of the corpus callosum are present (white arrows), but the posterior body and splenium are absent.

▶ Coronal T2-weighted image shows an isointense mass adjacent and just superior to the corpus callosum (black arrows). The hypointense band along its inferior margin represents chemical shift artifact.

Differential Diagnosis

▶ Pericallosal hemorrhage

▶ Intracranial dermoid

▶ Intracranial teratoma

▶ Lipomatous elements in other tumors (meningiomas, neuroectodermal tumors)

Teaching Points

▶ Intracranial lipomas result from abnormal differentiation of intracranial primitive mesenchymal tissue (meninx primitiva) into fatty tissue.

▶ The most common location of intracranial lipomas is pericallosal. Pericallosal lipomas are almost always associated with dysgenesis or hypogenesis of the corpus callosum, and occasionally with midline craniofacial anomalies.

▶ Lipomas can also occur in the quadrigeminal plate, suprasellar cistern, interpeduncular cistern, cerebellopontine angles, and sylvian fissures.

▶ Intracranial lipomas are often incidental. Symptoms, if present, are usually related to associated brain anomalies. If lipomas are adjacent to cranial nerves, they may cause cranial nerve dysfunction.

▶ On CT they are of fatty density and are sharply demarcated. Pericallosal lipomas may have foci of calcification.

▶ On MRI, they may demonstrate chemical shift artifact. Fat-saturated sequences will confirm the diagnosis.

▶ Pericallosal hemorrhage is readily distinguished from lipoma on many MR sequences (e.g., T2* imaging, fat suppression) or on CT.

▶ Intracranial dermoid is usually of slightly higher density than fat on CT and on MRI has more heterogeneous signal than lipomas.

▶ Teratoma has a more heterogeneous appearance and can show enhancement.

Management

▶ Pericallosal lipomas generally do not require treatment. Lipomas in other intracranial regions need treatment only if causing mass effect or clear-cut symptoms.

Further Reading

Ickowitz V, Eurin D, Rypens F, et al. Prenatal diagnosis and postnatal follow-up of pericallosal lipoma: report of seven new cases. *Am J Neuroradiol.* 2001;22:767-772.

Kieslich M, Ehlers S, Bollinger M, et al. Midline developmental anomalies with lipomas in the corpus callosum region. *J Child Neurol.* 2000;15:85-89.

History

▶ 13-year-old boy with headaches

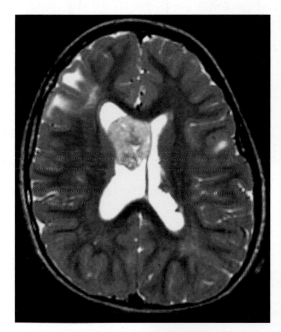
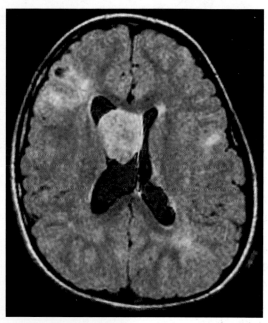
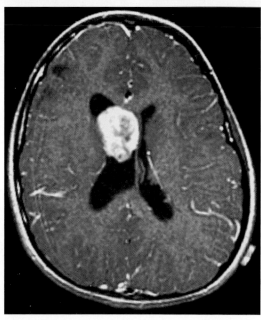

Case 81 Subependymal Giant Cell Astrocytoma (SEGA), Tuberous Sclerosis

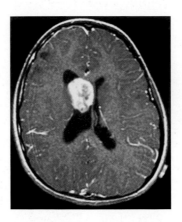

Findings

► There is an enhancing mass in the right lateral ventricle at the foramen of Monro.
► Also note the subependymal nodules lining the surface of the right lateral ventricle and the cortical tubers.

Differential Diagnosis

► With this constellation of findings, the practical differential diagnosis is limited and consists largely of subependymal hamartoma.

Teaching Points

► SEGA is a benign (WHO grade I) mixed glioneuronal tumor that is extremely rare in otherwise normal patients, but is more common in the setting of tuberous sclerosis (~10%).
► SEGA usually occurs in the first two decades. Clinical presentation is often related to hydrocephalus (headache, nausea/vomiting, papilledema, visual field deficit) or worsening seizures.
► The distinction between SEGA and subependymal nodule is based on behavior rather than histology. SEGA typically occurs in the region of the foramen of Monro, demonstrates contrast enhancement, and displays growth on serial imaging. Hydrocephalus from obstruction of the foramen of Monro is also considered a defining characteristic of SEGA, regardless of size.
► Contrast enhancement has limited utility for diagnosing SEGA, as some SEGAs do not enhance and some non-neoplastic subependymal nodules do enhance.

Management

► Patients with tuberous sclerosis should have surveillance imaging every 1 to 3 years until age 21 to screen for SEGA.
► SEGAs should be resected if they are enlarging or if there are new or progressive symptoms. Complete resection is curative.

Further Reading

Goh S, Butler WB, Thiele EA. Subependymal giant cell tumors in tuberous sclerosis complex. *Neurology*. 2004;63:1457-1461.
Koeller KK, Sandberg GD. Cerebral intraventricular neoplasms: radiologic-pathologic correlation. *Radiographics*. 2002;22:1473-1505.

History

► 53-year-old man with metastatic renal cell carcinoma presents with headaches, confusion, and vomiting. Blood pressure 210/120 mmHg

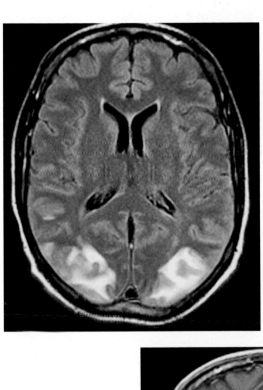
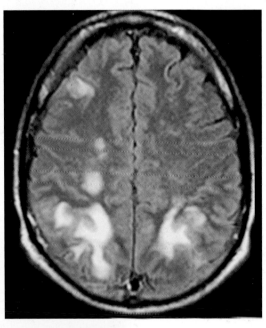
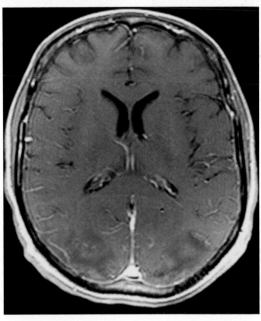

Case 82 Posterior Reversible Encephalopathy Syndrome (PRES)

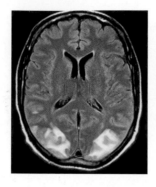 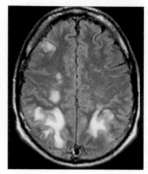

Findings

► The FLAIR sequence shows hyperintense lesions in the bilateral parietal and occipital lobes as well as less extensive lesions in the right frontal lobe. The subcortical white matter is more severely affected than adjacent cortex.
► The lesions do not enhance on the postcontrast T1-weighted images.
► The basal ganglia appear normal.

Differential Diagnosis

► Acute disseminated encephalomyelitis (ADEM)
► Hypoxic-ischemic injury
► Toxic or metabolic encephalopathy
► Progressive multifocal leukoencephalopathy

Teaching Points

► PRES is a disorder of cerebrovascular autoregulation. There are multiple etiologies, most of which are associated with acute hypertension. These include pre-eclampsia/eclampsia, immunosuppressant therapy (e.g., cyclosporine, tacrolimus), and autoimmune diseases.
► Elevated blood pressure exceeds the cerebral vascular autoregulatory abilities and damages the endothelium. This results in extravasation of proteins and fluid into the interstitial spaces, producing the vasogenic edema seen on imaging. PRES, as the name implies, predominately affects the posterior circulation because, in theory, it has less sympathetic innervation and does not autoregulate as well as the anterior circulation.
► Patients present with headache, seizures, altered mental status, and visual disturbance.
► On MRI the typical parieto-occipital lesions are hyperintense on T2-weighted and FLAIR images and involve cortex and, to a greater extent, subcortical white matter. Less commonly lesions may occur in the frontal and temporal lobes, basal ganglia, cerebellum, and deep white matter.
► The lesions usually have neither enhancement nor decreased diffusion. In severe cases, decreased diffusion may be present; this heralds the presence of irreversible injury.

Management

► Treatment/removal of the offending agent and control of blood pressure should be instituted quickly. The cerebral injuries in PRES are usually reversible when treatment is instituted early.

Further Reading

Bartynski WS. Posterior reversible encephalopathy syndrome. Part 1. Fundamental imaging and clinical features. *AJNR Am J Neuroradiol.* 2008;29:1036-1042.
Bartynski WS, Boardman JF. Distinct imaging patterns and lesion distribution in posterior reversible encephalopathy syndrome (PRES). *AJNR Am J Neuroradiol.* 2007;28:1320-1327.

History

▶ 10-year-old with an asymmetric face as well as numbness and weakness in extremities and skin lesions

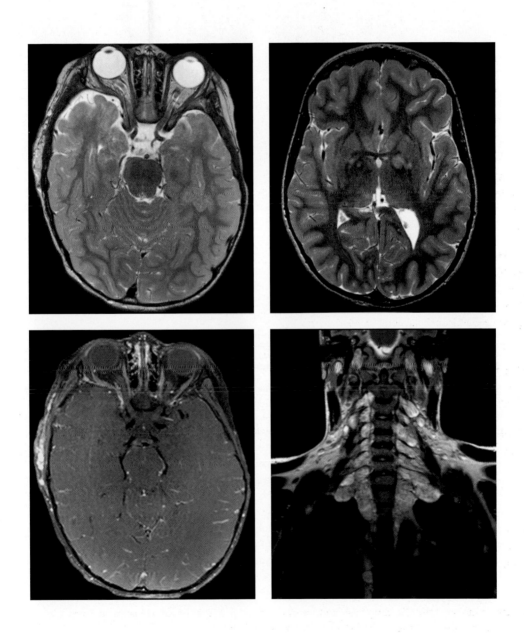

Case 83 Neurofibromatosis Type 1 (NF-1)

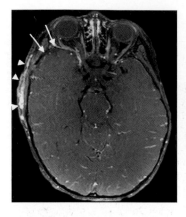 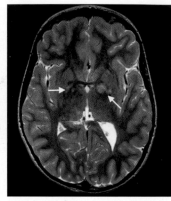 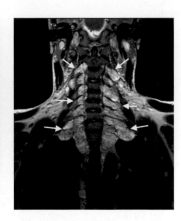

Findings

► Axial T2-weighted and postcontrast T1-weighted images demonstrate abnormal shape of the right sphenoid wing (arrows).
► There is irregular thickening and enhancement in the right temporal skin and subcutaneous tissues (arrowheads).
► Axial T2-weighted image shows small foci of T2 hyperintensity in the bilateral basal ganglia (arrows).
► Coronal T2-weighted image through the neck and upper chest shows multiple bilateral lobular masses within the neural foramina and along the cervical and thoracic nerve roots (arrows).

Differential Diagnosis

► This constellation of abnormalities is virtually pathognomonic for NF-1. For the isolated findings:
  ▪ NF-1 "bright spots"—demyelinating disorders, viral encephalitis, mitochondrial diseases, small glial neoplasms
  ▪ Thickened nerves—schwannomas, chronic inflammatory demyelinating polyneuropathy (CIDP), hereditary motor sensory neuropathies

Teaching Points

► NF-1 (von Recklinghausen's disease) is an autosomal dominant phakomatosis with responsible genes on chromosome 17.
► Patients often have spongiform changes in the brain manifesting as hyperintense areas on T2 or FLAIR imaging. They are most common in basal ganglia, thalami, brain stem, and cerebellar white matter. These lesions, colloquially referred to as unidentified bright objects (UBOs), often regress in late childhood.
► Patients may develop gliomas of the CNS, most commonly along the optic pathway, hypothalamus, and brain stem.
► Patients may have discrete nodular or extensive plexiform neurofibromas in the skin or deep tissues, or develop extensive neurofibromas along spinal nerve roots or peripheral nerves. The neurofibromas may present as diffuse thickening of the nerves, focal discrete lesions, or conglomerate masses.
► Other craniospinal manifestations of NF-1 include sphenoid wing dysplasia, iris hamartomas (Lisch nodules), dural ectasia in the spine, and vascular dysplasias (including focal intracranial stenosis and moyamoya).

Management

► Serial imaging is needed to assess changes and for development of glial neoplasms.
► Growing resectable tumors are treated by surgical resection. Chemotherapy and radiation are options for some tumors.

Further Reading

Fortman BJ, Kuszyk BS, Urban BA, et al. Neurofibromatosis type 1: a diagnostic mimicker at CT. *Radiographics*. 2001;21:601-612.
Lin DD, Barker PB. Neuroimaging of phakomatoses. *Semin Pediatr Neurol.* 2006;13:48-62.

History

▶ 46-year-old man with seizure activity

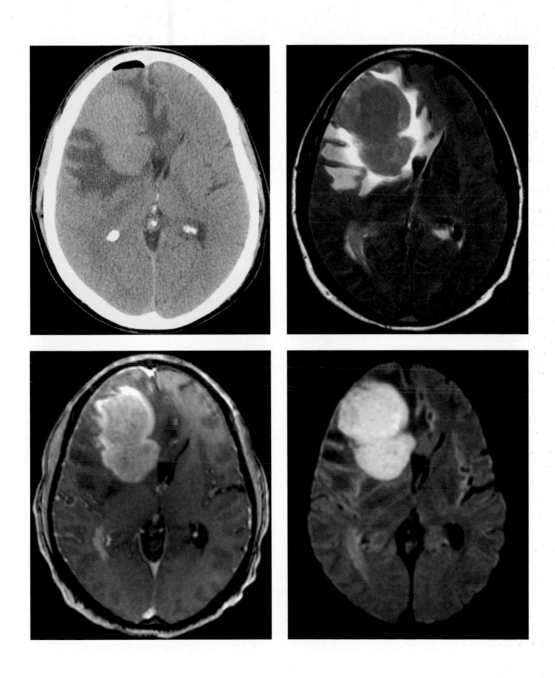

Case 84 Primary CNS Lymphoma

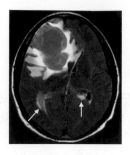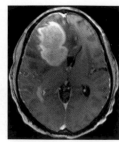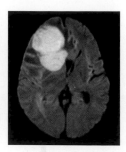

Findings

► There is a large, bilobed, intra-axial mass in the right frontal lobe. There is marked vasogenic edema and mass effect with effacement of the frontal horn of the right lateral ventricle and subfalcine herniation.
► On noncontrast CT, the mass is homogeneously hyperdense. A small amount of pneumocephalus is present due to recent biopsy.
► On MRI, the mass demonstrates T2 iso- to hypointense signal, homogeneous enhancement, and hyperintense signal on DWI.
► Additional lesions are seen within the atria of the bilateral ventricles (arrows).

Differential Diagnosis

► Glioblastoma multiforme
► Metastatic neoplasm

Teaching Points

► Primary CNS lymphomas (PCNSLs) are typically non-Hodgkin's lymphomas of B-cell origin.
► PCNSLs account for up to 15% of primary brain tumors. Immunocompromised patients are at higher risk, but the incidence is increasing in immunocompetent patients.
► PCNSLs are predominantly located in the supratentorial brain parenchyma, with frequent involvement of the periventricular white matter, deep gray nuclei, and corpus callosum. Seeding of the ependymal surfaces is common.
► Secondary lymphoma (from other sites) more often involves the leptomeninges and dura.
► Classic imaging findings related to dense cellularity include hyperattenuation on CT and T2 hypointensity and restricted diffusion on MRI.
► Imaging findings are influenced by patient immune status.
  ▪ PCNSLs usually demonstrate homogenous enhancement in immunocompetent patients.
  ▪ Hemorrhage and necrosis are more common in immunocompromised patients, resulting in heterogeneous ring enhancement. In HIV patients, this appearance is similar to that of toxoplasmosis.
► PCNSLs can also appear on imaging as a nonenhancing, infiltrative mass (in up to 10% of cases).

Management

► The suspicion of lymphoma on imaging studies alters the diagnostic and therapeutic approach. Rather than planned resection, diagnosis is made via stereotactic biopsy or positive CSF cytology.
► Primary treatment includes radiation and chemotherapy. While these tumors often respond rapidly, recurrence is common and median survival is only about 4 years.

Further Reading

Erdag N, Bhorade RM, Alberico RA, et al. Primary lymphoma of the central nervous system: typical and atypical CT and MR imaging appearances. *AJR Am J Roentgenol.* 2001;176:1319-1326.

Koeller KK, Smirniotopoulos JG, Jones RV. Primary central nervous system lymphoma: radiologic-pathologic correlation. *Radiographics.* 1997;17:1497-1526.

Soussain C, Hoang-Xuan K. Primary central nervous system lymphoma: an update. *Curr Opin Oncol.* 2009;21:550-558.

History

▶ 14-year-old otherwise healthy girl with amenorrhea

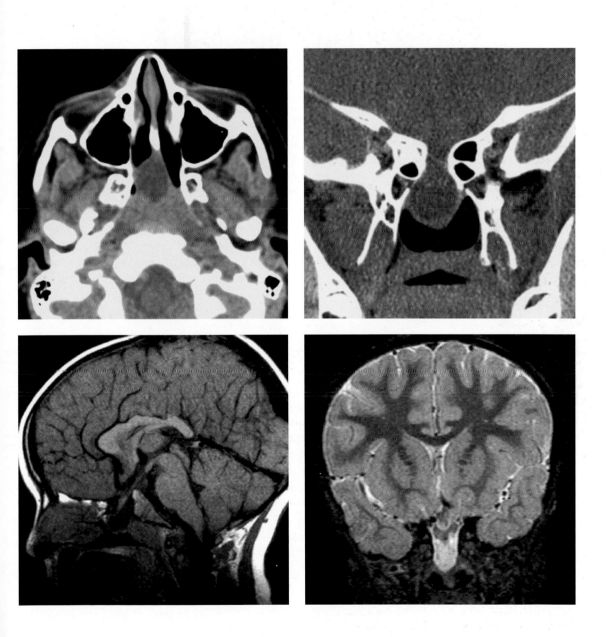

Case 85 Cephalocele (Sphenoidal)

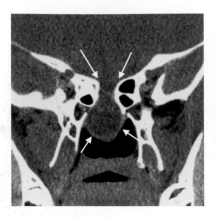 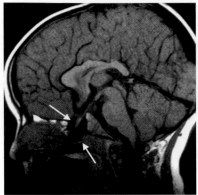

Findings

▶ Axial and coronal CT images demonstrate a gap within the central aspect of the sphenoid bone through which a low-attenuation pouch is protruding inferiorly into the nasopharynx (arrows).

▶ Sagittal T1-weighted and coronal T2-weighted images show that this protrusion of the intracranial contents is composed of CSF signal fluid (T1-dark, T2-bright), and parts of the pituitary infundibulum and optic chiasm are displaced inferiorly (arrows).

Differential Diagnosis

▶ Frontonasal and frontoethmoidal cephaloceles: nasal glioma, dermoid, hemangioma
▶ Sphenoidal: nasopharyngeal tumors with skull base involvement
▶ Orbital: orbital neurofibromas
▶ Occipital: destructive tumors of the skull

Teaching Points

▶ Cephalocele is a general term referring to extracranial extension of intracranial contents through defects in the bone and dura. Meningocele refers to herniation of meninges and CSF only. Meningoencephalocele or encephalocele refers to herniation of brain tissue, meninges, and CSF. Cephaloceles may be congenital or acquired.

▶ Cephaloceles can occur anywhere but common locations are frontoethmoidal, frontonasal, sphenoidal, occipital, and parietal. Other locations include the temporal bone, Meckel's cave, orbital apex, and other skull base foramina.

▶ Presentation of cephaloceles depends on their location. They may present with an obvious mass, seizures, CSF leak, meningitis, nasal stuffiness, nasopharyngeal mass, visual disturbances, and pituitary dysfunction, or they may even be asymptomatic only to be incidentally discovered on imaging.

▶ Cephaloceles are sometimes associated with midface anomalies, hypertelorism, and various brain anomalies such as abnormalities of the corpus callosum, Chiari II, and Dandy-Walker malformation.

Management

▶ Surgical repair is often undertaken for obvious encephaloceles or those with mass effect or symptoms. Small skull base cephaloceles may be left alone. Vascular imaging is occasionally needed for preoperative planning to avoid vascular injury during surgical repair.

Further Reading

Connor SE. Imaging of skull-base cephalocoeles and cerebrospinal fluid leaks. *Clin Radiol.* 2010;65:832-841.
Naidich TP, Altman MR, Braffman BH, et al. Cephaloceles and related malformations. *AJNR Am J Neuroradiol.* 1992;13:655-690.

History

▶ 52-year-old woman with epilepsy refractory to medications

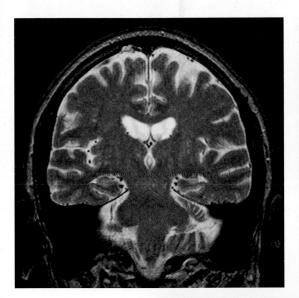
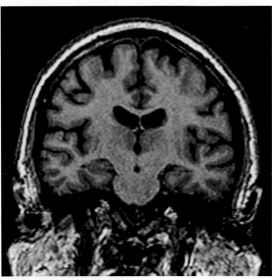

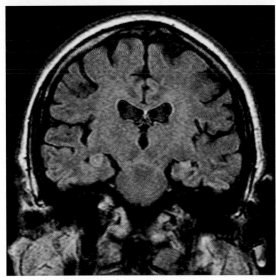

Case 86   Mesial Temporal Sclerosis

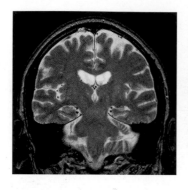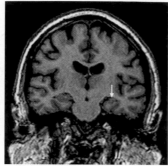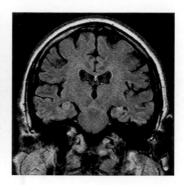

Findings

▶ Coronal MR images show asymmetry of the hippocampus, normal on the right and atrophic on the left (arrow).

▶ The atrophic left hippocampus has abnormal hyperintense signal on T2-weighted and FLAIR sequences.

Differential Diagnosis

▶ Chronic injury (e.g., old trauma)

▶ Encephalitis

▶ Glial neoplasm

▶ Seizure edema

Teaching Points

▶ Mesial temporal sclerosis (MTS), also known as hippocampal sclerosis, is an acquired disorder characterized by gliosis and tissue loss in the hippocampus, resulting in development of an epileptogenic focus. It is the most common cause of chronic epilepsy.

▶ The cause is rarely established, but this entity can be the result of febrile seizures or encephalitis or can occur as the result of chronic seizures from another anatomic source. Even when MTS is evident, one must perform a careful search for other seizure foci.

▶ The two primary imaging findings are:
  ▪ Atrophy of the hippocampus
  ▪ Hyperintense hippocampal signal on T2-weighted and FLAIR sequences

▶ Other findings include loss of hippocampal interdigitations and volume loss in the ipsilateral fornix, mammillary body, thalamus, and temporal lobe.

▶ Thin-section coronal imaging is needed to best examine the hippocampus.

▶ The FLAIR sequence, with its suppression of hyperintense signal in the adjacent CSF, is the most sensitive sequence for detecting the characteristic signal abnormality.

▶ The changes are present bilaterally in 15% of patients.

Management

▶ In persons whose seizures are refractory to medication, unilateral resection of the hippocampus and anterior temporal lobe is usually effective.

Further Reading

Connor SEJ, Jarosz JM. Magnetic resonance imaging of patients with epilepsy. *Clin Radiol.* 2001;56:787-801.

History

▸ 33-year-old man with history of multiple abdominal surgeries, now presenting with headache and seizures

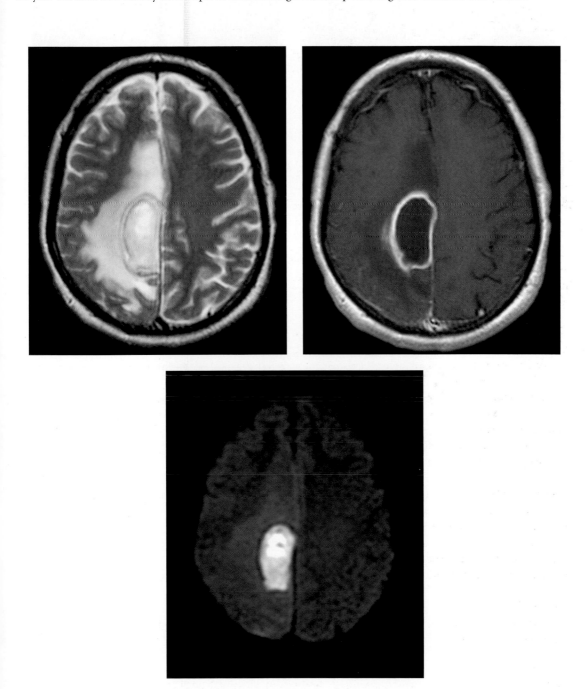

Case 87   Pyogenic Cerebral Abscess (*Streptococcus Mulleri*)

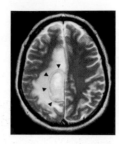 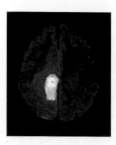

Findings

▸ Postcontrast T1-weighted images show a right-sided rim-enhancing mass. The rim of enhancing tissue is relatively smooth and uniform.

▸ T2-weighted images show a thin rim of hypointense material corresponding to the margins of the enhancing rim (arrowheads).

▸ On DWI, the majority of material in the non-enhancing center of the mass is hyperintense.

Differential Diagnosis

▸ Fungal, mycobacterial, or amebic abscess

▸ Metastatic neoplasm

▸ Primary CNS neoplasm

▸ Tumefactive demyelination

Teaching Points

▸ The most common cause of cerebral abscesses is direct spread of infections from the paranasal sinuses, oropharynx, and ear. Hematogenous spread is another important route.

▸ The most common organisms are streptococci and anaerobes, but the most likely organism for any particular abscess depends on the source and host immune system.

▸ Clinical symptoms include headache, focal neurologic deficit, impaired cognition, and fever. Fever is present in only 50% of patients.

▸ The imaging appearance of a brain abscess changes over weeks to months. The key stages of imaging evolution are:
   ▪ Early cerebritis—poorly marginated signal abnormality and patchy enhancement
   ▪ Late cerebritis—thick and irregular enhancing rim, non-enhancing center
   ▪ Early abscess—thick and irregular capsule with non-enhancing central fluid collection
   ▪ Late abscess—thin and uniform capsule with non-enhancing central fluid collection

▸ Key features that help to distinguish pyogenic abscess from neoplasm include:
   ▪ Thin, uniform enhancing margins
   ▪ A well-defined rim of hypointense signal on T2-weighted images
   ▪ The presence of uniform decreased diffusion in the non-enhancing abscess cavity
   ▪ Proton MRS detection of the products of bacterial metabolism (e.g., succinate, acetate) in the abscess cavity

Management

▸ Initially patients may be treated with empiric antibiotics, but sampling of the abscess facilitates the choice of optimal antibiotic coverage.

▸ Stereotactic drainage or surgical excision is generally needed for abscesses larger than 2.5 cm or not responding to initial antibiotic therapy.

Further Reading

Falcone S, Post MJ. Encephalitis, cerebritis, and brain abscess. *Neuroimaging Clin North Am.* 2000;10:333-353.

Luthra G, Parihar A, Nath K, et al. Comparative evaluation of fungal, tubercular, and pyogenic abscesses with conventional and diffusion MR imaging and proton MR spectroscopy. *AJNR Am J Neuroradiol.* 2007;28:1332-1338.

History

▶ 63-year-old man with vertigo and incidental imaging finding

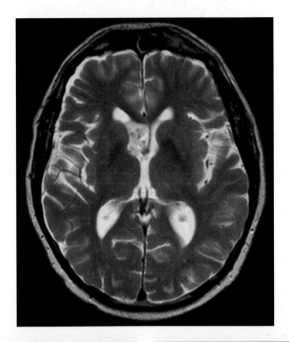

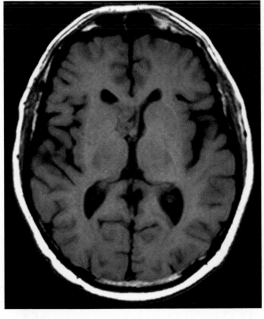

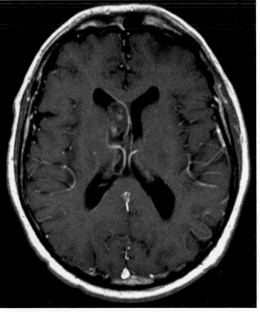

Case 88 Subependymoma

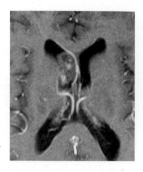

Findings

▶ There is a T1 iso- to hypointense, T2 hyperintense mass in the frontal horn of the right lateral ventricle, adjacent to the foramen of Monro and abutting the septum pellucidum.
▶ It has small internal foci enhancement.

Differential Diagnosis

▶ Central neurocytoma
▶ Subependymal giant cell astrocytoma
▶ Choroid plexus papilloma/carcinoma
▶ Metastasis
▶ For subependymomas occurring in the fourth ventricle (a more common location), the differential includes ependymoma, choroid plexus papilloma/carcinoma, hemangioblastoma, and metastasis.

Teaching Points

▶ Subependymoma is a rare (0.5% of intracranial tumors), slow-growing, benign (WHO grade I) neoplasm. It is thought to arise from subependymal glial cells.
▶ Patient demographics provide an important diagnostic clue: subependymoma occurs primarily in older adults (50 to 60 years), with a male predominance.
▶ Most are asymptomatic and discovered incidentally. Symptoms may arise from ventricular obstruction (headache, nausea, obtundation) or neural compression (focal deficits).
▶ The most common locations are the inferior fourth ventricle (60%) and the lateral ventricle (35%, usually in the frontal horn and abutting the septum pellucidum). Less common sites include the spinal cord and supratentorial brain parenchyma.
▶ On CT, calcification may be present.
▶ On MRI, subependymomas typically demonstrate T1 iso- to hypointensity and T2 hyperintensity. Enhancement is absent or partial. Tumors in the fourth ventricle are more likely to have enhancing elements.

Management

▶ Asymptomatic lesions should be followed with serial imaging (due to potential growth and possibility of mixed subependymoma–ependymoma).
▶ Surgical resection is usually curative and recurrence is uncommon.

Further Reading

Chiechi MV, Smirniotopoulas JG, Jones RV. Intracranial subependymomas: CT and MR imaging features in 24 cases. *AJR Am J Roentgenol.* 1995;165:1245-1250.
Ragel BT, Osborn AG, Whang K, et al. Subependymomas: An analysis of clinical and imaging features. *Neurosurgery.* 2006;58:881-890.

▶ 22-year-old graduate student found unresponsive in apartment

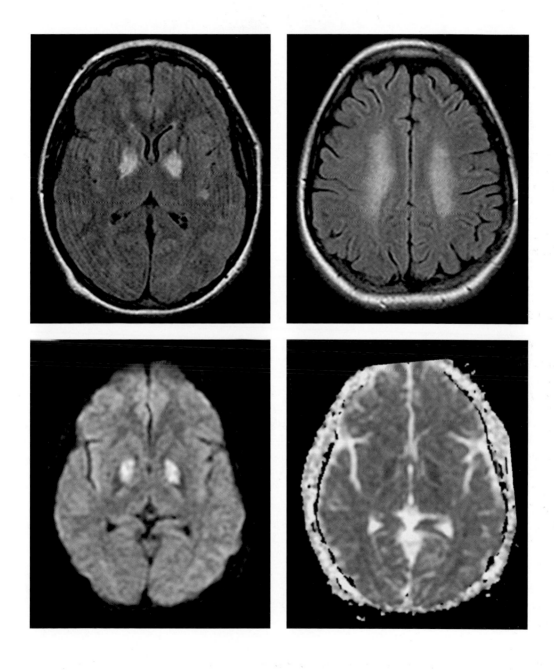

Case 89   Carbon Monoxide Poisoning

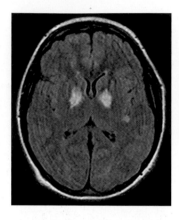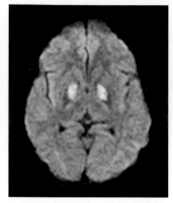

Findings

- ► Axial FLAIR and DWI sequences (with ADC maps) show symmetric hyperintensity and restricted diffusion, respectively, in the globus pallidus.
- ► There is ill-defined hyperintense signal in the centrum semiovale bilaterally.

Differential Diagnosis

- ► Hypoxic-ischemic injury
- ► Cocaine encephalopathy
- ► Wilson disease

Teaching Points

- ► CO poisoning is the most common cause of accidental poisoning in Europe and North America. CO is odorless and tasteless. Most cases result from fires, malfunctioning stoves and heaters, exhaust systems, and suicide attempts. CO binds 200 times more avidly to hemoglobin than does O_2.
- ► Patients present with confusion, loss of consciousness, headache, and nausea/vomiting.
- ► CO poisoning results in necrosis and edema in the globus pallidi.
- ► On MRI the globus pallidus develops hyperintense signal on T2-weighted and FLAIR sequences, variable signal abnormality on T1-weighted images, and restricted diffusion on DWI.
- ► Similar signal abnormality in the centrum semiovale is common. Other areas that may be affected include the medial temporal lobes, insula, and cerebellar hemispheres.
- ► Some patients experience sudden neurologic deterioration and coma several weeks after the initial insult. This correlates with the development of T2-hyperintense signal abnormality in the deep white matter, representing acute demyelination. The etiology for this delayed response is unclear but is thought to be autoimmune-mediated.

Treatment

- ► Despite treatment with high-concentration hyperbaric O_2, most patients have permanent neurologic deficits. Early treatment with oxygen portends a better prognosis.

Further Reading

Ernst A, Zibrak JD. Carbon monoxide poisoning. *N Engl J Med.* 1998;339:1603-1608.

O'Donnell P, Buxton PJ, Pitkin A, Jarvis LJ. The magnetic resonance imaging appearances of the brain in acute carbon monoxide poisoning. *Clin Radiol.* 2000;55:273-280.

History

▶ 26-year-old woman with severe headaches and left eye pain

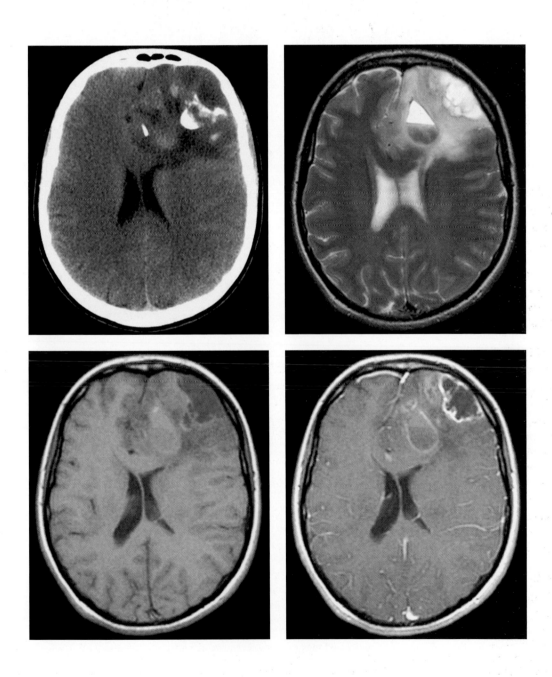

Case 90   Oligodendroglioma

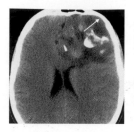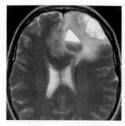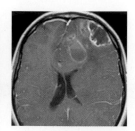

Findings

- ► Noncontrast CT demonstrates an area of hypoattenuation, mass effect, and coarse calcifications in the left frontal lobe.
- ► There is thinning of the adjacent calvarium (white arrow).
- ► MRI reveals a heterogeneous, T1-hypointense and T2-hyperintense mass that involves the cortex and white matter. There are two rim-enhancing cystic areas, the medial one having a fluid–fluid level consistent with hemorrhage.

Differential Diagnosis

- ► Astrocytoma
- ► Ganglioglioma
- ► Dysembryoplastic neuroepithelial tumor
- ► Pleomorphic xanthoastrocytoma

Teaching Points

- ► Oligodendrogliomas are slow-growing, infiltrative glial neoplasms that represent 5% to 20% of gliomas. They are WHO grade II tumors, with a median survival of 10 years. Anaplastic oligodendrogliomas (WHO grade III) have a median survival of 5 years.
- ► They occur most frequently in the fourth to sixth decades. The clinical presentation includes seizures (most common), headaches, and focal neurologic deficits.
- ► The most common locations are the frontal and temporal lobes. They occur rarely in the posterior fossa, spinal cord, and ventricles.
- ► On CT, the most helpful imaging findings are the presence of intratumoral calcification, cortical involvement, and remodeling of the adjacent calvarium (reflecting the slow growth pattern).
- ► MRI findings are often nonspecific. Common features include:
  - ▪ T1-hypointense and T2-hyperintense signal
  - ▪ Well-circumscribed margins (despite its infiltrative nature)
  - ▪ Involvement of the cortex and subcortical white matter
  - ▪ Variable enhancement
  - ▪ +/- cystic and hemorrhagic components
- ► Unlike astrocytomas, contrast enhancement does not reliably differentiate low-grade oligodendrogliomas from anaplastic tumors.
- ► The loss of chromosomes 1p and 19q may be seen in up to 70% of oligodendrogliomas and is associated with an improved response to chemotherapy and a better prognosis.

Management

- ► Surgical resection is the treatment of choice and may produce several years of disease-free survival.
- ► Radiation and chemotherapy are reserved for residual or recurrent disease.

Further Reading

Koeller KK, Rushing EJ. Oligodendroglioma and its variants: Radiologic-pathologic correlation. *Radiographics*. 2005;25:1669-1688.
Van den Bent MJ. Diagnosis and management of oligodendroglioma. *Semin Oncol*. 2004;31:645-652.

History

► 6-year-old boy presenting with a one-week history of nausea, vomiting, and headaches

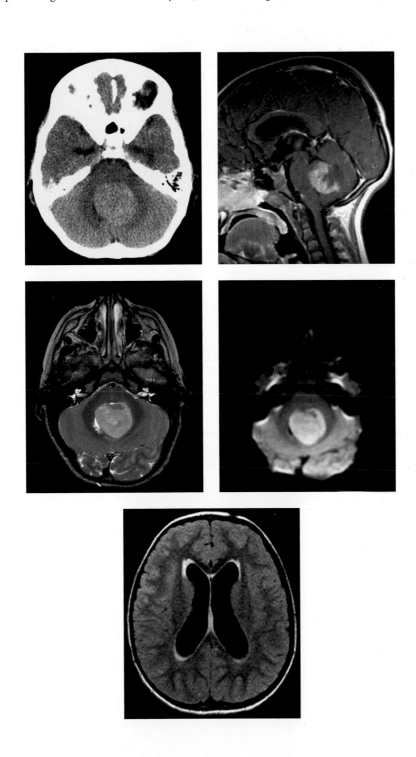

Case 91 Medulloblastoma

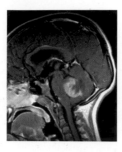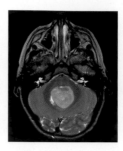

Findings

▶ On noncontrast CT, there is a large, high-attenuation mass centered within the fourth ventricle.

▶ On MRI the intraventricular mass is mildly hyperintense on T2-weighted images and hyperintense on DWI. It shows heterogeneous enhancement.

▶ Obstructive hydrocephalus with transependymal edema is demonstrated on the FLAIR sequence.

Differential Diagnosis

▶ Ependymoma
▶ Atypical teratoid rhabdoid tumor (ATRT)
▶ Pilocytic astrocytoma
▶ Choroid plexus papilloma/carcinoma
▶ Brain-stem glioma

Teaching Points

▶ Medulloblastomas are primitive neuroectodermal (small round blue cell) tumors that arise posterior to the fourth ventricle from the external granular layer of the superior medullary velum or vermis.

▶ They account for 30% to 50% of pediatric posterior fossa tumors. They are aggressive neoplasms (WHO grade IV) with a propensity for leptomeningeal spread.

▶ The typical age range is 5 to 12 years, although 30% of cases occur in patients 15 to 35 years old.

▶ Patients present with hydrocephalus or signs of brain-stem and cerebellar dysfunction.

▶ Imaging studies typically reveal a well-circumscribed mass adjacent to the cerebellar vermis.

▶ On CT they are of relatively high attenuation secondary to high cellular density. Calcification and cysts are present in 20% of cases.

▶ On MRI they demonstrate heterogeneous enhancement and internal decreased diffusion.

▶ MR spectroscopy is nonspecific and demonstrates low NAA and elevated choline.

▶ In contrast to medulloblastomas, ependymomas arise from the floor of the fourth ventricle, are more likely to have calcification and hemorrhage, and have a plastic growth pattern. ATRTs are indistinguishable by imaging criteria but typically occur in patients younger than 3 years of age.

▶ Medulloblastomas often arise within the lateral cerebellar hemispheres when presenting in older patients.

Management

▶ Preoperative imaging of the entire neuraxis is essential prior to surgical treatment due to the potential for CSF dissemination.

▶ Treatment options include surgery and chemotherapy. Radiation therapy is reserved for patients older than 3 years. The prognosis is generally good, with a 5-year survival approaching 75% to 85%.

Further Reading

Dhall G. Medulloblastoma. *J Child Neurol.* 2009;24:1418-1430.

Koeller KK, Rushing EJ. Medulloblastoma: a comprehensive review with radiologic-pathologic correlation. *Radiographics.* 2003;23:1613-1637.

History

► 43-year-old woman found unresponsive

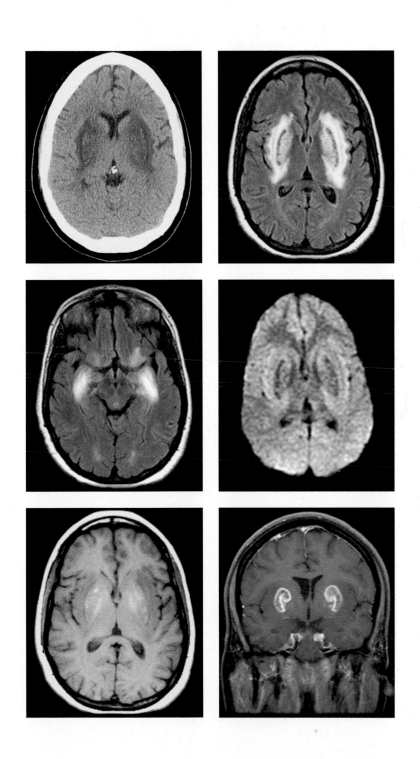

Case 92   Methanol Poisoning

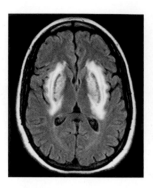

Findings

- ▶ Noncontrast CT scan shows symmetric heterogeneous hypoattenuation in the lentiform nucleus. Foci of increased attenuation likely represent petechial hemorrhage.
- ▶ On MRI the abnormality is largely hyperintense on T2-weighted images. Abnormal signal extends into both medial temporal lobes. There is no restricted diffusion.
- ▶ Areas with hypointensity on T2-weighted images and hyperintensity on T1-weighted images likely represent hemorrhage.
- ▶ Intense peripheral enhancement is present.

Differential Diagnosis

- ▶ Leigh disease
- ▶ Kearns-Sayre syndrome
- ▶ Wilson disease
- ▶ Osmotic demyelination
- ▶ Creutzfeldt-Jakob disease

Teaching Points

- ▶ Methanol is usually intentionally ingested as a suicide attempt or as a substitute for alcohol. It is found in many household products, including antifreeze and windshield wiper fluid.
- ▶ A latent period of 12 to 24 hours is seen as the methanol is metabolized to formaldehyde and formic acid, each of which is more toxic than methanol.
- ▶ Visual disturbances, secondary to optic nerve demyelination, are the most common symptom. Other CNS symptoms include headache, dizziness, nausea, weakness, and malaise. Metabolic acidosis may be severe. Death ensues in approximately one third of cases.
- ▶ Typical MRI findings are those of bilateral putaminal hemorrhagic necrosis with or without subcortical hemorrhagic necrosis. Restricted diffusion (absent in this case) is commonly present early. Enhancement, if present, is usually subtle.
- ▶ Other findings may include extensive cerebral edema, cerebellar necrosis, and optic nerve necrosis.

Management

- ▶ Ethanol administration is a mainstay of therapy. It has an affinity for alcohol dehydrogenase that is much greater than that of methanol, preventing methanol conversion to the more toxic metabolites.
- ▶ Other treatments include correction of metabolic imbalances and, in severe poisoning, hemodialysis.

Further Reading

Blanco M, Casado R, Vázquez F, et al. CT and MR imaging findings in methanol intoxication. *AJNR Am J Neuroradiol.* 2006;27:452-454.
Sharma P, Eesa M, Scott JN. Toxic and acquired metabolic encephalopathies: MRI appearance. *AJR Am J Roentgenol.* 2009;193:879-886.

History

▶ 2-year-old with seizures and left hemiparesis

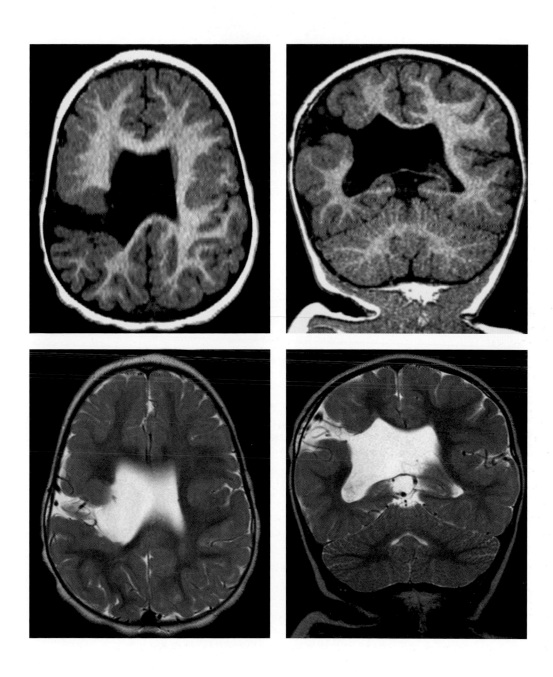

Case 93 Schizencephaly

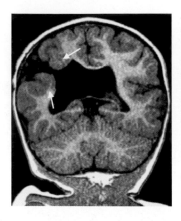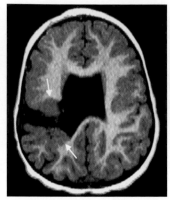

Findings

▸ T1- and T2-weighted images show a fluid (CSF)-filled cleft extending from the surface of the right hemisphere to the left lateral ventricle. The margins of the cleft are lined by dysplastic/polymicrogyric gray matter (arrows).

Differential Diagnosis

▸ Porencephaly
▸ Postoperative cavities and clefts
▸ Gray-matter heterotopia

Teaching Points

▸ Schizencephaly is a disorder in which there is a cleft between the surface of the brain and the ventricle. The cleft is lined by dysplastic or polymicrogyric brain.
▸ The etiology of schizencephaly is controversial. Most cases are thought to be due to an early destructive insult occurring before neuronal migration. Later, when neuronal migration occurs from the germinal matrix, the cleft becomes lined with gray matter. In rare cases, a genetic mutation may be responsible.
▸ Patients may have seizures, motor deficits, spasticity, or developmental delay. Clinical severity is related to the extent and location of the cleft(s) and the associated malformations.
▸ The cleft may be wide open and filled with CSF (open-lip schizencephaly) or narrow/closed (closed-lip schizencephaly). The clefts may be unilateral or bilateral.
▸ In closed-lip schizencephaly, a "dimple" along the wall of the lateral ventricle may point to the abnormality.
▸ Schizencephaly is associated with other malformations, such as septo-optic dysplasia and corpus callosum anomalies.
▸ Some porencephalic or postoperative cavities may also represent a CSF-filled connection between the brain surface and the ventricle, but these will not be lined by gray matter.

Management

▸ Treatment is supportive and may include anticonvulsants for seizures.

Further Reading

Granata T, Freri E, Caccia C, et al. Schizencephaly: clinical spectrum, epilepsy, and pathogenesis. *J Child Neurol.* 2005;20:313-318.
Hayashi N, Tsutsumi Y, Barkovich AJ. Morphological features and associated anomalies of schizencephaly in the clinical population: detailed analysis of MR images. *Neuroradiology.* 2002;44:418-427.

History

▶ 5-year-old boy with mild developmental delay

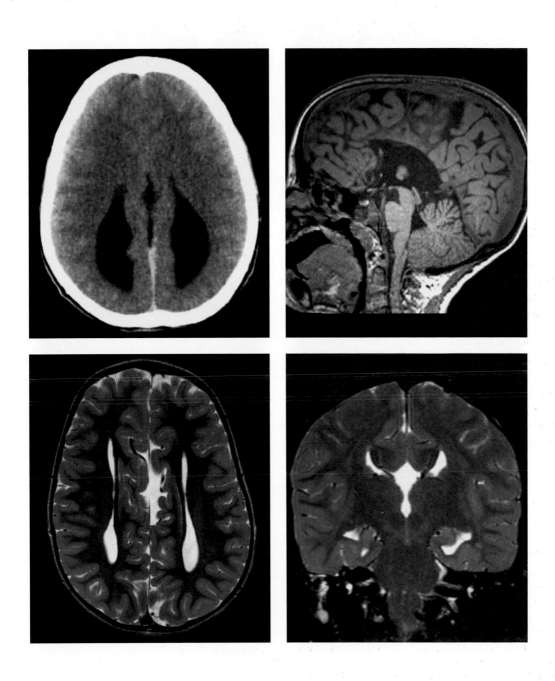

Case 94   Agenesis of the Corpus Callosum (ACC)

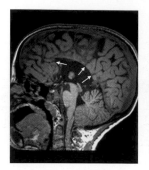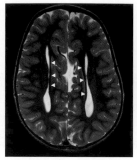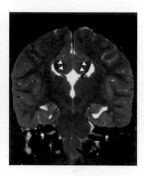

Findings

▶ On noncontrast CT, there is prominence of the posterior aspect of the lateral ventricles (colpocephaly).

▶ On the sagittal T1-weighted MR image, there is absence of the corpus callosum, and the medial sulci of the hemisphere radially extend all the way to the margins of the third ventricle (arrows).

▶ On the T2-weighted images, the corpus callosum is absent at midline. The lateral ventricles have a parallel configuration, and there is small bundle of white matter (bundle of Probst) running anteroposteriorly along the medial aspect of the lateral ventricles (arrowheads). On the coronal image, the configuration of the ventricles resembles a "Texas Longhorn."

Differential Diagnosis

▶ Hydrocephalus (with stretching and thinning of the corpus callosum)

▶ Neonatal corpus callosum (can be very thin)

▶ Periventricular leukomalacia with associated white matter and corpus callosum volume loss

▶ Postsurgical (callosotomy)

Teaching Points

▶ ACC may be isolated but is very commonly associated with a variety of additional brain malformations or syndromes.

▶ Associated syndromes include gray matter heterotopia, Chiari II malformation, lissencephaly, Dandy-Walker, cytomegalovirus infection, and fetal alcohol syndrome.

▶ Associated findings in ACC include:

  ▪ Colpocephaly

  ▪ Partial deficiency of the falx cerebri

  ▪ Vertical orientation of the hippocampus

  ▪ Probst bundles: dense white matter tracts that were normally destined to cross the midline, but in patients with ACC are situated in an anteroposterior orientation medial to the lateral ventricles

▶ There is a high prevalence of interhemispheric cysts and lipomas of the corpus callosum. Azygous anterior cerebral arteries and midline venous anomalies (persistent falcine sinus) are occasionally seen.

Management

▶ Evaluate imaging carefully for other brain anomalies and malformations. Isolated ACC may produce minimal symptoms. Intelligence may be normal. Prognosis and management depend on the presence of other associated abnormalities.

Further Reading

Hetts SW, Sherr EH, Chao S, et al. Anomalies of the corpus callosum: an MR analysis of the phenotypic spectrum of associated malformations. *AJR Am J Roentgenol.* 2006;5:1343-1348.

Küker W, Mayrhofer H, Mader I, et al. Malformations of the midline commissures: MRI findings in different forms of callosal dysgenesis. *Eur Radiol.* 2003;13:598-604.

History

▶ 22-year-old woman with weakness in all four extremities

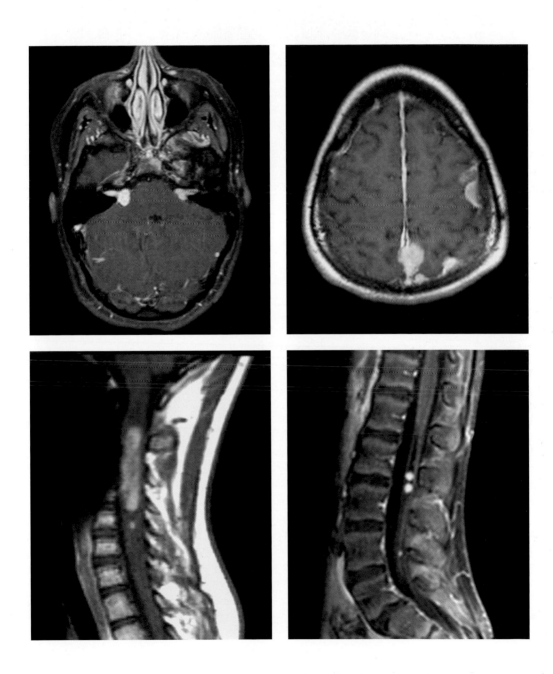

Case 95 Neurofibromatosis Type 2 (NF-2)

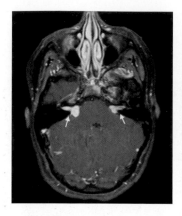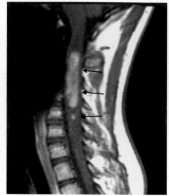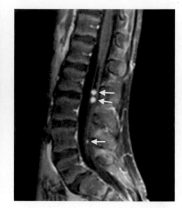

Findings

▸ Postcontrast T1-weighted images of the brain show bilateral enhancing masses in the internal auditory canals and cerebellopontine angles (short arrows).

▸ There are multiple dural-based extra-axial masses over the cerebral convexities.

▸ Contrast-enhanced T1-weighted sagittal image of the cervical spine shows enhancing intramedullary masses within the spinal cord (black arrows).

▸ Contrast-enhanced T1-weighted sagittal image of the lumbar spine shows multiple small enhancing nodular masses along the cauda equina (arrows).

Differential Diagnosis

▸ Metastases

▸ Multiple meningiomas (e.g., postradiation)

▸ Schwannomatosis

▸ Lymphoma

▸ Neurosarcoidosis

Teaching Points

▸ NF-2 is an autosomal dominant tumor-producing phakomatosis with responsible genes on chromosome 22.

▸ NF-2 is mainly characterized by multiple inherited schwannomas, meningiomas, and ependymomas (MISME syndrome). Bilateral vestibular schwannomas are diagnostic of the disease. Patients with unilateral vestibular schwannomas and either a positive family history, or other schwannomas, meningiomas, ependymomas, gliomas, or juvenile posterior subcapsular cataracts can be presumed to have NF-2.

▸ Clinical presentation may be hearing loss, other cranial neuropathies, or extremity weakness and pain.

▸ Schwannomas in NF-2 patients can be seen along the other cranial or spinal nerves. Both the brain and the spine should be evaluated with MRI in patients with findings suspicious of NF-2.

Management

▸ Treatment is surgical resection of tumors, if feasible.

Further Reading

Lin DD, Barker PB. Neuroimaging of phakomatoses. *Semin Pediatr Neurol.* 2006;13:48-62.

Rodriguez D, Young Poussaint T. Neuroimaging findings in neurofibromatosis type 1 and 2. *Neuroimaging Clin North Am.* 2004;14:149-170.

History

► Neonate with large head size

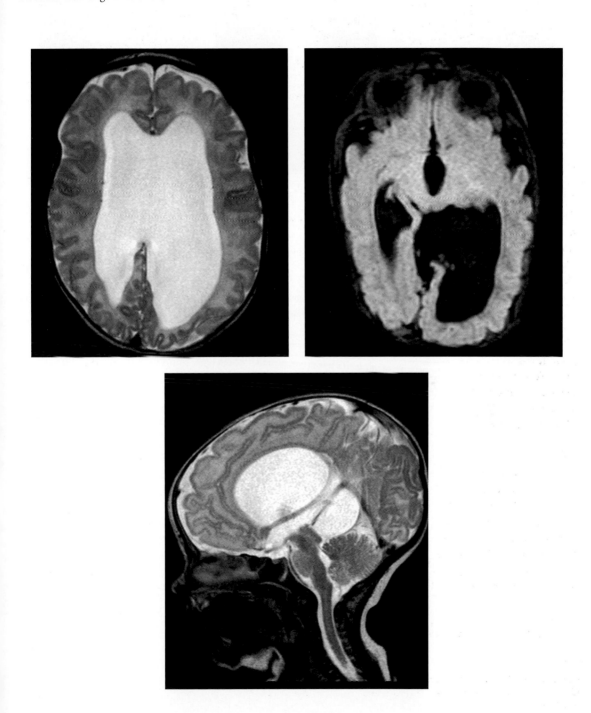

Case 96 Aqueductal Stenosis

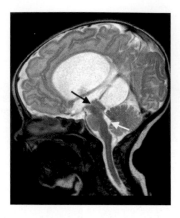

Findings

▶ The lateral and third ventricles are enlarged. The corpus callosum is stretched and thin. The fourth ventricle is normal in size (white arrow).

▶ The cerebral aqueduct is very narrow (black arrow). No mass is present.

Differential Diagnosis

▶ Neoplasms or cysts around aqueduct (pineal region tumors, tectal glioma, arachnoid cysts)

▶ Postinflammatory aqueductal gliosis after hemorrhage or infection

Teaching Points

▶ Aqueductal stenosis is due to narrowing or occlusion of the aqueduct of Sylvius connecting the third and fourth ventricles. It is a common cause of congenital hydrocephalus, although it may present later in life, including in adulthood.

▶ Clinical signs and symptoms depend on severity and may include macrocephaly, bulging fontanelle in infants, headache, papilledema, and sixth nerve palsy.

▶ Ultrasound, CT, or MRI will show enlargement of the lateral and third ventricles. The fourth ventricle is normal in size. Sometimes communicating hydrocephalus too may present with a normal-sized fourth ventricle.

▶ Thin, high-resolution T2-weighted images may show obliteration of the aqueduct or small areas of web-like narrowing in the aqueduct.

▶ When the hydrocephalus is compensated, there will be no sign of periventricular edema (transependymal flow of CSF).

▶ Carefully scrutinize the tectal plate and periaqueductal region to look for subtle masses, such as tectal glioma, that may mimic aqueductal stenosis.

Management

▶ If left untreated, it will result in loss of brain substance over time. Treatment is CSF diversion, either by endoscopic third ventriculostomy through the floor of the third ventricle, or ventriculoperitoneal shunting.

Further Reading

Chahlavi A, El-Babaa SK, Luciano MG. Adult-onset hydrocephalus. *Neurosurg Clin North Am.* 2001;12:753-760.
Partington MD. Congenital hydrocephalus. *Neurosurg Clin North Am.* 2001;12:737-742.

History

▶ 84-year-old man with lung cancer. Screening MRI for metastasis

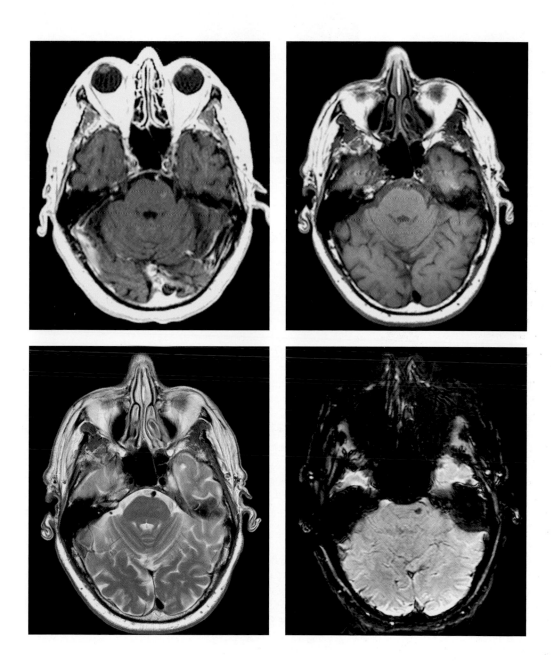

Case 97   Capillary Telangiectasia

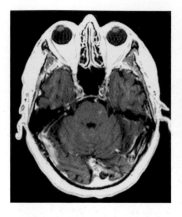 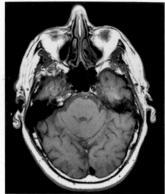 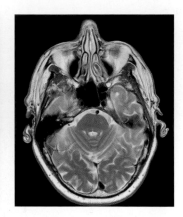

Findings

► On the postcontrast T1-weighted MRI, there is a small focus of enhancement in the left basis pontis.
► There is minimal hyperintense signal at this site on T2-weighted images, and there is no mass effect.
► On T2*-weighted imaging there is a corresponding focus of hypointense signal consistent with susceptibility-related signal loss

Differential Diagnosis

► Pontine hemorrhage
► Metastasis
► Demyelinating disease

Teaching Points

► Capillary telangiectasias represent circumscribed collections of dilated capillaries within normal cerebral parenchyma. There is no arteriovenous shunting.
► They are an incidental finding (usually at autopsy) and generally produce no symptoms or hemorrhage. However, they may be found in association with cavernous malformations, developmental venous anomalies, or arteriovenous malformations.
► The pons is by far the most common location.
► MRI demonstrates a focus of intraparenchymal enhancement. However, unlike hemorrhage or neoplasms, there is little or no signal abnormality on precontrast T1-weighted, T2-weighted, or FLAIR sequences.
► On heavily T2*-weighted (gradient echo) sequences the blood pool within the lesions may create marked hypointensity.

Management

► Capillary telangiectasias are not treated. A typical imaging appearance is considered diagnostic.

Further Reading

Hallam DK, Russell EJ. Imaging of angiographically occult cerebral vascular malformations. *Neuroimag Clin North Am.* 1998;8:323-347.
Yoshida Y, Satoshi T, Kudo K, et al. Capillary telangiectasia of the brain stem diagnosed by susceptibility-weighted imaging. *J Comput Assist Tomogr.* 2006;30:980-982.

History

▶ 5-year-old girl with two-week history of ataxia

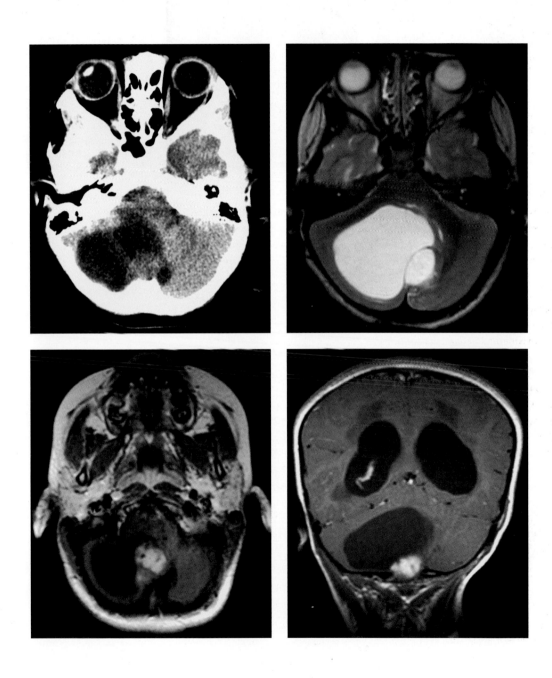

Case 98   Pilocytic Astrocytoma

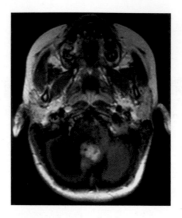

Findings

▶ Multiloculated, cystic mass of the right cerebellar hemisphere with an enhancing mural nodule.
▶ Compression of the fourth ventricle results in obstructive hydrocephalus.
▶ There is no calcification or hemorrhage.

Differential Diagnosis

▶ Hemangioblastoma
▶ Medulloblastoma
▶ Ependymoma
▶ Atypical teratoid/rhabdoid tumor (ATRT)
▶ Dorsal exophytic brain-stem glioma

Teaching Points

▶ Juvenile pilocytic astrocytoma (JPA) is the most common pediatric cerebellar tumor (80% to 90%) and typically occurs in the first two decades. It is a low-grade (WHO grade I) tumor with excellent prognosis (>90% 10-year survival).
▶ The classic appearance (two thirds of cases) is a cystic mass with an enhancing mural nodule, usually within the cerebellar hemisphere. It also may arise in the vermis (midline).
▶ Patients present with hydrocephalus (fourth ventricular compression) and/or cerebellar signs.
▶ Other common locations for JPA are the optic pathway, hypothalamus, and brain stem.

Management

▶ Surgery is the treatment of choice for cerebellar JPA. Gross total resection is considered curative.
▶ Surgical risk may be too high for JPA located in the optic pathway, hypothalamus, or brain stem. In these cases, patients are followed clinically or with imaging. Progressive disease can be treated with chemotherapy or radiation therapy.

Further Reading

Koeller KK, Rushing EJ. Pilocytic astrocytoma: radiologic-pathologic correlation. *Radiographics.* 2004;24:1693-1708.
Nejat F, El Khashab M, Rutka JT. Initial management of childhood brain tumors: neurosurgical considerations. *J Child Neurol.* 2008;23:1136-1148.

History

▶ 54-year-old man with dysphasia and right-hand weakness

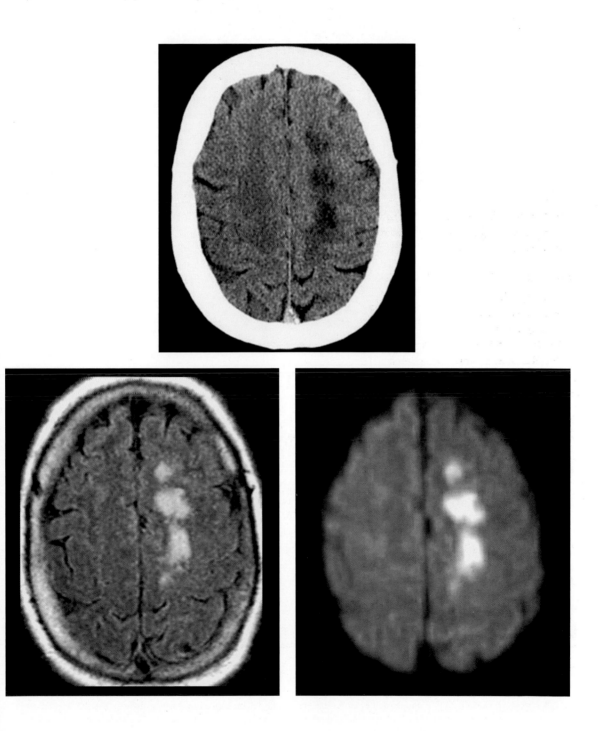

Case 99 Border-Zone Infarction

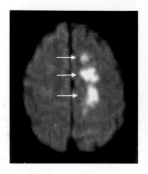 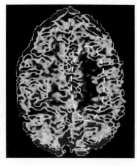 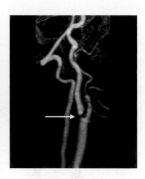

Findings

▶ Noncontrast CT scan demonstrates hypoattenuation within the left centrum semiovale and adjacent subcortical white matter.

▶ MRI reveals foci of restricted diffusion (white arrows) and hyperintense signal on the FLAIR sequence consistent with acute or subacute infarction. Note the parasagittal arrangement of the infarcts. This distribution conforms to the border zone between the middle and anterior cerebral arterial territories.

▶ Perfusion-weighted MRI demonstrates a regional reduction in cerebral blood flow in the same region (dotted oval, middle).

▶ Gadolinium-enhanced MRA reveals severe (>70%) focal stenosis at the left internal carotid artery origin (white arrow).

Differential Diagnosis

▶ Embolic infarction

▶ Lacunar infarction

▶ Vasculitis/vasculopathy

▶ Demyelination

Teaching Points

▶ Border-zone infarcts arise from insufficient perfusion at the distal capillary beds between arterial systems.

▶ They represent 10% of cerebral infarcts. The most common cause is severe internal carotid artery stenosis or occlusion accompanied by systemic hypotension. Microembolization from cardiac surgery or unstable plaques can produce a similar appearance, possibly since microemboli can be poorly cleared in these areas.

▶ The positions of the arterial border zones vary with large vessel vascular anatomy. Cortical border zones are usually found anteriorly at the borders of the anterior and middle cerebral arteries and posteriorly at the junction of the anterior, middle, and posterior cerebral arteries. Internal border zones are present in the corona radiata (between lenticulostriate perforators and the superficial perforators from middle cerebral artery cortical branches) and centrum semiovale (between the superficial perforators of the anterior and middle cerebral arteries). Internal border zones have a characteristic anterior-posterior linear distribution that may be confluent or multifocal ("rosary bead" appearance).

▶ Cerebrovascular reserve studies and PET oxygen extraction fraction may predict which patients with vascular stenosis/occlusion will go on to develop infarction.

Management

▶ Head and neck vascular imaging is essential to identify a causative stenosis/occlusion that may be amenable to revascularization.

Further Reading

Momjian-Mayor I, Baron JC. The pathophysiology of watershed infarction in internal carotid artery disease. *Stroke.* 2005; 35:567-577.
Rovira A, Grivé E, Rovira A, et al. Distribution territories and causative mechanisms of ischemic stroke. *Eur Radiol.* 2005; 15:416-426.

History

▶ 3-year-old boy with small head circumference and developmental delay

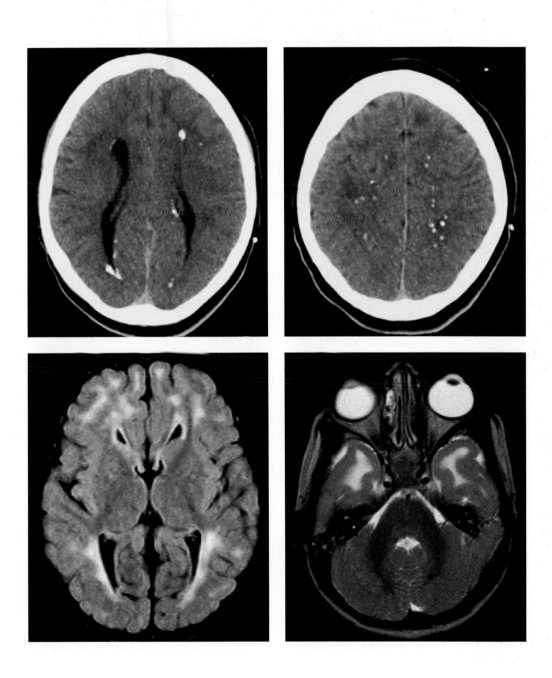

Case 100 Congenital Infection (Cytomegalovirus)

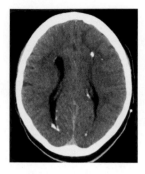 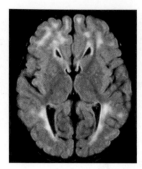

Findings

► CT images demonstrate numerous punctuate calcifications in the brain, many of them in a periventricular distribution. There are also subtle scattered areas of white matter hypoattenuation.
► Axial FLAIR and T2-weighted MRI images show patchy areas of abnormal hyperintensity in the white matter, including in the temporal lobe.

Differential Diagnosis

► Tuberous sclerosis
► Congenital toxoplasmosis
► Megalencephalic leukoencephalopathy with subcortical cysts
► Pseudo-TORCH syndromes

Teaching Points

► TORCH (toxoplasmosis, other, rubella, CMV, herpes) infections are a group of perinatal infections that can lead to a variety of cerebral injuries in newborns.
► Congenital cytomegalovirus (CMV) infection is the most common intrauterine TORCH infection. Fetal harm is more common in mothers with primary CMV infection during pregnancy compared to those with recurrent infection.
► Clinical symptoms are variable and the diagnosis is sometimes made later in life. Developmental delay, motor deficits, and sensorineural hearing loss are common manifestations. The disease is often a static, nonprogressive encephalopathy.
► The most common imaging finding of congenital CMV infection is intracranial calcification, which is commonly periventricular but may be present in other areas of the brain, including the basal ganglia. These calcifications are well demonstrated on CT but often invisible on MRI.
► Other abnormalities, better demonstrated on MRI, include:
  ▪ Microcephaly, small volume of the brain and cerebellum, and ventriculomegaly
  ▪ White matter signal abnormalities due to delayed myelination, myelin destruction, or gliosis
  ▪ Cystic changes in the temporal lobe tips or periventricular region
  ▪ Neuronal migrational abnormalities such as focal or diffuse polymicrogyria, agyria, or pachygyria

Management

► There is no direct treatment other than supportive measures and rehabilitation for children diagnosed beyond infancy. Antiviral therapy can be used in young infants.

Further Reading

Fink KR, Thapa MM, Ishak GE et al. Neuroimaging of pediatric central nervous system cytomegalovirus infection. *Radiographics*. 2010;30:1779-1796.
van der Knaap MS, Vermeulen G, Barkhof F, et al. Pattern of white matter abnormalities at MR imaging: use of polymerase chain reaction testing of Guthrie cards to link pattern with congenital cytomegalovirus infection. *Radiology*. 2004;230:529-536.

History

▶ 8-year-old boy with progressive learning and behavioral disorders and worsening vision and hearing

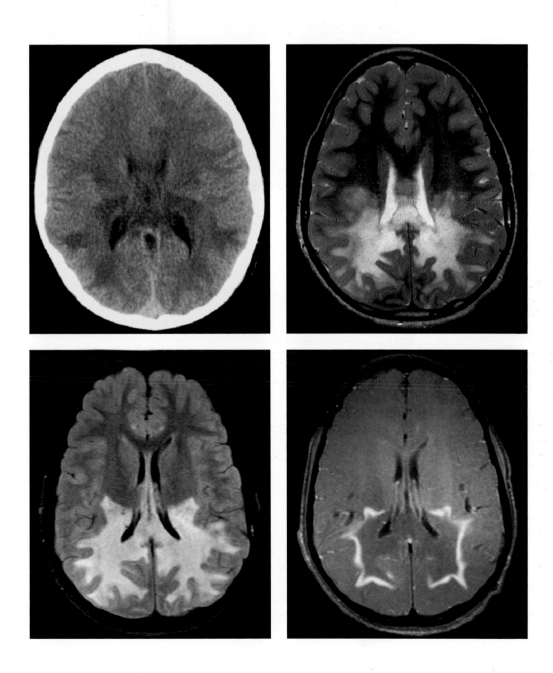

Case 101   X-linked Adrenoleukodystrophy (X-ALD)

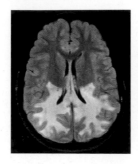 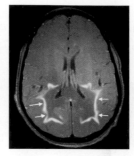

Findings

▶ CT shows decreased attenuation in the splenium of the corpus callosum and posterior white matter.

▶ In the same areas there is hyperintensity on the T2-weighted and FLAIR images.

▶ On the postcontrast T1-weighted image, there is a "leading edge" of enhancement along the periphery of the white matter area of signal abnormality (arrows).

Differential Diagnosis

▶ Alexander's disease

▶ Metachromatic leukodystrophy

▶ Neonatal hypoglycemia

▶ Periventricular leukomalacia

Teaching Points

▶ Adrenoleukodystrophy is an inherited disorder where impaired β-oxidation of very-long-chain fatty acids leads to a severe inflammatory demyelination and axonal degeneration in the brain and spinal cord. There are many different mutations and variants of adrenoleukodystrophy, the most common being classic X-linked disease.

▶ Clinical signs and symptoms include learning difficulties, behavioral problems, abnormal skin pigmentation, adrenal insufficiency, and disorders of gait, vision, and hearing commonly in preteen boys.

▶ Classic late-stage X-ALD has a characteristic imaging appearance with predominantly posterior white matter signal abnormality and often a leading edge of enhancement. Early in the disease, the abnormalities may be limited to the splenium of the corpus callosum.

▶ Alexander's disease produces similar demyelination and may enhance but typically has anterior predominance.

▶ Metachromatic leukodystrophy produces demyelination that typically involves both anterior and posterior white matter. It often produces a "tigroid" appearance to the white matter and does not enhance.

▶ Neonatal hypoglycemia also has a posterior predominance and shows restricted diffusion but occurs in a different clinical setting and does not enhance.

▶ Periventricular leukomalacia is an ischemic injury in premature children. It has posterior predominance but is marked by tissue loss and gliosis.

Management

▶ Serial MRIs with contrast are used to assess CNS involvement. The disease is fatal without treatment.

▶ Therapy includes dietary restriction and adrenal hormone replacement. Lorenzo's oil may increase the symptom-free period before clinical or MRI abnormalities are detected. Early bone marrow transplant may stabilize demyelination.

Further Reading

Kim JH, Kim HJ. Childhood X-linked adrenoleukodystrophy: clinical-pathologic overview and MR imaging manifestations at initial evaluation and follow-up. *Radiographics.* 2005;25:619-631.

Melhem ER, Barker PB, Raymond GV, et al. X-linked adrenoleukodystrophy in children: review of genetic, clinical, and MR imaging characteristics. *AJR Am J Roentgenol.* 1999;173:1575-1581.

History

▶ 12-year-old with chronic headache and paresthesias in the hands bilaterally

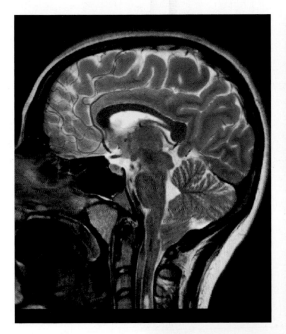
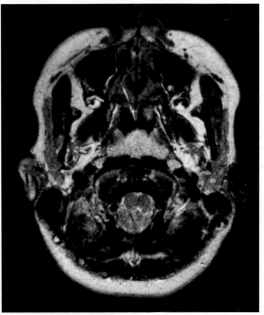
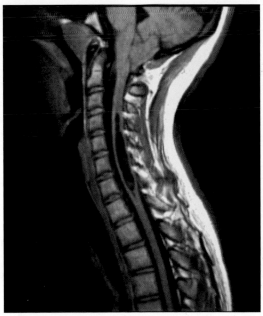

Case 102 Chiari I Malformation

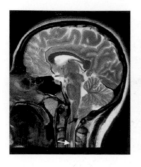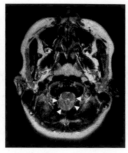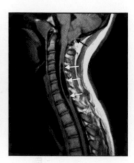

Findings

▶ Sagittal T2-weighted image demonstrates extension of the cerebellar tonsils below the foramen magnum, to the level of the posterior arch of C1 (black arrow). There is a pointed configuration of the tonsils.

▶ Axial T2-weighted image shows crowding at the foramen magnum and effacement of the CSF spaces around the cervicomedullary junction (arrowheads).

▶ Sagittal T1- and T2-weighted images show syringohydromyelia in the cervical spinal cord (white arrows).

Differential Diagnosis

▶ Normal tonsillar displacement below foramen magnum, without Chiari I malformation

▶ Chiari II malformation

▶ Acquired cerebellar tonsillar herniation (from intracranial mass effect)

Teaching Points

▶ Chiari I malformation refers to abnormal descent of the cerebellar tonsils into the cervical spinal canal, with a pointed or "peg-shaped" configuration of the tonsils.

▶ Protrusion of the cerebellar tonsils into the cervical spinal canal is asymptomatic in about half of patients. The most common symptom in Chiari I malformation is headache. Many other clinical signs and symptoms have been described, including cranial nerve symptoms, ocular disturbances, hearing and vestibular symptoms, and gait disturbances, among others. Symptoms referable to syringohydromyelia may also be present.

▶ Imaging criteria for the diagnosis are controversial. Classic imaging findings are:
  ▪ Descent of the cerebellar tonsils below the foramen magnum by 5 mm or more
  ▪ Pointed configuration of the tonsils
  ▪ Crowding at the foramen magnum

▶ Other findings include a short clivus and syringohydromyelia in the cervical or thoracic spinal cord. Occasionally hydrocephalus is seen.

▶ Sometimes MRI phase-contrast cine CSF flow studies are performed to demonstrate decreased CSF flow at the foramen magnum, but the utility of this technique is controversial.

▶ Look for signs of increased intracranial pressure and intracranial hypotension, as they may manifest by acquired descent or herniation of the cerebellar tonsils.

Management

▶ In symptomatic patients or in those with syringohydromyelia, surgical decompression is considered. Surgery includes suboccipital craniectomy +/- resection of the posterior arch of C1 and duraplasty to expand the dura at this level.

Further Reading

Schijman E, Steinbok P. International survey on the management of Chiari I malformation and syringomyelia. *Childs Nerv Syst.* 2004; 20:341-348.

Tubbs RS, Lyerly MJ, Loukas M, et al. The pediatric Chiari I malformation: a review. *Childs Nerv Syst.* 2007;23:1239-1250.

History

► 5-month-old girl status post fall off a couch

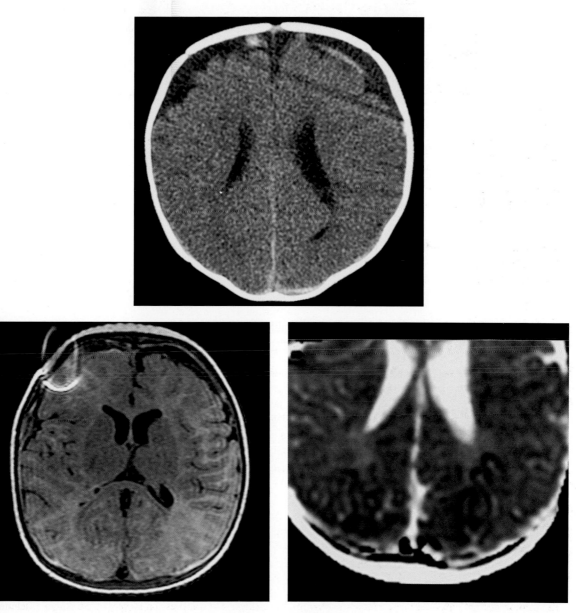

ADC map

Case 103 Nonaccidental Trauma

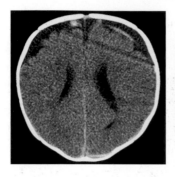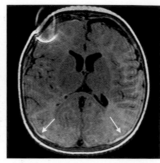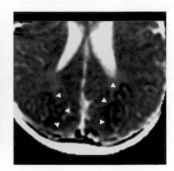

Findings

- ▶ The CT scan shows bifrontal prominent extra-axial spaces containing curvilinear high-attenuation material representing subdural blood. A small amount of subdural blood also layers along the posterior falx and left occipital lobe.
- ▶ The FLAIR image is normal except for a small amount of hyperintense extra-axial blood overlying the parietal lobes (arrows).
- ▶ The ADC map demonstrates low signal within the bilateral occipital cortices (arrowheads) not seen on the other sequence.

Differential Diagnosis

- ▶ Acute or subacute subdural hematomas with cortical ischemic injury

Teaching Points

- ▶ Head trauma is the most common cause of morbidity and mortality in abused children, especially in children under the age of 2 years. Risk factors for abuse include developmental disorders, prior history of abuse, young parents, low socioeconomic status, and prematurity.
- ▶ The injuries in nonaccidental trauma can be the result of shaking, strangulation, direct trauma, or a combination thereof. The clinical presentation is variable and includes irritability, loss of appetite, vomiting, lethargy, and apneic episodes. Victims can also present with seizures, which range from an isolated seizure to status epilepticus.
- ▶ A history of relatively minor trauma that does not match the severity of documented injury raises suspicion for nonaccidental injury.
- ▶ Subdural hematomas are the most common intracranial manifestations in nonaccidental trauma. Hemorrhages of different ages further raise suspicion. Other findings visualized on CT include skull fractures, subarachnoid blood, and acute cerebral contusions.
- ▶ Hypoxic-ischemic changes are best diagnosed with MRI using diffusion-weighted imaging. Injured tissue that appears normal on CT and conventional MRI sequences will often show diffusion-weighted abnormalities.
- ▶ In the subacute setting, when hemorrhage becomes isodense to brain or CSF on CT, MRI is more sensitive for detecting subacute blood. Gradient sequences with long TEs are very sensitive to the presence of blood products.

Management

- ▶ Notification of child protective services is mandatory in all 50 states when a physician suspects child abuse.
- ▶ The presence of brain injury usually prompts additional imaging, including skeletal survey.

Further Reading

Barkovich AJ. Brain and spine injuries in infancy and childhood. In: Barkovich AJ, ed. Pediatric Neuroimaging, 4th ed. Philadelphia: Lippincott, Williams & Wilkins, 2005:273-279.

Barkovich AJ, Sargent SK. Profound asphyxia in the preterm infant: imaging findings. *AJNR Am J Neuroradiol.* 1995;16:1837-1846.

History

▶ 9-year-old boy with progressive gait abnormality, spasticity, dystonia, abnormal movements, and dysarthria

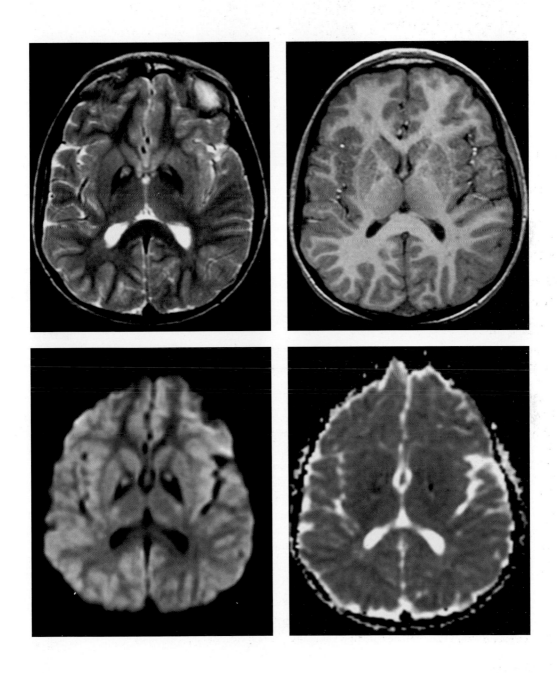

Case 104 Pantothenate Kinase-Associated Neurodegeneration (PKAN)

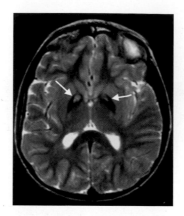

Findings

▶ T2-weighted image shows abnormal symmetric bilateral T2 hypointensity in the globus pallidus (arrows), with a more central focus of T2 hyperintensity, producing an "eye of the tiger."
▶ T1-weighted image show only slight T1 hypointensity in the globus pallidus.
▶ Diffusion images (DWI and ADC maps) do not show areas of reduced diffusion.

Differential Diagnosis

▶ Hypoxic injury
▶ Carbon monoxide toxicity
▶ Kernicterus
▶ Physiologic globus pallidus T2 hypointensity in adults and older teenagers
▶ Other metabolic disorders such as Kearns-Sayre and neuronal ceroid lipofuscinosis

Teaching Points

▶ PKAN, formerly called Hallervorden-Spatz syndrome, is an autosomal recessive disorder with its most commonly identifiable cause being a mutation in the pantothenate kinase 2 (PANK2) gene. Other similar disorders have been grouped under the term neurodegeneration with brain iron accumulation (NBIA).
▶ Patients present in childhood, usually younger than 10. They develop gait difficulty and pyramidal and extrapyramidal symptoms. They also often develop a pigmentary retinopathy. Over time they develop speech problems and cognitive deterioration. The disease is progressive over many years.
▶ MRI is the imaging study of choice and demonstrates abnormal, symmetric T2 hypointensity in the globus pallidus secondary to iron accumulation. Within this area of low signal there is often a smaller focus of T2 hyperintensity due to destructive changes and gliosis. This appearance has been called an "eye-of-the-tiger" sign.
▶ The globus pallidus often develops hypointense signal on T2-weighted images in older teenagers and adults, but this finding is not normal in younger children.

Management

▶ There is currently no cure for this disease. Treatment is symptomatic and supportive.

Further Reading

Baumeister FA, Auer DP, Hortnagel K, et al. The eye-of-the-tiger sign is not a reliable disease marker for Hallervorden-Spatz syndrome. *Neuropediatrics.* 2005;36:221-222.
Hayflick SJ, Hartman M, Coryell J, et al. Brain MRI in neurodegeneration with brain iron accumulation with and without PANK2 mutations. *AJNR Am J Neuroradiol.* 2006;27:1230-1233.

History

▶ 38-year-old woman with sudden onset of severe, recurrent headaches 5 days ago

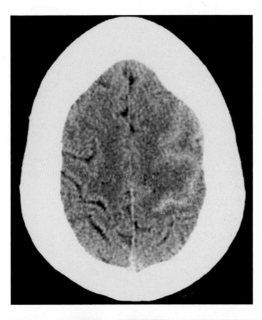

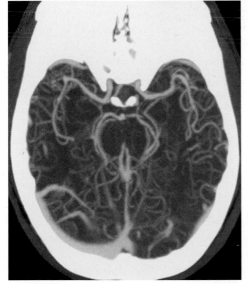

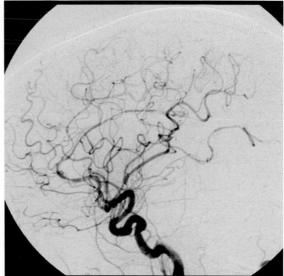

Internal carotid artery injection

Case 105 Reversible Cerebral Vasoconstriction Syndrome (RCVS)

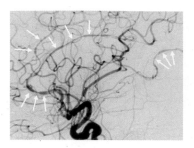

Findings

- The noncontrast CT shows high-attenuation subarachnoid hemorrhage within the sulci of the left cerebral convexity.
- MIP reconstruction from CT angiography demonstrates irregular stenoses of the middle and posterior cerebral arteries.
- On digital subtraction angiography (DSA) there are extensive segmental areas of alternating focal stenosis and dilatation ("beading") of the large and medium-sized branches of the anterior and middle cerebral arteries (arrows).

Differential Diagnosis

- Primary CNS vasculitis
- Vasculitis related to systemic autoimmune disease (e.g., systemic lupus erythematosus) or infection
- Mycotic aneurysms

Teaching Points

- RCVS is a group of disorders characterized by prolonged but reversible vasoconstriction of the cerebral arteries. Etiologies are diverse and include migrainous, postpartum, and drug-related. Offending medications include selective serotonin reuptake inhibitors as well as illicit drugs (e.g., cocaine, Ecstasy).
- Patients with RCVS classically present with acute onset of severe headache ("thunderclap headache") that is often recurrent. There are associated neurologic findings in up to 30% of cases.
- Brain imaging is frequently normal in RCVS but can reveal cortical subarachnoid hemorrhage, focal cortical or border-zone infarction, or intracerebral hemorrhage.
- Angiography reveals a classic pattern of diffuse, segmental narrowing with alternating areas of focal dilatation (beaded pattern). CTA and MRA are often able to demonstrate the vascular abnormalities, but their sensitivity and specificity are not established. Catheter angiography is the gold standard.
- The imaging and angiographic findings cannot be differentiated from those seen with cerebral vasculitis. Therefore, clinical context and laboratory studies, including CSF analysis (normal in RCVS), must be performed for accurate diagnosis.

Management

- Treatment is empiric and includes immediate discontinuation of potential causative medications. Vasodilator therapy with calcium channel blockers (nimodipine or verapamil) is the mainstay of therapy. Magnesium sulfate and possibly high-dose corticosteroids may also be administered.
- Although the vast majority of patients have a benign course, 10% of patients may develop permanent deficits, usually related to ischemic stroke.

Further Reading

Ducros A, Boukobza M, Porcher R, et al. The clinical and radiological spectrum of reversible cerebral vasoconstriction syndrome. A prospective series of 67 patients. *Brain.* 2007;130:3091-3101.
Schwedt TJ, Matharu MS, Dodick DW. Thunderclap headache. *Lancet Neurol.* 2006;5:621-631.

History

▶ 54-year old man with 3-week progressive vision loss

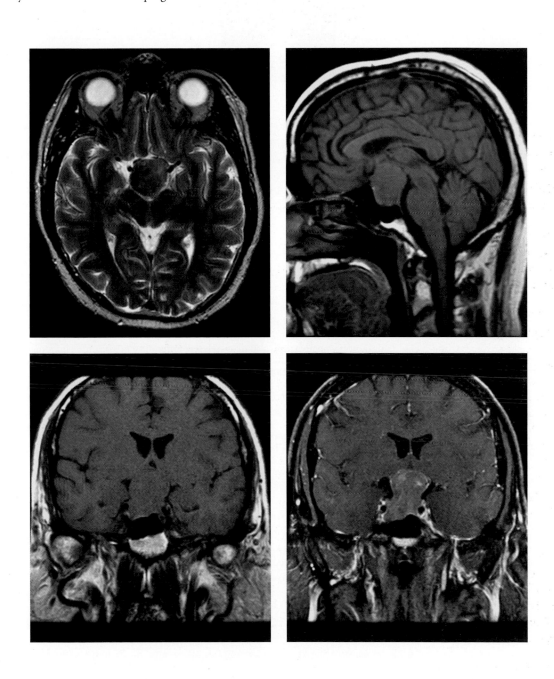

Case 106   Pituitary Macroadenoma

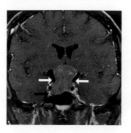

Findings

- ▶ There is a large sellar and suprasellar mass. The tumor has a waist at the level of the diaphragma sellae (white arrows).
- ▶ The mass is T1 iso-intense and T2 hypointense and demonstrates mild enhancement.
- ▶ There is possible extension into the right cavernous sinus (black arrow).

Differential Diagnosis

- ▶ Meningioma
- ▶ Germ cell tumor
- ▶ Craniopharyngioma
- ▶ Glial neoplasm
- ▶ Lymphocytic hypophysitis
- ▶ Metastasis

Teaching Points

- ▶ Pituitary adenoma is an epithelial neoplasm of pituitary origin. It is the most common adult intrasellar tumor, and it is usually benign.
- ▶ 75% of pituitary adenomas are functional, and they can have various clinical manifestations:
  - ▪ Prolactin (most common): amenorrhea, infertility, impotence
  - ▪ Growth hormone: acromegaly/gigantism
  - ▪ ACTH: Cushing disease
  - ▪ TSH: hyperthyroidism
- ▶ Mass effect from macroadenomas (i.e., adenomas >10 mm) can produce bitemporal hemianopsia (optic chiasm compression), hydrocephalus (third ventricle compression), hypopituitarism (pituitary compression), and cranial nerve palsies (cavernous sinus involvement).
- ▶ Macroadenomas have a characteristic waist at the diaphragma sellae and may have cystic degeneration, hemorrhage, and variable enhancement.
- ▶ Meningiomas in this region are more likely to encase and narrow the carotid arteries. Germ cell tumors are more common in young patients, grow rapidly, and may be multiple. Craniopharyngiomas are more often cystic and calcified. Metastases are more likely to involve the posterior pituitary, produce diabetes insipidus, and may destroy bone.
- ▶ Microadenomas (<10 mm) enhance less rapidly than normal pituitary and can be identified on early post-gadolinium imaging as a small circumscribed mass with hypoenhancement relative to pituitary tissue.

Management

- ▶ Medical therapy with dopamine agonists is the mainstay of therapy for prolactinoma.
- ▶ Transsphenoidal surgery is the primary treatment for the remainder of pituitary adenomas, including macroadenomas.
- ▶ Radiation therapy is reserved for residual tumor and is limited by the risk of potential injury to the optic apparatus and the risk of hypopituitarism.

Further Reading

Fitzpatrick M, Tartaglino L, Hollander M, et al. Imaging of sellar and parasellar pathology. *Radiol Clin North Am.* 1999;37:101-121.
Kreutzer J, Fahlbusch R. Diagnosis and treatment of pituitary tumors. *Curr Opin Neurol.* 2004;17:693-703.

History

▶ 21-year-old man with lower extremity pain and weakness

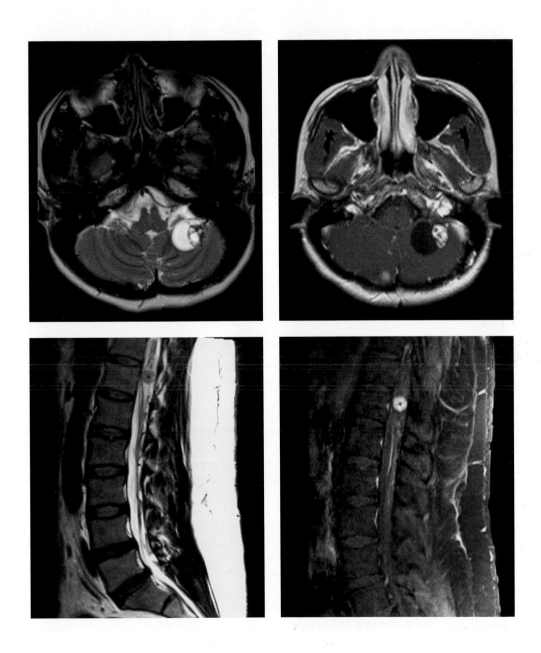

Case 107 Von Hippel-Lindau Disease (VHL)

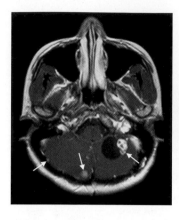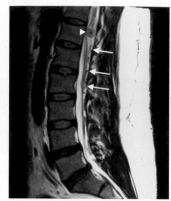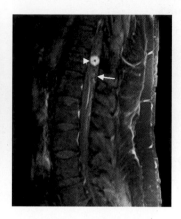

Findings

▶ T2-weighted and postcontrast T1-weighted images of the brain show multiple enhancing lesions in the cerebellum (arrows). The largest lesion on the left has a cyst with enhancing mural nodule appearance.

▶ T2-weighted and postcontrast T1-weighted images of the lumbar spine show an enhancing intradural mass (arrowheads). There are associated vascular flow voids (arrows), suggestive of a highly vascular lesion.

Differential Diagnosis

▶ Metastases

▶ Pilocytic astrocytoma

Teaching Points

▶ VHL is an autosomal dominant syndrome with multiple hemangioblastomas, ocular angiomas, pancreatic and renal cysts, renal cell carcinoma, pheochromocytoma, cystadenomas, islet cell tumors, and endolymphatic sac tumors. It is caused by mutations in the VHL tumor suppressor gene.

▶ In the brain, the hemangioblastomas occur primarily in the cerebellum and brain stem. They appear as either a cystic mass with enhancing mural nodule or as a nodular enhancing mass. When a cyst is present, its walls typically do not enhance.

▶ On T2-weighted images, flow voids may be visible in and around the mass secondary to the highly vascular nature of these lesions. On catheter angiography, the lesions appear as vascular masses with enlarged feeding arteries and arteriovenous shunting; they may mimic arteriovenous malformations.

▶ In the spine, single or multiple enhancing nodules may be seen within or along the surface of the spinal cord and nerve roots. Syringohydromyelia can also occur secondary to some of these tumors.

▶ Endolymphatic sac tumor is a rare papillary adenocarcinoma arising from the endolymphatic sac in the temporal bone and is seen with higher incidence in patients with VHL.

Management

▶ Surgical resection of symptomatic tumors is often performed, sometimes with preoperative embolization. Stereotactic radiosurgery of smaller lesions may be attempted.

▶ Periodic follow-up with imaging and ophthalmoscopic examination is suggested, as new lesions often develop over time.

Further Reading

Leung RS, Biswas SV, Duncan M, et al. Imaging features of von Hippel-Lindau disease. *Radiographics.* 2008;28:65-79.
Lin DD, Barker PB. Neuroimaging of phakomatoses. *Semin Pediatr Neurol.* 2006;13:48-62.

Part 2   **Spine**

History

▶ 48-year-old woman with lower back pain

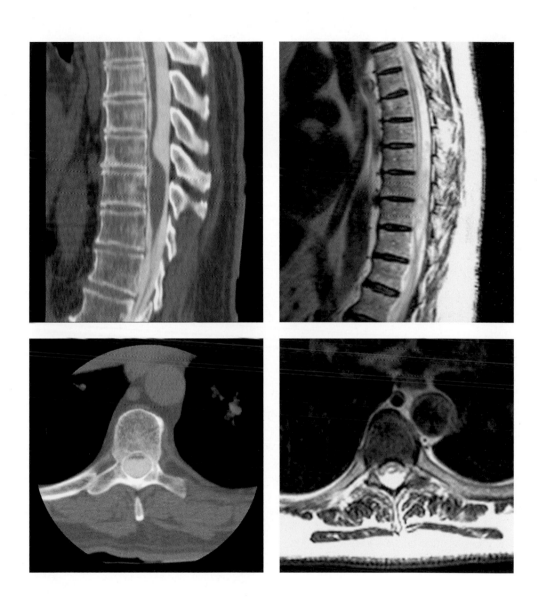

Case 108 Arachnoid Cyst

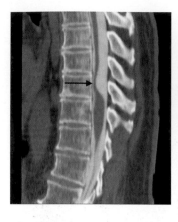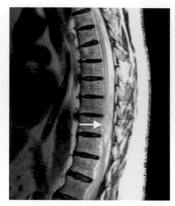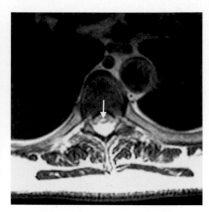

Findings

► CT myelogram with sagittal reformatting shows ventral displacement and compression of the spinal cord at T8–T10 with dorsal expansion of the subarachnoid space (black arrow).
► Sagittal and axial T2-weighted images show similar displacement.
► Within the central spinal cord above the level of cord compression there is an area of signal similar to CSF, consistent with syrinx (white arrow).

Differential Diagnosis

► Dural herniation of the spinal cord
► Dural ectasia

Teaching Points

► Arachnoid cysts are extramedullary, well-circumscribed CSF-filled collections. They can be extradural or intradural. Intradural cysts are less common.
► Arachnoid cysts can be congenital or acquired and occur when the arachnoid herniates through a dural defect.
► 80% are located in the thoracic region and most are dorsal in location.
► The mass effect may cause neurologic symptoms by compressing the spinal cord and nerve roots. Patients usually present with back pain or myelopathy.
► On MRI, the arachnoid cyst should follow CSF signal intensity on all sequences.
► The cyst wall is rarely complete, and on myelography the cyst usually fills with injected contrast. Careful fluoroscopic observation of the region during contrast instillation is needed. The cyst is sometimes slow to fill and delayed images may be necessary for diagnosis.
► Pressure remodeling of the adjacent bone may be present.

Management

► Prognosis is excellent with surgical excision or shunting.

Further Reading

Nabors MW, Pait TG, Byrd EB, et al. Updated assessment and current classification of spinal meningeal cysts. *J Neurosurg.* 1988;68: 366-377.
Silbergleit R, Brunberg JA, Patel SC, et al. Imaging of spinal intradural arachnoid cysts: MRI, myelography and CT. *Neuroradiology.* 1998;40:664-668.

History

▶ 15-year-old boy with non-germinomatous germ cell tumor status post chemotherapy and radiation

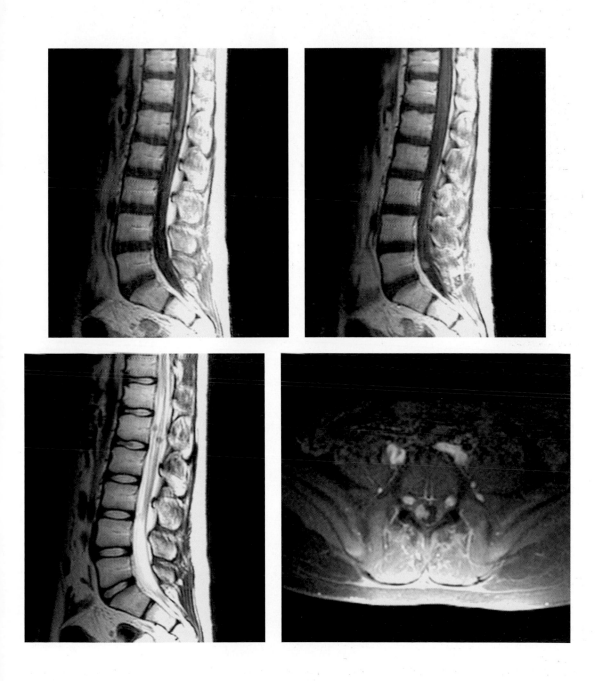

Case 109   Drop Metastasis

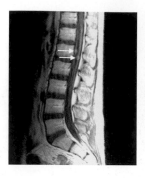 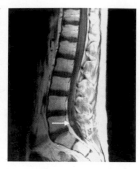 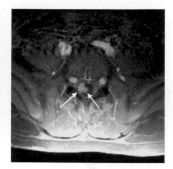

Findings

- There are multiple nodular lesions along the cauda equina (arrows). They are present at the L1, L4, and L5 levels. The enhancement is best demonstrated on the axial postcontrast T1-weighted images with fat saturation.
- Bone marrow signal is normal.

Differential Diagnosis

- Lymphoma
- Infectious/inflammatory meningitis (herpes, Lyme disease, sarcoid, CMV)
- Neurofibromatosis type 2 (multiple schwannomas and/or meningiomas)
- Multiple neurofibromas
- Arachnoiditis

Teaching Points

- Spinal drop metastases, also known as leptomeningeal metastases, occur when the spinal subarachnoid space is seeded by tumor. They most commonly occur in the lumbosacral spine but can occur anywhere along the neuraxis. Their presence portends a poor prognosis.
- Typical symptoms include headache, nausea, vomiting, cranial nerve palsies, back pain, and radicular pain.
- Primary intracranial neoplasms are the most likely to produce drop metastases. The neoplasm with the greatest predilection for this spread is medulloblastoma. Other primary CNS tumors that may produce drop metastases include ependymoma, glioblastoma, and pineal region tumors.
- Tumors outside the CNS may also seed the spinal subarachnoid space; breast, lung, and lymphoma are the most common.
- Contrast-enhanced MRI is most sensitive imaging study for detection of leptomeningeal metastases. On imaging, the disease is typically localized or diffuse.
- Localized disease is visible as multiple enhancing nodules along the surface of the cord or cauda equina.
- In the diffuse form, a fine layer of enhancement coats the cord and nerve roots; this is sometimes referred to as "sugarcoating." This pattern can also be seen as the result of infectious/inflammatory processes.

Management

- The diagnosis of leptomeningeal metastases is confirmed with CSF cytology.
- Treatment usually consists of radiation and/or intrathecal methotrexate. Most often systemic tumors are treated with both, while primary intracranial tumors are treated with radiation therapy.

Further Reading

Pawha P, Sze G. Neoplastic disorders of the spine and spinal cord. In Atlas S, ed. Magnetic Resonance Imaging of the Brain and Spine, 4th ed. Philadelphia: Lippincott Williams, 2000:1545-1546.

History

▶ 77-year-old woman with the sudden onset of lower extremity paralysis and loss of sensation below the umbilicus

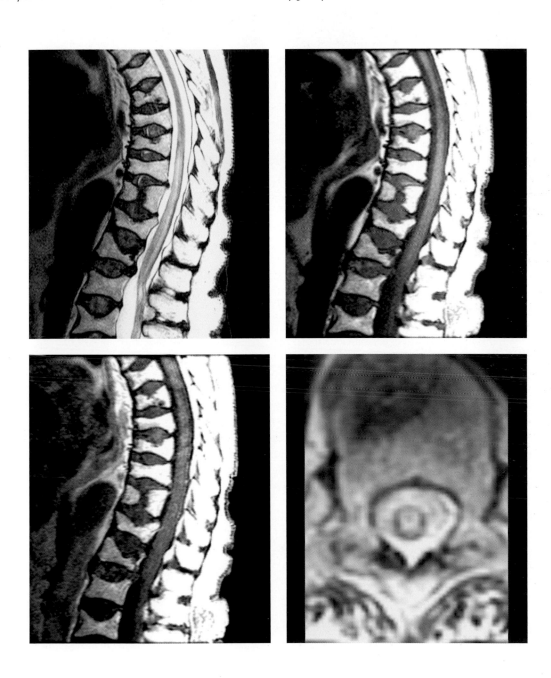

Case 110 Spinal Cord Infarction

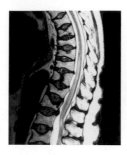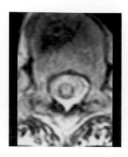

Findings

▶ T2-weighted images demonstrate hyperintense signal within the central aspect of the lower thoracic cord extending across multiple segments to just above the conus.

▶ There is no enhancement on postcontrast images.

▶ There are multiple old vertebral compression fractures (unrelated).

Differential Diagnosis

▶ Transverse myelitis

▶ Multiple sclerosis

▶ Spinal dural AV fistula

▶ Spinal cord astrocytoma

Teaching Points

▶ Spinal cord infarction is rare. Etiologies include spinal and aortic surgery, vertebral or aortic dissection, atherosclerosis, hypotension, and vasculitis.

▶ Due to the pial collateral network and the paired posterior spinal arteries, spinal cord infarction is most common in the anterior spinal artery territory (anterior two thirds of the cord). The gray matter, located centrally, has the highest metabolic demand, making it more susceptible to ischemia. The thoracic cord is most susceptible to ischemia because of limited collateral flow.

▶ Patients present with abrupt onset of paralysis and loss of pain and temperature sensation below the lesion. Posterior column function (vibration and position sense) is usually preserved.

▶ MRI abnormalities are nonspecific and consist of hyperintensity on T2-weighted images within the central aspect of the spinal cord. In more severe cases the entire cross-section of the cord can be involved. There is no abnormal enhancement. Mass effect, when present, is mild.

▶ In subacute ischemia, postcontrast enhancement can be present, and this may persist for months. In the chronic stage, cord atrophy develops.

▶ The longitudinal extent of infarction usually involves more than one vertebral body segment. When the infarct results from occlusion of a segmental artery, the ipsilateral half of the vertebral body may also infarct, which can be a clue to the diagnosis.

▶ DWI of the spinal cord, while technically difficult, can demonstrate decreased diffusion.

Management

▶ Treatment is supportive with anticoagulation and steroids. Prognosis is dismal, with most patients having permanent paralysis.

Further Reading

Kring T, Lausjaunias PL, Hans F, et al. Imaging in spinal vascular disease. *Neuroimaging Clin North Am*. 2007;17:57-72.
Maward ME, Rivera V, Crawford S, et al. Spinal cord ischemia after resection of thoracoabdominal aortic aneurysms: MR findings in 24 patients. *AJNR Am J Neuroradiol*. 1990;11:987-991.

History

▶ 60-year-old woman with back pain

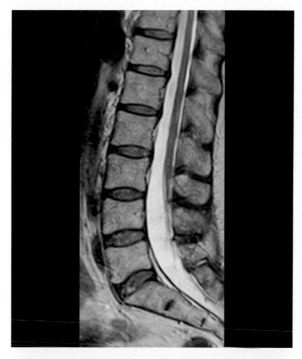

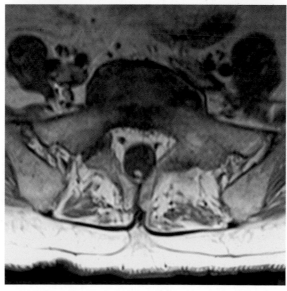

Case 111 Tethered Cord

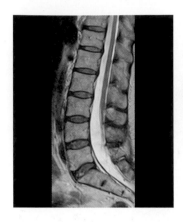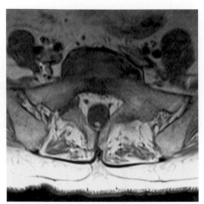

Findings

► The conus terminates at the L4 level and has a smoothly tapered configuration.
► The conus merges with a thickened and fatty filum terminale (hyperintense signal on the T1 axial image).

Differential Diagnosis

► This appearance is characteristic of this entity. However, one must evaluate for the presence of other associated abnormalities of the spinal cord and vertebrae (see below).

Teaching Points

► Tethered cord syndrome (tight filum terminale syndrome) refers to a constellation of symptoms and imaging findings that are likely the result of incomplete involution of the terminal cord or failure of the filum to properly lengthen during embryogenesis.
► Presentation is most common in children during periods of rapid growth, but symptoms can begin at any age. They include lower extremity weakness and abnormal reflexes, bladder dysfunction, and back pain. Symptoms are thought to result from abnormal perfusion to the stretched conus and associated nerve roots.
► The normal conus medullaris should terminate at or above the inferior endplate of L2.
► The normal filum terminale should measure 1 mm or less at the L5/S1 level. The short filum terminale is commonly thickened and contains a lipoma.
► Associated abnormalities include syringohydromyelia, myelomalacia, diastematomyelia, spinal dysraphism, scoliosis, or VATER syndrome.
► MRI is the modality of choice for evaluating tethered cord syndrome. Axial T1-weighted images are best for demonstrating lipomas of the filum terminale and axial T2-weighted images best demonstrate the thickened filum. Axial images should be obtained from the conus medullaris through the bottom of the thecal sac.
► In a minority of cases, the spinal cord may be tethered but terminate at a normal level. Conversely, some patients with a low-lying conus medullaris may be asymptomatic.

Management

► In symptomatic patients, surgical untethering is performed. The recurrence rate is as high as 25%.

Further Reading

Barkovich AJ. Congenital anomalies of the spine. In: Barkovich AJ, ed. Pediatric Neuroimaging, 4th ed. Philadelphia: Lippincott, Williams & Wilkins, 2005:709-710, 732-735.
Lew SM, Kothbauer KF. Tethered cord syndrome: An updated review. *Pediatr Neurosurg*. 2007;43:236-248.

History

▶ 58-year-old man with back pain progressing to quadriplegia over the course of two weeks

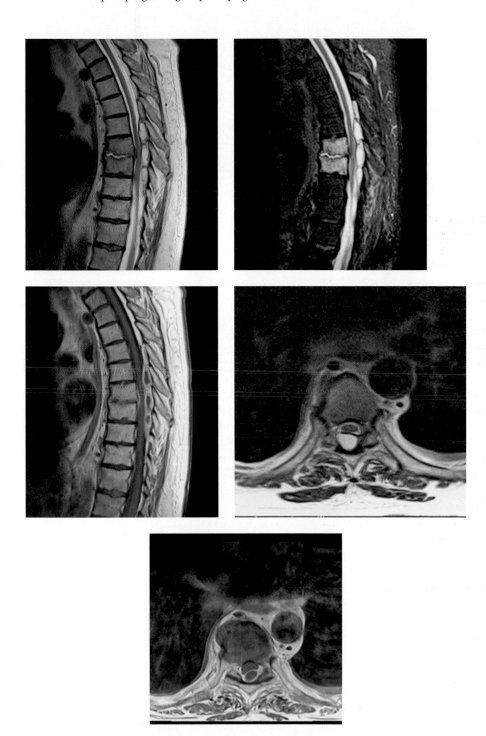

Case 112 Epidural Abscess and Spondylodiscitis

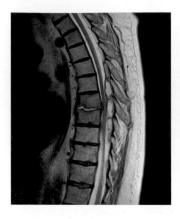 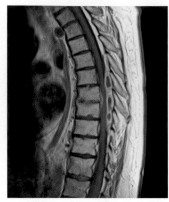

Findings

► Sagittal T2-weighted and STIR sequences show a T2-hyperintense, loculated dorsal epidural collection in the midthoracic spine.
► Postcontrast T1-weighted images show peripheral enhancement about the collection. There is a small site of ventral epidural enhancement.
► The adjacent midthoracic intervertebral disc demonstrates abnormal signal and irregular height loss. This is associated with extensive marrow edema within the adjacent vertebral bodies.

Differential Diagnosis

► Epidural hematoma
► Extradural neoplasm (e.g., metastasis)

Teaching Points

► Epidural abscesses are pyogenic collections of the epidural space. They most commonly occur as a result of direct extension of bacterial spondylodiscitis but can result from extension of other paraspinal infections or by hematogenous seeding
► Patients present with back pain and fever with or without neurologic deficit.
► Risk factors include IV drug use, diabetes mellitus, immunodeficiency, poor dentition, and alcoholism. *Staphylococcus aureus* is the causative agent in 50% to 70% of cases. 15% of these organisms are methicillin-resistant.
► Spinal epidural abscesses occur in all segments of the spinal canal, with a predilection for the lower thoracic and upper lumbar spine.
► MRI is the best imaging tool for depicting spinal epidural abscess. On T2-weighted imaging the collections are centrally hyperintense and are outlined by the darker dura. There is often thin, peripheral enhancement about the margin of the collection. However, granulation tissue may predominate and result in more diffuse enhancement.
► Larger abscesses may produce spinal cord or cauda equina compression. Hyperintense signal within the spinal cord on T2-weighted images may represent vasogenic edema or cord infarction.

Management

► Abscesses producing cord or cauda equina compression generally require immediate surgical drainage of the abscess. Smaller abscesses may be treated with a prolonged course of antibiotics alone.

Further Reading

Ruiz A, Post MJ, Sklar EM, et al. MR imaging of infections of the cervical spine. *Magn Reson Imaging Clin North Am.* 2000;8:561-580.

History

▶ 36-year-old woman with slowly progressive bilateral leg weakness

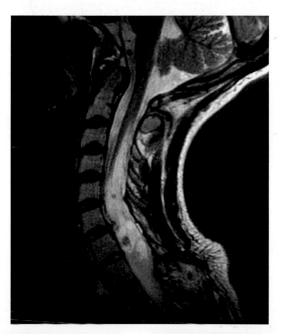

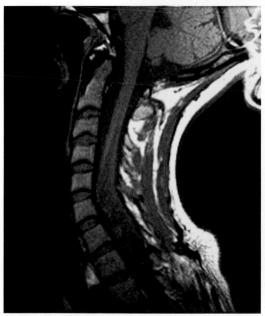

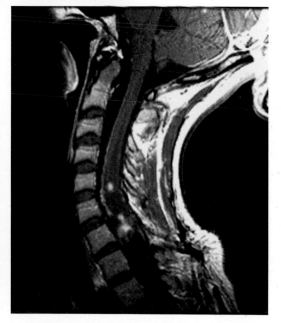

Case 113 Spinal Cord Hemangioblastoma (HB)

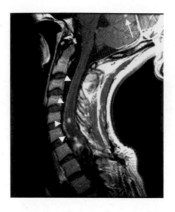

Findings

- There is extensive signal abnormality in the cervical spinal cord, T2 hyperintense and T1 hypointense. There is marked cord expansion.
- There is a small nodular, intramedullary mass at the C5 level and a heterogeneously enhancing intramedullary mass at C7.
- There is a prominent vessel arising from the neoplasm and extending along the ventral aspect of the cord (arrowheads).
- There is a very small enhancing nodule in the cerebellum at the upper margins of the image (arrow).

Differential Diagnosis

- Metastasis
- Astrocytoma
- Ependymoma
- Lymphoma
- Inflammatory/infectious diseases (e.g., sarcoid, fungus)

Teaching Points

- Spinal HBs are rare, WHO grade I vascular neoplasms accounting for 3% of all intramedullary tumors. They represent the third most common enhancing intramedullary spinal cord neoplasm (after ependymomas and astrocytomas).
- Most spinal HBs are sporadic, but 25% to 30% occur in patients with von Hippel-Lindau syndrome (VHL).
- Symptoms are related to local mass effect, hydrosyringomyelia, or hemorrhage.
- HBs typically become apparent in the second decade. For this reason, routine screening of the brain and spine with MRI is recommended for patients with VHL starting at age 10.
- HBs of the spinal cord can be solitary or multiple. Multiple tumors are more common in VHL. A dorsal position along the surface of the cervical or thoracic cord is the most common location.
- On MRI, spinal HBs demonstrate intense homogenous enhancement. Larger masses (>24 mm) tend to have heterogeneous enhancement as well as adjacent prominent vascular signal voids (which are highly suggestive of the diagnosis). Cord edema spanning multiple vertebral body segments is a common finding.

Management

- Surgical excision (often with preoperative embolization) is often curative but in cases of inaccessible or multiple HBs, stereotactic radiosurgery may be preferred.

Further Reading

Chu BC, Terae S, Hida K, et al. MRI findings in spinal hemangioblastomas: correlation with symptoms and with angiographic and surgical findings. *AJNR Am J Neuroradiol.* 2001;22:206-217.

History

► 22-year-old man with decreased strength in his left arm after a motorcycle accident

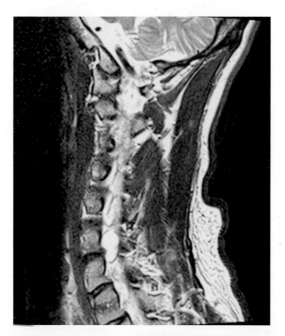

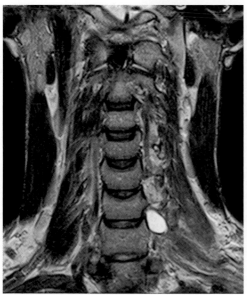

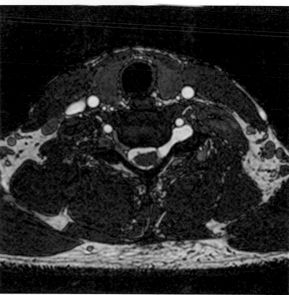

Case 114 Nerve Root Avulsion and Pseudomeningocele

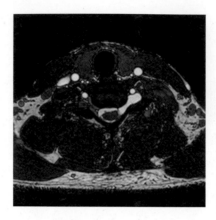

Findings

▶ There is a well-demarcated collection with signal characteristics similar to those of CSF extending through the left C6-7 neural foramen. No nerve root is present within the collection.

▶ The spinal cord is shifted towards the avulsed nerve root.

▶ On the coronal T2-weighted image there is signal abnormality in the left scalene muscles, consistent with denervation.

Differential Diagnosis

▶ Meningocele

▶ Nerve sheath tumor

Teaching Points

▶ Brachial plexus injuries occur in the setting of a severe traction injury with forced abduction or downward displacement of the arm. This results in functional impairment of the upper extremity.

▶ The most common cause of injury is motorcycle accidents in young men. MRI plays an important role in assessing the integrity of the nerve roots and in distinguishing between pre- and post-ganglionic injuries, which is important for treatment planning.

▶ Pre-ganglionic injuries typically take the form of nerve root avulsion. These avulsions are commonly associated with pseudomeningocele formation and discontinuity of the nerve root.

▶ Secondary findings of nerve injury include spinal cord edema, and edema and enhancement of the nerve roots and the paraspinal muscles. Chronic changes are characterized by nerve and muscle atrophy.

▶ Post-ganglionic injuries (distal to the sensory ganglion) take the form of avulsion or stretch injury. Stretch injuries are characterized by T2 hyperintense signal within the neural elements.

▶ CT myelography is as sensitive as MRI for detecting nerve root avulsion.

Management

▶ Treatment may be conservative or surgical depending on the severity of the injury. Prospects of regaining full function are poor, but surgical procedures (e.g., neurolysis, nerve grafting, and nerve transfer) may be attempted.

Further Reading

Yoshikawa T, Hayashi N, Yamamoto S, et al. Brachial plexus injury: clinical manifestations, conventional imaging findings, and the latest imaging techniques. *RadioGraphics*. 2006;26:S133-S143.

History

▶ 77-year-old man with progressive lower extremity weakness and positive Babinski sign. A CT myelogram is obtained because the patient has a pacemaker

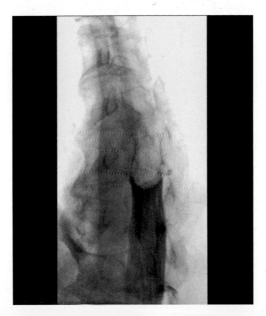

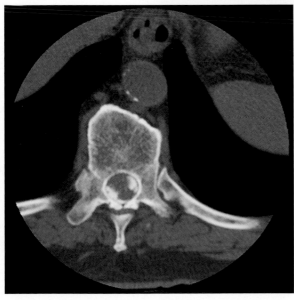

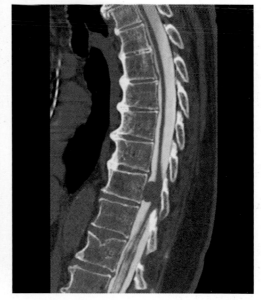

Case 115 Spinal Meningioma

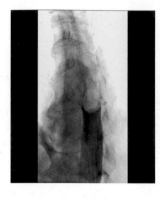
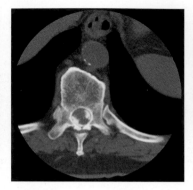
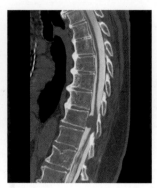

Findings

► The myelogram images show a large filling defect in the spinal canal. The acute angles of the contrast column mark this as an intradural mass.
► The CT myelogram shows that the mass is ventrally located, displacing the spinal cord posteriorly.
► A sharp meniscus of contrast caps the lesion and there is enlargement of the ipsilateral subarachnoid space, best seen on the sagittal CT reconstructions. These features indicate an extramedullary, intradural location.

Differential Diagnosis

► Schwannoma
► Metastasis
► Lymphoma

Teaching Points

► Meningiomas are the second most common intraspinal neoplasms, after nerve sheath tumors. Meningiomas arise from persistent arachnoid remnants and usually adhere to the dura.
► The average age of presentation is in the fifth and sixth decades, and 60% to 80% occur in women. Radicular pain and myelopathic pain are typical presentations.
► Spinal meningiomas usually occur as intradural extramedullary masses that occur most frequently in the posterolateral thoracic spine. The ventral position of the meningioma in this case is somewhat unusual.
► They are well encapsulated and displace the cord and nerve roots without invasion.
► On CT they are typically hyperattenuating and may be calcified.
► Myelography will delineate the extramedullary (and usually intradural) nature of the mass and show its extent.
► MRI characteristics include iso-intensity to the cord on T1- and T2-weighted sequences. There is dense homogenous enhancement.
► It can be difficult to distinguish a meningioma from a nerve sheath tumor, but several discriminators can be helpful. Nerve sheath tumors are more commonly anteriorly positioned, neurofibromas are usually multiple, and schwannomas are characteristically hyperintense on T2-weighted images.

Management

► Symptomatic meningiomas are surgically resected. Prognosis is excellent and the recurrence rate is low.

Further Reading

Beall DP, Googe DJ, Emery RL, et al. Extramedullary intradural spinal tumors: a pictorial review. *Curr Prob Diagn Radiol.* 2007;36:185-198.
Pawha P, Sze G. Neoplastic disorders of the spine and spinal cord. In: Atlas S. Magnetic Resonance Imaging of the Brain and Spine, 4th ed. Philadelphia: Lippincott Williams, 2008:1539-1543.

History

▶ 52-year-old man with one-week history of progressive ataxia, weakness, and hyperreflexia

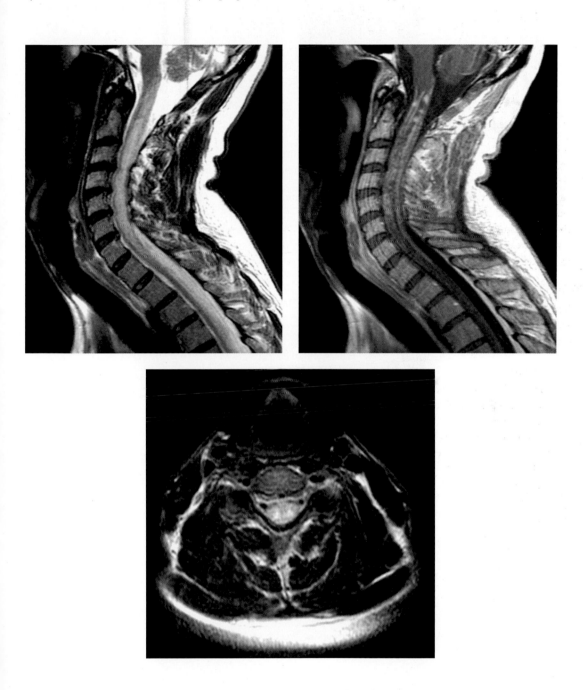

Case 116 Acute Transverse Myelitis

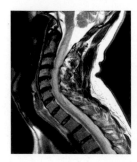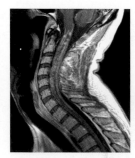

Findings

▶ There is a single large band of signal abnormality within the spinal cord, hyperintense on T2-weighted images.
▶ Postcontrast T1-weighted images show patchy enhancement, much of it peripheral.
▶ The lesion produces relatively little mass effect.

Differential Diagnosis

▶ Multiple sclerosis (MS)
▶ Spinal cord neoplasm (e.g., astrocytoma)
▶ Spinal cord infarction

Teaching Points

▶ Acute transverse myelitis is an inflammatory disorder of the spinal cord. It may be idiopathic or occur secondary to an underlying illness.
▶ Secondary causes include:
  ▪ Systemic autoimmune disease (systemic lupus erythematosus, Sjögren disease, sarcoidosis)
  ▪ Viral and bacterial infection (direct involvement vs. autoimmune attack)
  ▪ Post-vaccination
  ▪ Paraneoplastic syndrome
  ▪ Vascular (vasculitis)
▶ Symptoms develop rapidly over several hours to days. Transverse myelitis is generally a monophasic illness, but a small percentage of patients may suffer a recurrence, especially if there is a predisposing underlying illness. Recovery is variable, with 30% to 50% showing complete recovery.
▶ MRI shows T2 hyperintensity within the central spinal cord, mild cord expansion, and peripheral enhancement. Lesions may be solitary or multifocal.
▶ Differentiation from MS may be difficult. The lesions of transverse myelitis typically extend over at least two vertebral lengths (in contrast to the smaller plaques of MS).
▶ 2% to 8% of patients thought to have acute transverse myelitis go on to develop MS. Patients with severe transverse myelitis are less likely to develop MS than those with mild cases. Patients who have abnormal brain MRIs are much more likely to develop MS.

Management

▶ Treatments for idiopathic and immune-mediated etiologies include corticosteroids, intravenous immunoglobulins, and plasmapheresis. For secondary causes treatment is directed toward the underlying disease.

Further Reading

Harzheim M, Schlegel U, Urbach H, et al. Discriminatory features of acute transverse myelitis: a retrospective analysis of 45 patients. *J Neurol Sci.* 2004;217:217-223.
Jeffery DR, Mandler RN, Davis LE. Transverse myelitis: retrospective analysis of 33 cases, with differentiation of cases associated with multiple sclerosis and parainfectious events. *Arch Neurol.* 1993;50:532.

History

▶ 73-year-old man with longstanding dizziness

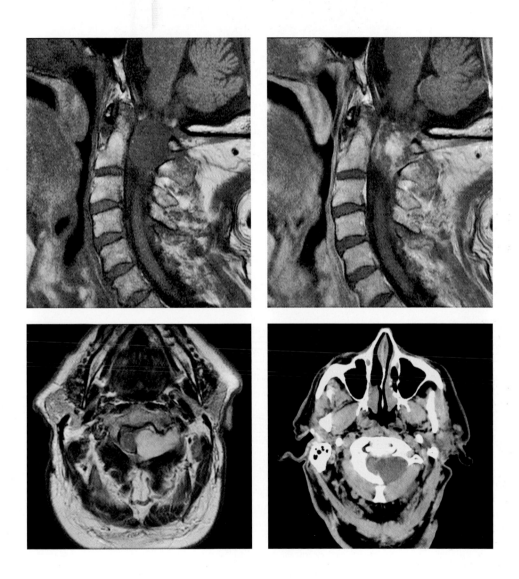

Case 117 Spinal Nerve Sheath Tumor

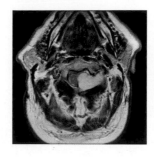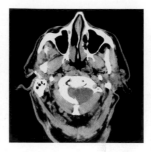

Findings

- ► A large, dumbbell-shaped, well-marginated, extradural mass extends through the C1-2 neural foramen. It compresses the cervical spinal cord.
- ► The mass is hyperintense on T2-weighted images and shows heterogeneous postcontrast enhancement.
- ► The posterior arch of C1 is remodeled, indicating a longstanding process.

Differential Diagnosis

- ► Schwannoma
- ► Neurofibroma
- ► Meningioma
- ► Metastasis
- ► Primary osseous neoplasm

Teaching Points

- ► Nerve sheath tumors, which include both neurofibromas and schwannomas, are the most common extramedullary spinal tumors. Although these tumors are histologically distinct, their imaging appearance is similar.
- ► Multiple enhancing nerve sheath tumors is a hallmark of the neurofibromas that occur in the setting of neurofibromatosis type 1 (NF-1). Up to 65% of patients with NF-1 have spinal neurofibromas. Some neurofibromas, however, occur in patients without NF-1. Multiple schwannomas are associated with NF-2.
- ► Symptoms associated with nerve sheath tumors are variable but most commonly are pain and radiculopathy.
- ► Most nerve sheath tumors have an intradural extramedullary location. The remainder have both intradural and extradural components or are completely extradural. Tumors with both intradural and extradural components typically are dumbbell-shaped.
- ► Nerve sheath tumors are well-circumscribed masses that are typically isoattenuating to the spinal cord on CT. Larger tumors may undergo cystic change and become hypoattenuating. Bone remodeling and expansion of the neural foramen are common findings and reflect the slow growth of these tumors.
- ► On MRI, they are typically hyperintense on T2-weighted images and show postcontrast enhancement. Enhancement is uniform or heterogeneous depending on the degree of cystic change.
- ► A target sign (central T2 hypointensity, peripheral T2 hyperintensity) and multiplicity of lesions are more common with neurofibromas.
- ► Malignant degeneration of spinal nerve sheath tumors, although rare, is characterized by rapid growth.

Management

- ► Symptomatic nerve sheath tumors are treated with surgical resection. In cases of malignant transformation, adjunctive radiation and chemotherapy may be employed.

Further Reading

Beall DP, Googe DJ, Emery RL, et al. Extramedullary intradural spinal tumors: a pictorial review. *Curr Prob Diagn Radiol.* 2007;36:185-198.

Pawha P, Sze G. Neoplastic disorders of the spine and spinal cord. In: Atlas S. Magnetic Resonance Imaging of the Brain and Spine, 4th ed. Philadelphia: Lippincott Williams, 2008:1538-1539.

History

▶ 10-year-old boy with hairy patch in lumbosacral region

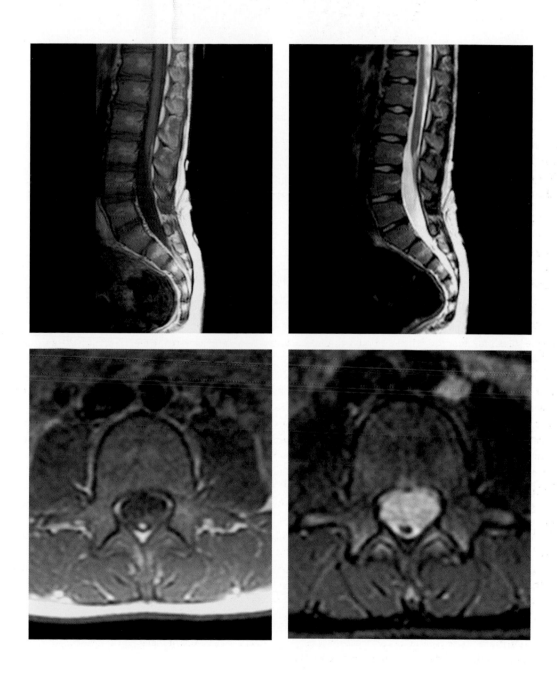

Case 118 Dorsal Dermal Sinus

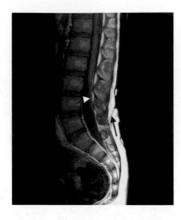 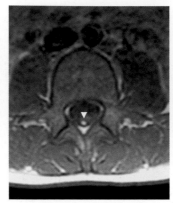

Findings

▶ The conus medullaris terminates at the level of the L3 vertebral body, lower than normal, consistent with tethered cord.

▶ A thin tract, hypointense to fat, extends through the subcutaneous tissues from the skin surface at L4 to the dorsal spinal column at L5 (black arrow).

▶ A fibrofatty stalk, hypointense on T2-weighted images and hyperintense on T1-weighted images (white arrowhead), extends from the conus medullaris to the dorsal spinal canal at the level of L5.

Differential Diagnosis

▶ Sacrococcygeal dimple

Teaching Points

▶ Dorsal dermal sinuses are epithelium-lined sinus tracts that extend from the skin surface for a variable distance. They result from focal incomplete disjunction of cutaneous from neural ectoderm. The tract may end in the subcutaneous fat or extend into the spinal canal. 50% to 70% terminate in the spinal canal.

▶ Sinus tracts that extend into the canal terminate on CNS structures that include the dura, spinal cord, conus, or filum terminale. 50% of dorsal dermal sinus tracts are associated with dermoids and epidermoid tumors. When present, the tracts frequently terminate on these lesions.

▶ Most dorsal dermal sinus tracts are located in the lumbosacral region (>50%). Presentation varies from early childhood to the third decade. Acute presentation is seen in the setting of infection, which includes meningitis and spinal abscesses. Patients may also present because of nerve root and/or spinal cord compression by a dermoid or epidermoid tumor.

▶ Osseous abnormalities vary from none to multilevel spinal dysraphism.

Management

▶ Excision of tract and cord untethering is performed when these lesions are symptomatic.

Further Reading

Barkovich AJ. Congenital anomalies of the spine. In: Barkovich AJ. Pediatric Neuroimaging, 4th ed. Philadelphia: Lippincott Williams & Wilkins, 2005:717-719.

Radmanesh F, Nejat F, El Khashab M. Dermal sinus tract of the spine. *Childs Nerv Syst.* 2010;26:349-357.

History

▶ 71-year-old woman with recurrent thoracolumbar pain on her right side

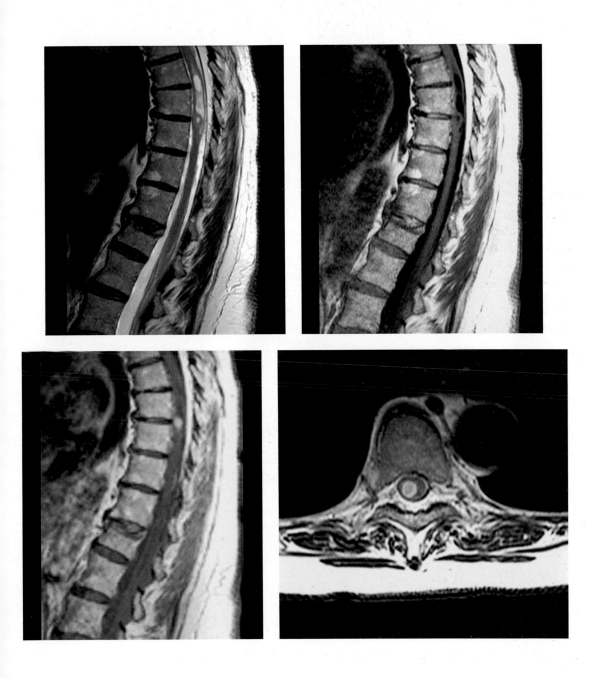

Case 119 Ependymoma

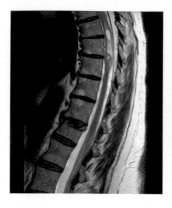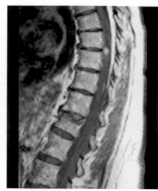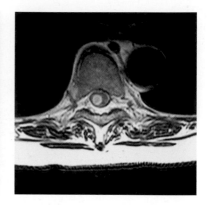

Findings

▶ A well-circumscribed cystic and solid intramedullary mass is present in the lower thoracic spine.

▶ The solid nodule homogenously enhances.

Differential Diagnosis

▶ Astrocytoma

▶ Hemangioblastoma

▶ Metastasis

Teaching Points

▶ Ependymomas are neoplasms arising from ependymal cells lining the central canal of the spinal cord. They are the most common primary tumor of the spinal cord in adults, closely followed by astrocytomas. In children astrocytomas are more common than ependymomas.

▶ Ependymomas of the spinal cord usually occur in the fourth and fifth decades, far older than intracranial ependymomas. The most common presenting symptom is back or neck pain.

▶ Ependymomas often have a heterogeneous appearance secondary to their predilection for hemorrhage and cyst formation. Typically, ependymomas are T1 hypointense and T2 hyperintense with irregular enhancement. Hemosiderin deposited around the margin of the tumor may give the tumor a T2-hypointense ring. Other findings include cord expansion with osseous remodeling, syrinx formation, and cord edema.

▶ It can be very difficult to distinguish ependymomas from astrocytomas on imaging, but there are several helpful criteria:

  ▪ Ependymomas arise from ependymal cells that line the central spinal canal. This accounts for the central location of ependymomas, in contrast to the typically eccentric position of astrocytomas.

  ▪ Hemorrhage and cyst formation make ependymomas more heterogeneous than astrocytomas.

  ▪ Classically, ependymomas are well-circumscribed, encapsulated tumors, in contrast to the infiltrative astrocytomas.

  ▪ Ependymomas are more commonly found in the lower cord.

Management

▶ Spinal ependymomas are treated by surgical resection. There is a 15% rate of recurrence. Postoperative MRI is important since only patients with residual or recurrent neoplasm receive adjuvant radiation therapy.

Further Reading

Pawha P, Sze G. Neoplastic disorders of the spine and spinal cord. In: Atlas S. *Magnetic Resonance Imaging of the Brain and Spine*, 4th ed. Philadelphia: Lippincott Williams, 2008:1547-1553.

Van Goethem JWM, van den Hauwe L, Ozsarlak O, et al. Spinal tumors. *Eur J Radiol.* 2004;50:159-176.

History

▶ 55-year-old man with right-sided sciatica

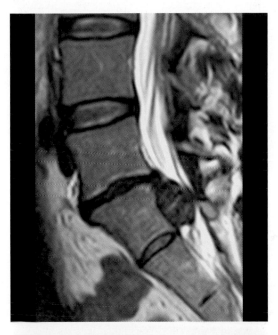

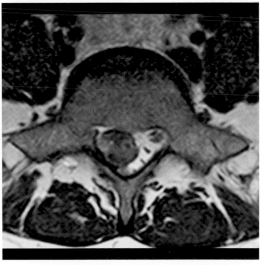

Case 120 Disc Extrusion

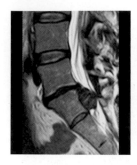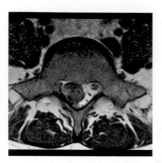

Findings

▶ Sagittal and axial T2-weighted images demonstrate a hypointense ventral epidural mass dorsal to the S1 vertebral body and eccentric to the right. It is continuous with the L5-S1 intervertebral disc.

▶ The mass deforms the thecal sac and displaces right-sided sacral nerve roots.

Differential Diagnosis

▶ Sequestered disc
▶ Disc protrusion
▶ Nerve sheath tumor

Teaching Points

▶ Disc herniation is the displacement of material from the nucleus pulposus through a tear or defect in the annulus fibrosus.

▶ The imaging definitions of disc pathology parallel but are different from those of surgical pathology. Standards for the description of disc pathology in the lumbar spine on MRI have been published (see below).

▶ Disc herniation is the localized (<50% of disc circumference) displacement of disc material beyond the confines of the disc space. A disc bulge is the displacement of disc material involving more than 50% of the disc circumference.

▶ Herniated discs continuous with the parent disc are focal or broad-based disc protrusions or extrusions. An extrusion is present if the width of disc material at its base measures less than its depth on axial images or if the material extends cranially or caudally beyond the disc on sagittal images.

▶ The herniated disc material is described as central, paracentral, foraminal, or extraforaminal depending on its location in the axial plane.

▶ A sequestered disc is an extrusion that has migrated and no longer has continuity with the parent disc.

▶ On MRI, herniated disc material may be iso-intense or hyperintense to the disc material within the disc space on T2-weighted images and is usually iso-intense on T1-weighted images.

▶ Enhancement is typically limited to the margins of the herniated disc material.

Management

▶ Imaging findings must be correlated with history and clinical examination. Many imaging abnormalities do not produce clinical symptoms.

▶ 90% of patients improve with conservative management (NSAIDs, rest, physical therapy).

▶ Surgery should be reserved for those who fail to respond to conservative management, have cauda equina syndrome, or have worsening neurologic deficits.

Further Reading

http://www.asnr.org/spine_nomenclature

Carvi y Nievas MN, Hoellerhage HG. Unusual sequestered disc fragments simulating spinal tumors and other space-occupying lesions. *J Neurosurg Spine.* 2009;11:42-48.

Millette PC, Fardon DL. Nomenclature and classification of lumbar disc pathology. *Spine.* 2001;26;E93-E113.

History

▶ 26-year-old man with low back pain

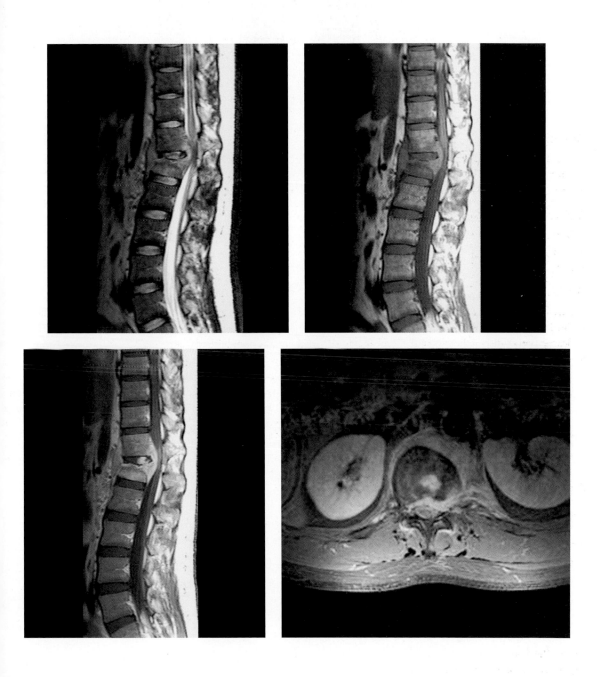

Case 121 Tuberculous Spondylitis

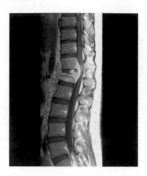

Findings

▶ MRI of the lumbar spine shows superior endplate compression deformity at L1. There is a soft tissue mass surrounding the T12 and L1 vertebral bodies and intervening disc space. It is hyperintense on T2-weighted images and enhances uniformly after contrast administration. The ventral epidural component displaces the thecal sac.
▶ The posterior aspect of the intervertebral disc contains enhancing material, but its involvement is less extensive than that of the vertebral bodies.

Differential Diagnosis

▶ Pyogenic spondylitis
▶ Metastatic neoplasm
▶ Lymphoma or myeloma

Teaching Points

▶ Tuberculous spondylitis occurs by hematogenous dissemination. It is most commonly found in the thoracic and lumbar spine.
▶ Signs and symptoms include back pain, fever, kyphosis, and neurologic deficits. The onset is insidious, with duration of symptoms ranging from months to years. This contrasts with the acute/subacute onset of pyogenic spondylitis.
▶ The initial site of infection is usually the anterior-inferior aspect of the vertebral body. The spread of infection occurs beneath the anterior longitudinal ligament to involve the adjacent vertebrae. The intervening disc space is relatively spared because *M. tuberculosis* lacks the proteolytic enzymes needed to penetrate the disc. Disc space narrowing is seen with collapse and destruction of the adjacent vertebrae, which allows disc material to herniate into the endplate.
▶ MRI is the imaging modality of choice. The classic imaging findings are contiguous vertebrae involvement with relative sparing of the intervening disc space, vertebral body destruction with a gibbus deformity, paraspinal abscess/phlegmon, and epidural involvement.
▶ The posterior elements are rarely involved, a feature that helps distinguish TB from metastasis.
▶ The relative lack of disc involvement helps distinguish TB from pyogenic spondylitis.

Management

▶ Treatment includes long-term anti-tuberculosis medication.
▶ When necessary, surgical decompression and instrumentation are used to treat vertebral collapse and neurologic complications.

Further Reading

Gouliamos AD, Kehagias DT, Lahanis S, et al. MR imaging of tuberculous vertebral osteomyelitis: pictorial review. *Eur Radiol.* 2001;11:575-579.
Mendonca R. Spinal infections and inflammatory disorders. In: Atlas S. *Magnetic Resonance Imaging of the Brain and Spine*, 4th ed. Philadelphia: Lippincott Williams, 2008:1702-1704.

History

▶ Newborn boy with intrauterine abnormalities noted on prenatal ultrasound

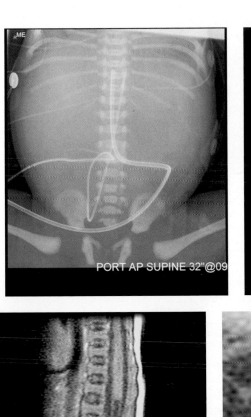

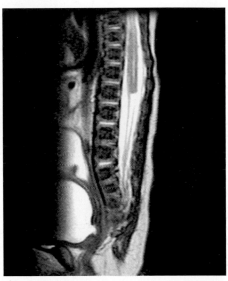

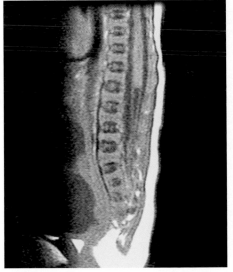

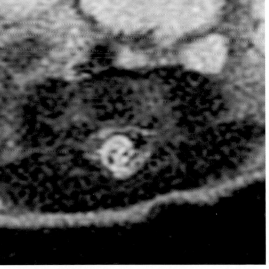

Case 122 Caudal Regression

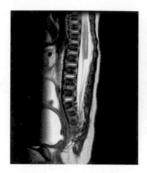

Findings

▶ AP radiograph demonstrates absence of the coccyx and fifth sacral element.

▶ On sagittal MRI sequences, the distal spinal cord has a blunted appearance and terminates at the mid-L2 level.

▶ The nerve roots of the cauda equina appear normal.

Differential Diagnosis

▶ Tethered spinal cord

Teaching Points

▶ Caudal regression syndrome is a spectrum of anomalies ranging from partial absence of the coccyx to complete lumbosacral agenesis. Most cases are sporadic, but 15% to 20% of infants with caudal regression syndrome have diabetic mothers.

▶ The severity of the osseous abnormalities correlates with the degree of distal spinal cord hypoplasia.

▶ Associated abnormalities include OEIS (omphalocele, cloacal exstrophy, imperforate anus, and spinal deformities) and VACTERL (vertebral anomalies, anorectal malformations, cardiac malformations, tracheoesophageal fistula, renal anomalies, and limb anomalies).

▶ Clinical presentation is highly variable depending on the degree of hypogenesis. Mild cases may have isolated deformities of the foot and minor lower extremity muscle weakness. Severe cases have fusion of the lower extremities (sirenomelia) with sensorimotor paralysis. Regardless of the severity, almost all patients have a neurogenic bladder. Spinal canal stenosis, if present, is most common at the level above the last intact vertebral body.

▶ Spinal cord tethering is most commonly found in milder cases of sacral hypogenesis. Termination of the spinal cord below L1 is highly correlated with sacral malformations below S1. Termination of the spinal cord above L1 is highly correlated with more severe sacral hypogenesis.

▶ Plain radiographs are helpful for diagnosing the osseous abnormalities.

▶ MRI demonstrates the spinal cord hypoplasia and associated spinal cord tethering if present. In more severe cases (where cord tethering is generally not found) the distal spinal cord has a characteristic "blunted" appearance.

▶ In very mild cases, only the tip of the conus may be absent, without cord tethering.

Management

▶ If symptomatic cord tethering is present, surgical untethering is performed.

▶ Laminectomy and duroplasty are performed for any associated spinal stenosis.

Further Reading

Barkovich AJ. Congenital anomalies of the spine. In: Barkovich AJ. *Pediatric Neuroimaging*, 4th ed. Philadelphia: Lippincott Williams & Wilkins, 2005:709-710, 735-738.

Pang D. Sacral agenesis and caudal spinal cord malformations. *Neurosurgery.* 1993;32:755-779.

History

► 12-year-old boy with back pain

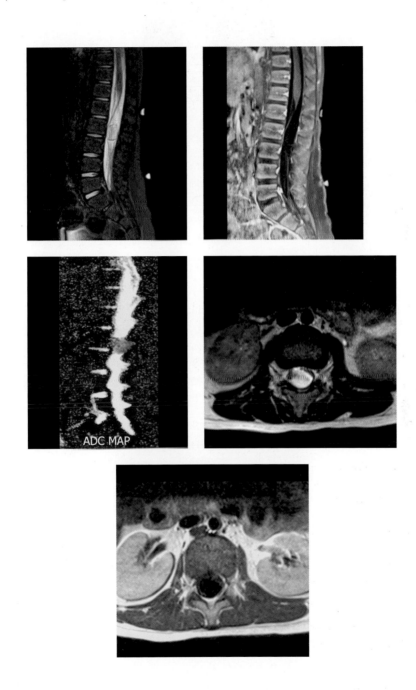

Case 123 Spinal Epidermoid Tumor

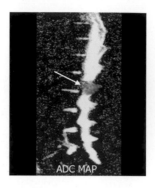

Findings

▶ A nonenhancing mass within the spinal canal at the level of L2 ventrally displaces the nerve roots of the cauda equina. It is largely iso-intense to CSF on T2-weighted and postcontrast T1-weighted images.

▶ The mass is hypointense to CSF on the ADC map (arrow).

Differential Diagnosis

▶ Dermoid tumor

▶ Arachnoid cyst

Teaching Points

▶ Epidermoid and dermoid tumors are benign spinal tumors derived from mesenchymal cells. Epidermoids are composed of only the epidermal elements of skin. Dermoids are composed of skin appendages, including hair follicles, sweat glands, and sebaceous glands. This composition influences their signal characteristics on MRI.

▶ Patients present with insidious myelopathy or, in the case of rupture, acute chemical meningitis. Dermoids usually present in childhood. Epidermoids tend to present later, in the third to fourth decade.

▶ Both tumors are well-circumscribed masses. Epidermoids closely follow CSF signal and may be difficult to detect on conventional MRI sequences. Dermoids that contain fat are conspicuous on T1 sequences, but this is an inconsistent finding. Commonly dermoids, like epidermoids, closely follow CSF signal.

▶ Both tumors are best diagnosed by identifying displacement of the spinal cord or nerve roots by a mass and by signal intensity that differs slightly from CSF. Similar to intracranial epidermoids, diffusion imaging helps distinguish spinal epidermoids from other "cystic"-appearing masses.

▶ Epidermoids are acquired 40% of the time, usually from iatrogenic implantation of epidermal cells during lumbar puncture. All spinal dermoids are congenital tumors arising from congenital dermal rests.

▶ 20% of dermoid and epidermoid tumors are associated with dermal sinuses. Dermoids are most commonly found in the lower spine, while epidermoids are fairly evenly distributed along the spine. Either lesion can be intra- or extramedullary.

Management

▶ Surgical excision. Recurrence, particularly of epidermoids, is a common problem.

Further Reading

Barkovich AJ. Congenital anomalies of the spine. In: Barkovich AJ. *Pediatric Neuroimaging*, 4th ed. Philadelphia: Lippincott Williams & Wilkins, 2005:757-758.

Kukreja K, Manzano G, Ragheb J, et al. Differentiation between spinal arachnoid and epidermoid-dermoid cysts: is diffusion-weighted MRI useful? *Pediatr Radiol.* 2007;37:556-560.

History

▶ 83-year-old woman with a 4-month history of worsening back pain not relieved by epidural steroid injections

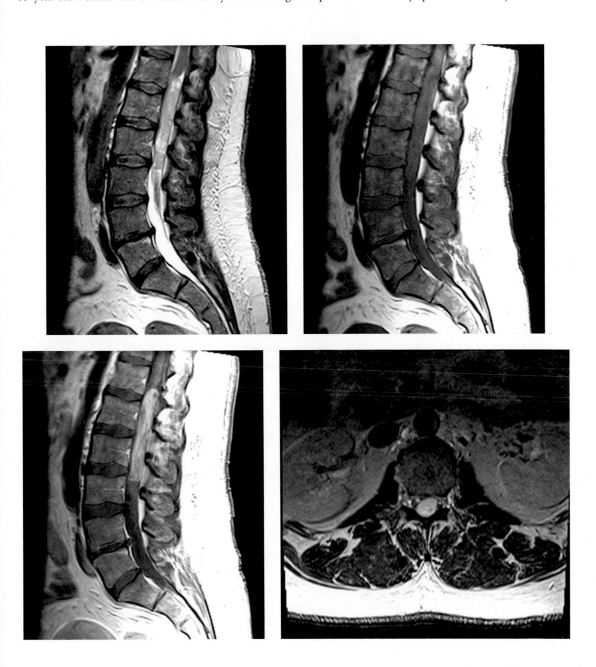

Case 124 Myxopapillary Ependymoma

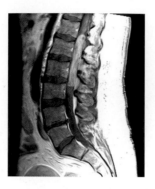

Findings

- ▶ A large ovoid mass fills and slightly expands the spinal canal just below the conus medullaris.
- ▶ The mass is largely hyperintense on T2-weighted images. There is a rim of T2 hypointensity about its margin.
- ▶ The mass enhances diffusely.

Differential Diagnosis

- ▶ Paraganglioma
- ▶ Nerve sheath tumor
- ▶ Meningioma
- ▶ Metastasis

Teaching Points

- ▶ Myxopapillary ependymomas of the filum terminale are distinct from the more common ependymomas found in the spinal cord. The myxopapillary subtype arises from ependymal cells of the filum terminale and is the most common tumor in this region.
- ▶ Myxopapillary ependymomas are well-circumscribed, soft, expansile masses. The tumor grows slowly and therefore is usually large at presentation (more than two vertebral body segments in length). The expanded spinal canal may be completely replaced by tumor.
- ▶ They most commonly present in the fourth decade but are reported over a broad range of ages. The most common presenting symptom is back pain.
- ▶ Radiographs and CT show osseous changes, including scalloping of the posterior vertebral bodies, widening of the interpedicular distance, and thinning of the pedicles and lamina.
- ▶ The myxopapillary subtype is the most likely ependymoma to hemorrhage. They can present as non-aneurysmal subarachnoid hemorrhage or as superficial siderosis of the brain stem and basilar cisterns. Hemosiderin (T2 hypointensity) at the margins of a filar tumor is characteristic of a myxopapillary ependymoma.
- ▶ Myxopapillary tumors are unique for their mucin production. Although most tumors are T1 hypointense, the protein content in mucin can result in T1 hyperintensity. If present, this is highly suggestive of the diagnosis.
- ▶ Other findings on MRI include intense enhancement after the administration of contrast and hyperintensity on T2-weighted images.

Management

- ▶ Surgical resection is usually curative.

Further Reading

Wippold FJ II, et al. MR imaging of myxopapillary ependymoma. *AJR Am J Roentgenol.* 1995;165:1263-1267.

History

▶ 44-year-old man with numbness and pain in the left foot and leg for 1 year

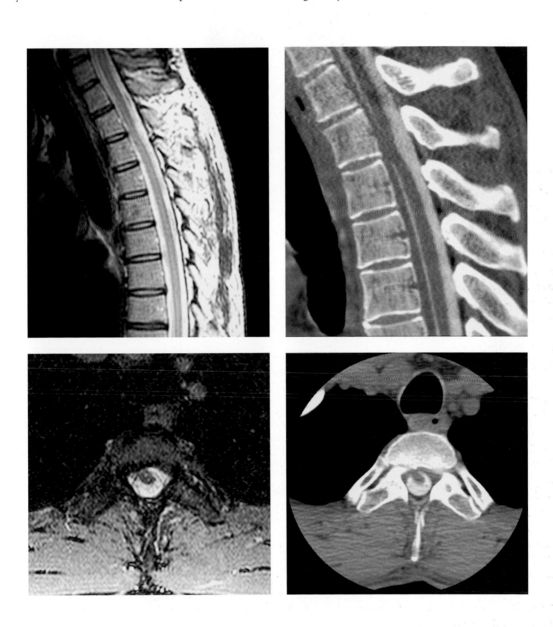

Case 125   Anterior Cord Herniation

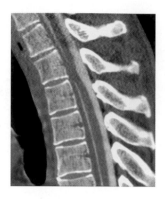

Findings

► Sagittal T2-weighted MRI and sagittal reconstructions from CT myelogram demonstrate focal anterior displacement of the spinal cord. The dorsal subarachnoid space is expanded.
► On axial T2-weighted images, the ventrally placed spinal cord is eccentric to the right and contacts the dura. Cord signal is normal.
► On CT myelogram there is no contrast anterior to the cord.

Differential Diagnosis

► Dorsal arachnoid cyst

Teaching Points

► Spinal cord herniation is a rare but increasingly recognized cause of myelopathy.
► It is the result of a ventral dural defect in the thoracic spine through which the spinal cord herniates. The etiology is controversial, with several hypotheses proposed, including congenital weakness of the ventral dura, dural injury secondary to disc herniations, and inflammatory processes.
► The herniated spinal cord becomes compromised as a result of adhesions, deformation, and vascular impairment.
► Middle-aged adults are most commonly affected and typically present with progressive lower limb sensorimotor deficits. In one series 75% presented with Brown-Séquard syndrome (decreased pain and temperature in one leg and motor weakness on the other side).
► The diagnosis is made by MRI and/or CT myelography. Typical imaging findings include:
  ▪ Focal cord kinking with anterior or anterolateral displacement
  ▪ Focal spinal cord thinning and enlargement of the dorsal subarachnoid space
► It may be difficult to differentiate spinal cord herniation from a dorsal intradural arachnoid cyst. In fact, they may coexist.
  ▪ On CT myelogram, a spinal cord herniation will have no contrast separating it from the ventral dura; a thin rim of contrast should be seen anterior to the cord with a dorsal arachnoid cyst.
  ▪ On phase-contrast cine MRI a normal CSF pulsatile pattern is observed within the dorsal subarachnoid space with spinal cord herniation. The pulsation is absent or attenuated with an arachnoid cyst.

Management

► Surgical reduction of the herniation with repair of the dural defect

Further Reading

Brugières P, Malapert D, Adle-Biassette H, et al. Idiopathic spinal cord herniation: value of MR phase-contrast imaging. *AJNR Am J Neuroradiol*. 1999;20:935-939.
Najjar MW, Baeesa SS, Lingawi SS. Idiopathic spinal cord herniation: a new theory of pathogenesis. *Surg Neurol*. 2004;62:161-171.

History

▶ 63-year-old woman with ataxia

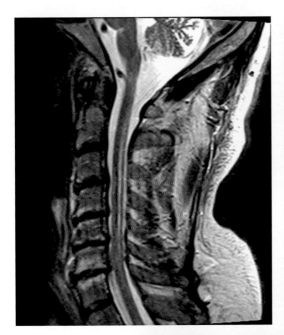
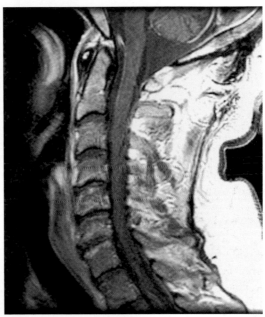
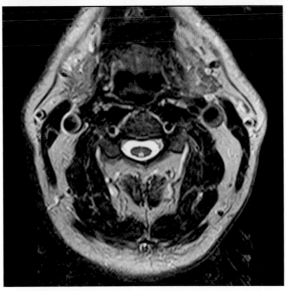

Case 126 Subacute Combined Degeneration (SCD)

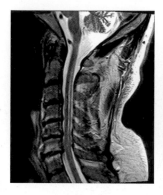 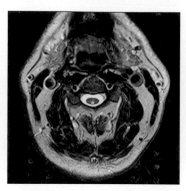

Findings

► There is hyperintense signal on T2-weighted MR images, limited to the posterior columns and extending from C2 to C7.
► There is no mass effect or enhancement on postcontrast T1-weighted images.
► On the axial T2-weighted images the signal has an inverted-V configuration.

Differential Diagnosis

► HIV myelitis
► Multiple sclerosis
► Cord ischemia
► Infectious myelitis

Teaching Points

► SCD results from vitamin B12 deficiency. There is accumulation of methylmalonic acid, which is toxic to myelin, causing demyelination of the posterior and lateral columns of the spinal cord.
► Pernicious anemia, the inability to absorb B12 because of intrinsic factor deficiency, is the most common cause of B12 deficiency in the United States. Dietary lack of B12 is rare. Another rare cause is nitrous oxide anesthesia or abuse; nitrous oxide can inactivate B12 in susceptible patients.
► Clinical presentation includes generalized weakness, paresthesias of the hands and feet, loss of position and vibratory sensation, and sensory ataxia.
► The cervical and upper thoracic portions of the spinal cord are most commonly affected.
► On MRI there is hyperintense signal on T2-weighted images in the dorsal cervical and thoracic cord. The abnormal signal in the dorsal columns frequently extends over multiple levels, which helps to distinguish SCD from other demyelinating diseases.
► Mild enhancement can be present.
► HIV myelitis can have an identical appearance.

Management

► Treatment of SCD from malabsorption consists of monthly lifetime injections of vitamin B12. When treated early, symptoms and imaging findings may resolve completely.

Further Reading

Ravina B, Loevner LA, Bank W. MR Findings in subacute combined degeneration of the spinal cord: a case of reversible cervical myelopathy. *AJR Am J Roentgenol.* 2000;174:863-865.
Thurner MM, Cartes-Zumelzu F, Mueller-Mang C. Demyelinating and infectious diseases of the spinal cord. *Neuroimaging Clin North Am.* 2007;17:37-55.

History

▶ 10-year-old boy with lower neck pain

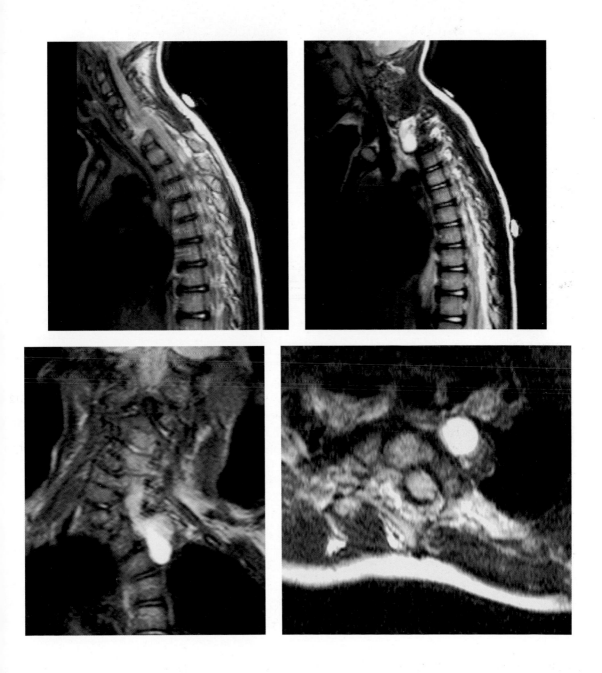

Case 127   Neuroenteric Cyst

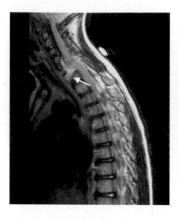 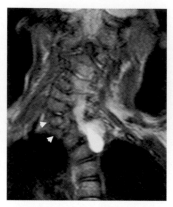

Findings

▶ Triplanar T2-weighted MR images demonstrate a cystic structure at the cervicothoracic junction. It is located in the prevertebral space.

▶ The lesion extends into the spinal canal through an osseous defect in the spine (arrow).

▶ There is marked focal scoliosis and anomalous vertebral body formation at the cervicothoracic junction (arrowheads).

Differential Diagnosis

▶ Arachnoid cyst

▶ Meningocele

Teaching Points

▶ Neuroenteric (or neurenteric) cysts are enteric-lined cysts found in the spinal canal that connect to the spinal cord or vertebrae. These rare congenital anomalies form when the notochord and foregut fail to separate.

▶ Clinical presentation is variable, ranging from asymptomatic to progressive myelopathy. Symptoms, when present, are usually insidious. Acute presentation can be seen in the setting of secondary infection.

▶ Most neuroenteric cysts are found at the cervicothoracic junction or about the conus medullaris. The vast majority are intradural-extramedullary in location and ventral to the cord.

▶ Associated vertebral anomalies, which include hemivertebrae, butterfly vertebrae, and spina bifida defects, are present in approximately 50% of patients. The spinal canal is commonly widened at the level of the cyst. The cysts may communicate with an extraspinal component through an associated vertebral anomaly.

▶ Relative to CSF, the cysts are iso- to hyperintense with T1 weighting and hypo- to iso-intense with T2 weighting. The signal variability depends on the protein content of the cysts.

▶ A neuroenteric cyst should always be considered in the differential diagnosis of a posterior mediastinal or abdominal cyst or intraspinal cystic mass seen in the setting of vertebral anomalies.

Management

▶ Complete surgical excision is curative in most cases.

Further Reading

Gao P, Osborn AG, Smirniotopoulos JG, et al. Neurenteric cysts: pathology, imaging spectrum, and differential diagnosis. *Int J Neuroradiol.* 1995;1:17-27.

History

► 52-year-old man with slowly progressive lower extremity weakness and paresthesias

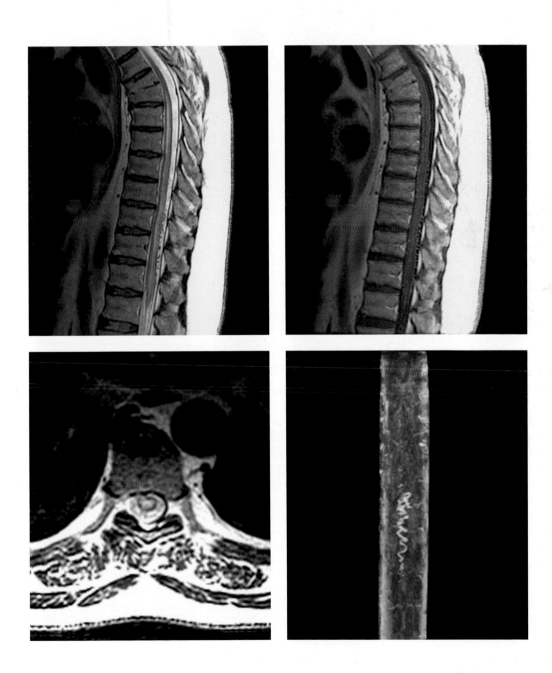

Case 128 Spinal Dural Arteriovenous Fistula

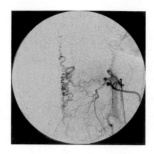

Findings

► T2-weighted MR images demonstrate extensive hyperintense intramedullary signal abnormality over a long segment of the thoracic spinal cord.

► Enlarged and serpiginous flow voids are present along the dorsal surface of the spinal cord.

► Contrast-enhanced MRA confirms the presence of dilated pial veins.

► Arterial-phase catheter angiography shows the dural arterial venous fistula with shunting into the pial venous system.

Differential Diagnosis

► Spinal cord astrocytoma

► Demyelination

► Spinal cord infarction

► Infectious myelitis

Teaching Points

► Spinal vascular malformations may be classified with the following scheme:
  ▪ Type I: spinal dural arteriovenous fistula (SDAVF)
  ▪ Type 2: glomus arteriovenous malformation (AVM) (resembles brain AVM)
  ▪ Type 3: juvenile AVM (a metameric lesion involving multiple tissues)
  ▪ Type 4: spinal cord pial arteriovenous fistula

► SDAVFs are thought to be acquired and usually the result of trauma. They account for 85% of spinal vascular malformations.

► Patients typically present with slowly progressive myelopathy.

► The fistula occurs within the dura of the nerve root sleeve, usually in the neural foramen. It connects to the pial veins along the spinal cord. The resultant venous hypertension produces cord edema.

► The fistula most commonly occurs in the thoracolumbar spine, but the cord edema, visible as central intramedullary T2 hyperintensity, may extend the full length of the cord.

► Prominent flow voids may be present along the dorsal aspect of the spinal cord on T2-weighted and postcontrast T1-weighted images.

► Dynamic contrast-enhanced MRA is often able to confirm the diagnosis by demonstrating the feeding artery and enlarged veins.

Management

► Spinal angiography is needed to confirm the diagnosis, establish the sites of fistulization, and identify any nearby arteries supplying the spinal cord (e.g., artery of Adamkiewicz).

► SDAVF is treated with transarterial embolization by liquid embolics or with surgical occlusion at the site of fistula. Complete treatment requires occlusion of the proximal aspect of the draining vein.

Further Reading

Anson J, Spetzler R. Classification of spinal arteriovenous malformations and implications for treatment. *BNI Q.* 1992;8:2-8.

Hurst R. Vascular disorders of the spine and spinal cord. In: Atlas S. *Magnetic Resonance Imaging of the Brain and Spine*, 4th ed. Philadelphia: Lippincott Williams, 2008:1628-1636.

History

► 13-year-old girl with headaches

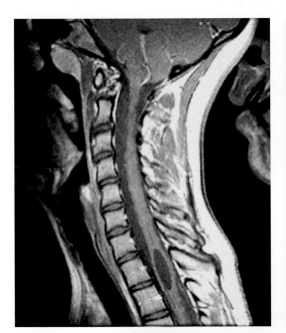
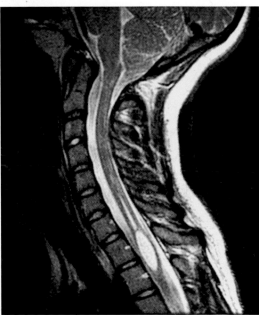
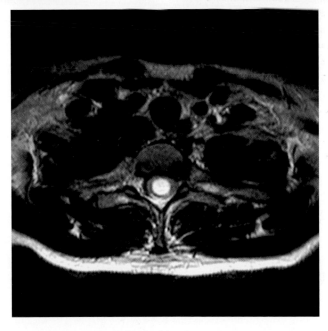

Case 129 Syringohydromyelia

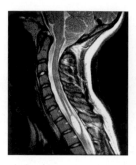

Findings

▶ T2-weighted and postcontrast T1-weighted MR images demonstrate an expansile intramedullary lesion of the lower cervical and upper thoracic spinal cord with signal characteristics similar to those of CSF.

▶ There is no abnormal enhancement.

▶ The cerebellar tonsils protrude through the foramen magnum and have a pointed configuration, consistent with a Chiari I malformation.

Differential Diagnosis

▶ Cystic intramedullary spinal cord neoplasm

Teaching Points

▶ Syringomyelia is a cystic spinal cord cavity separate from the central cord canal; it has no ependymal lining. Hydromyelia refers to cystic dilatation of the central canal with an ependymal lining. The imaging appearance of these entities is similar and can be termed syringohydromyelia. It is not clinically important to differentiate between the two entities, and the terms "syrinx" and "syringomyelia" are most commonly used to describe any simple cord cyst.

▶ Syringohydromyelia most commonly occurs in the setting of Chiari type 1 malformations. Other congenital causes include Klippel-Feil syndrome, tethered spinal cord, and myelomeningocele. Acquired causes include trauma, neoplasm, hemorrhage, and infection. 15% to 20% of cases are idiopathic.

▶ A syrinx can be asymptomatic and discovered incidentally on MRI. Symptoms, when present, are variable and include pain and temperature disturbances (in a cloak-like distribution), distal upper extremity weakness, severe pain, and spastic paraparesis.

▶ On MRI, syringohydromyelia has signal characteristics similar to CSF. The cyst can be septated or beaded, with variation in its size. Edema or gliosis may be present nearby. There is variable cord expansion.

▶ When an underlying etiology is present, no further imaging is needed. However, in the absence of a related congenital malformation, postcontrast imaging is recommended. Abnormal enhancement usually indicates the presence of a neoplastic or inflammatory process.

Management

▶ Treatment of the underlying process (Chiari decompression, cord untethering, surgical excision of tumor) will often result in resolution of the syringohydromyelia.

▶ In some cases direct surgical decompression of the cavity with fenestration or shunt placement is performed.

Further Reading

Barkovich AJ. Congenital anomalies of the spine. In: Barkovich AJ. *Pediatric Neuroimaging*, 4th ed. Philadelphia: Lippincott Williams & Wilkins, 2005:759-766.

Evans A, Stoodley N, Halpin S. Magnetic resonance imaging of intraspinal cystic lesions: a pictorial review. *Curr Probl Diagn Radiol.* 2002;21:79-94.

History

▶ 8-year-old with in-turning left foot and bladder dysfunction

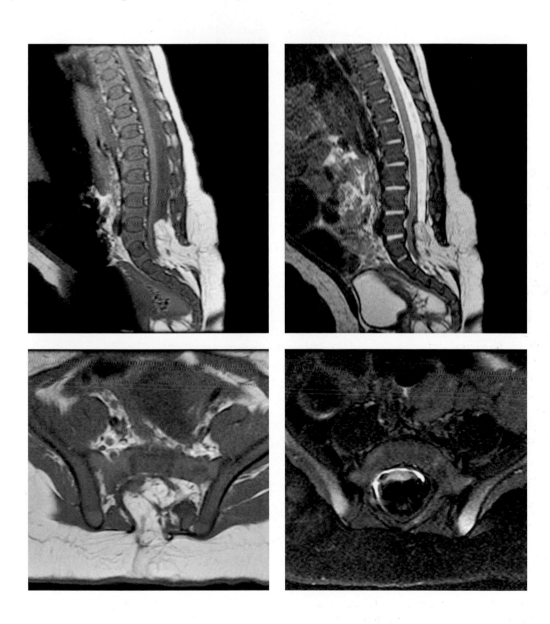

Case 130 Lipomyelocele

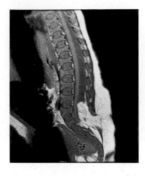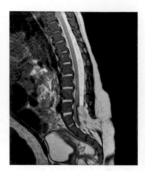

Findings

► Sagittal T1- and T2-weighted and axial T1-weighted images show a lobulated mass in the dorsal spinal canal with signal matching that of fat.
► The cauda equina has no clear termination, gradually thinning as it passes inferiorly and forming a neural placode.
► Axial T1-weighted images show a large dysraphic defect through which the lipoma is continuous with the subcutaneous fat.

Differential Diagnosis

► Intradural lipoma

Teaching Points

► Lipomyeloceles are part of a spectrum of disorders classified as spinal dysraphism or neural tube defects. The spectrum of spinal lipomas includes intradural lipomas, lipomyeloceles, and lipomyelomeningoceles.
► Intradural lipomas are juxtamedullary masses enclosed within an intact dural sac. They often lie dorsal to the cord and may expand the spinal canal. Two thirds occur in the cervical and thoracic spine.
► Both lipomyeloceles and lipomyelomeningoceles usually occur in the lumbosacral region. They are lipomas that attach to and tether a mass of dysplastic neural tissue (neural placode). The lipoma extends through an osseous defect in the dorsal spine.
► Lipomyeloceles have a normal-sized subarachnoid space. The meninges and neural elements are contained within the canal.
► Lipomyelomeningoceles have an expanded subarachnoid space with dorsal displacement of the placode and meninges through the site of spinal dysraphism.
► Approximately 50% of patients have butterfly vertebrae, segmentation anomalies, and sacral abnormalities. 5% to 10% have anorectal and GU abnormalities.
► When a mass is present, patients with lipomyeloceles and lipomyelomeningoceles are diagnosed within 6 months of age. Without a lumbosacral mass, patients present later, typically with neurologic or urologic symptoms during childhood.

Management

► Surgical untethering of the spinal cord

Further Reading

Barkovich AJ. Congenital anomalies of the spine. In Barkovich AJ. *Pediatric Neuroimaging*, 4th ed. Philadelphia: Lippincott Williams & Wilkins, 2005:724-731.
Rossi A, Biancheri R, Cama A, et al. Imaging in spine and spinal cord malformations. *Eur J Radiol.* 2004;50:177-200.

History

▶ 81-year-old woman who fell down three steps

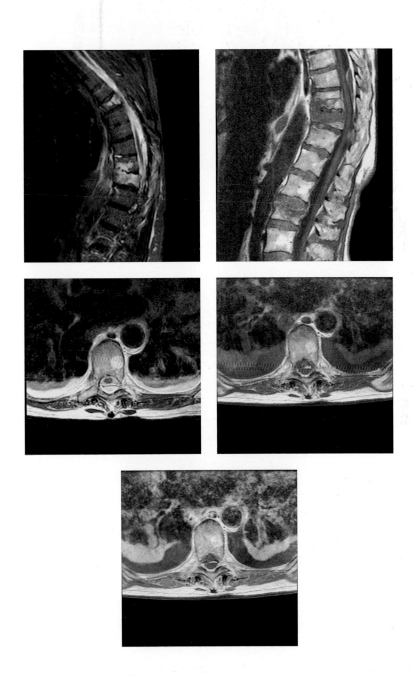

Case 131 Spinal Epidural Hematoma

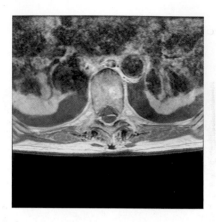

Findings

▸ There are compression fractures with height loss, wedge deformity, and marrow edema in several thoracic and lumbar vertebrae.

▸ In the lower thoracic spine, there is a dorsal epidural mass displacing the spinal cord anteriorly. It is hyperintense on T2-weighted images and hypointense on T1-weighted images, and shows no contrast enhancement.

Differential Diagnosis

▸ Epidural abscess
▸ Epidural neoplasm

Teaching Points

▸ Spinal epidural hemorrhages usually occur in the setting of trauma, recent instrumentation, vascular malformation, or anticoagulation. They may occur spontaneously. Lumbar punctures and spinal anesthesia are the most common procedures implicated in spinal epidural hematomas. Spontaneous epidural hematomas are usually of venous origin.

▸ Spinal epidural hematomas most commonly lie within the dorsal epidural space.

▸ MRI is the imaging modality of choice and will show an extramedullary mass displacing or encasing the cord. Compression of the epidural fat, thecal sac, and spinal cord is a common finding.

▸ The signal characteristics of the blood vary depending on its age.

▪ In the acute phase the blood is typically iso- to hypointense on T1-weighted images and heterogeneously hyperintense on T2-weighted images. These findings are nonspecific, which can make hematoma difficult to distinguish from other conditions in cases of complicated clinical history.

▪ Gradient-echo sequences may help by showing susceptibility-related signal loss in the hematoma.

▪ In the subacute period the blood becomes hyperintense on T1-weighted images, making the diagnosis more straightforward.

▪ In the chronic phase, enhancing granulation tissue can be seen.

Management

▸ Small hematomas may require only medical management, including treatment of any bleeding disorder. In the setting of symptomatic cord or nerve root compression, urgent surgical evacuation is necessary.

Further Reading

Fukui MB, Swarnkar AS, Williams RL. Acute spontaneous spinal epidural hematomas. *AJNR Am J Neuroradiol.* 1999;20:1365-1372.
Holta S, Heiling M, Lonntoft M. Spontaneous spinal epidural hematoma. Findings at MR imaging and clinical correlation. *Radiology.* 1996;199:409-433.

History

▸ 10-year-old girl with neurogenic bladder

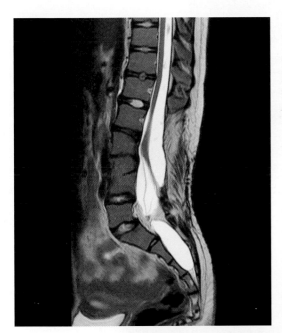
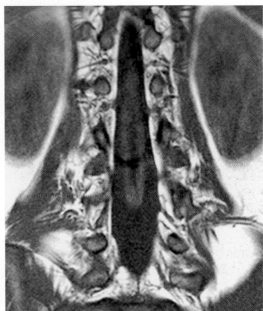
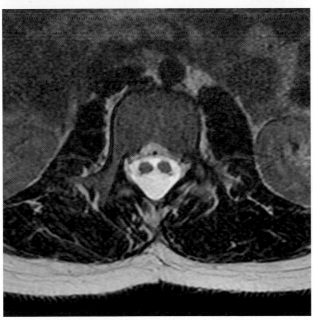

Case 132 Diastematomyelia

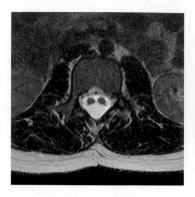

Findings

- There is a complex segmentation anomaly in the lumbar spine with fusion of L2, L3, and L4.
- On sagittal T2-weighted images, the spinal cord appears dysmorphic. It appears thin and has a gradually tapered configuration with the conus tip at L4. It appears bowed anteriorly and merges with the dorsal dura.
- Coronal and axial sequences demonstrate two equally sized hemicords.
- An intrasacral meningocele is present.

Differential Diagnosis

- Arachnoiditis

Teaching Points

- Diastematomyelia refers to a sagittal clefting of the spinal cord and/or conus medullaris into two symmetric or asymmetric hemicords. Each hemicord contains a central canal and a dorsal and ventral horn. The hemicords usually unite above and below the cleft. The clefting can be complete or incomplete.
- Diastematomyelia is most common in the lumbar spine and occurs much more frequently in females. Cutaneous lesions (nevi, hairy patch, dimples) overlie the spinal abnormality in most cases.
- Diastematomyelia is classified on the basis of the dura:
  - Type I: Two distinct dural sacs. Usually a bony or cartilaginous spur is present at the inferior aspect of the cleft. These patients are almost always symptomatic.
  - Type II: Single dural sac. A fibrous spur is often present, but there is no cartilaginous or bony spur. These patients are frequently asymptomatic.
- Common presenting complaints include bladder and bowel incontinence, clubfoot deformity with ipsilateral weakness, and scoliosis (especially in older children). 75% of patients have an associated tethered cord.
- Other associated abnormalities include myelomeningoceles, lipomas, dermoid or epidermoid tumors, vertebral body fusion abnormalities, and kyphoscoliosis.
- MRI is the imaging modality of choice. CT myelogram may be preferred in severely scoliotic patients.

Management

- Symptomatic patients are treated with surgical removal or bony, cartilaginous, or fibrous spur and untethering of the spinal cord.

Further Reading

Barkovich AJ. Congenital anomalies of the spine. In: Barkovich AJ. *Pediatric Neuroimaging*, 4th ed. Philadelphia: Lippincott Williams & Wilkins, 2005:744-752.
Rossi A, Biancheri R, Cama A, et al. Imaging in spine and spinal cord malformations. *Eur J Radiol*. 2004;50:177-200.

History

▸ 71-year-old woman with worsening back pain and lower extremity weakness. She is 4 months status post evacuation of lumbar intradural hematoma after traumatic lumbar puncture

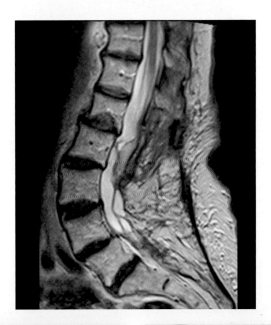

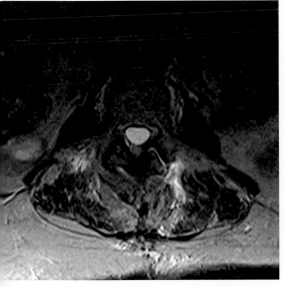

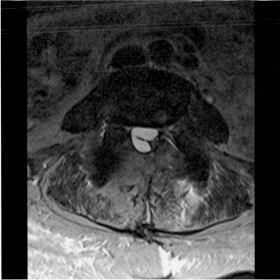

Case 133 Arachnoiditis

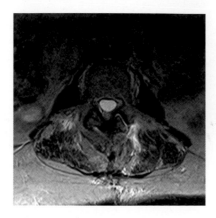

Findings

- ► T2-weighted MRI images show an abnormal thecal sac. The nerve roots of the cauda equina are positioned posteriorly and adherent to the posterior dura.
- ► Low-signal bands, representing adhesions, course through the thecal sac and create intradural cysts.

Differential Diagnosis

- ► Intradural mass (myxopapillary ependymoma, metastases)
- ► Spinal stenosis with apparent nerve-root clumping

Teaching Points

- ► Arachnoiditis is chronic inflammation of all three meningeal layers and the nerve roots. It may be local or diffuse, with the diffuse form being more severe and progressive.
- ► The most common cause of arachnoiditis is prior lumbar surgery. Other causes include intradural injections (steroids contrast agents, anesthetic agents), subarachnoid hemorrhage, trauma, and meningitis (rarely in the antibiotic era). Nonionic contrast agents are much less likely to cause arachnoiditis than lipid-based or ionic agents.
- ► Patients typically present with low back pain and weakness and sensory loss in the lower extremities. The symptoms of focal arachnoiditis typically affect a specific nerve root.
- ► MRI or CT myelography is the imaging study of choice. Contrast enhancement is not helpful in the diagnosis.
- ► The most common patterns are (a) peripheral adherent nerve roots with an empty central thecal sac and (b) centrally placed and clumped nerve roots.
- ► The clumped nerve roots can simulate a soft tissue mass. Cysts and loculations created by adhesions may also be present. Occasionally, syringomyelia results as a complication.

Management

- ► The management of arachnoiditis is difficult. Treatment is usually aimed at control of pain in a manner similar to other types of chronic pain, and may include analgesics, steroids, and electrical stimulation.

Further Reading

Mendonca R. Spinal infection and inflammatory disorders. In: Atlas S. *Magnetic Resonance Imaging of the Brain and Spine*, 4th ed. Philadelphia: Lippincott Williams, 2008:1671-1674.

Part 3   **Ear, Nose, and Throat**

History

▶ 58-year-old with acute breathing difficulty

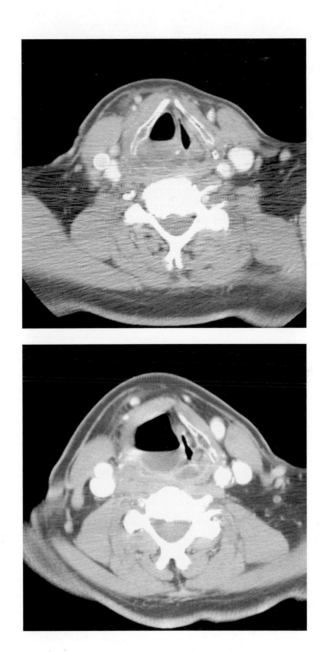

Case 134 Laryngocele, Infected (Pyolaryngocele)

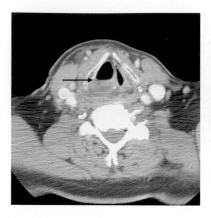 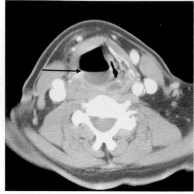

Findings

▶ There is a lesion in the right paraglottic space that contains a fluid–fluid level (arrow).
▶ The laryngeal airway is displaced to the left and narrowed.

Differential Diagnosis

▶ Saccule (ventricular appendix)
▶ Thyroglossal duct cyst
▶ Cystic neoplasm (e.g., squamous cell carcinoma)

Teaching Points

▶ Laryngoceles are air- or fluid-filled structures in the paraglottic space that communicate with the laryngeal ventricle.
▶ They are most commonly internal, being confined to the larynx. External laryngoceles extend through the thyrohyoid membrane to the anterior neck.
▶ Fifteen percent of laryngoceles are secondary laryngoceles, resulting from an obstructing lesion in the laryngeal ventricle. For this reason, patients with laryngoceles warrant endoscopic evaluation of the larynx to exclude an occult neoplasm.
▶ The normal saccule (ventricular appendix) can be visualized in some patients. These are termed laryngoceles only when they are large enough to distort the normal submucosal anatomy.
▶ When a laryngocele becomes infected, it is termed a pyolaryngocele. These lesions can cause life-threatening airway compromise.

Management

▶ When a laryngocele is identified, endoscopy is indicated to evaluate for an obstructing lesion in the laryngeal ventricle.
▶ If asymptomatic, laryngoceles do not need specific treatment. When symptomatic, surgical removal is curative.

Further Reading

Curtin HD. The larynx. In: Som PM, Curtin HD. *Head and Neck Imaging*, 4th ed. Philadelphia: Mosby, 2003:1652-1654.

History

▶ Patient presenting with three days of pain, redness, and slight swelling in the right eye

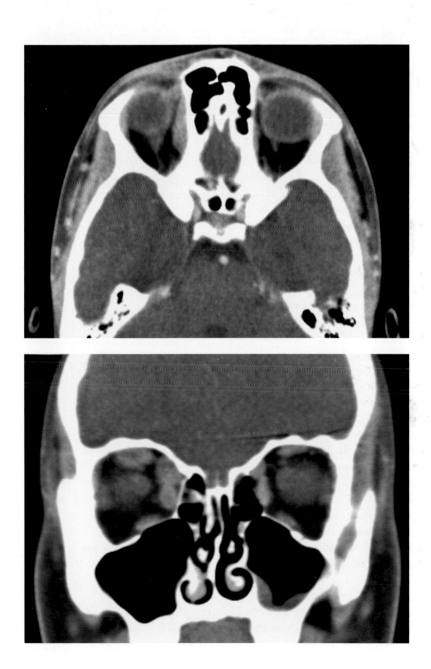

Case 135 Idiopathic Inflammatory Orbital Disease (Orbital Pseudotumor)

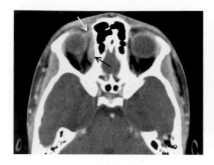 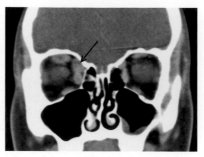

Findings

▶ There is enlargement and thickening of the superior oblique muscle (black arrow), including its tendon (white arrow), the superior rectus muscle, and the medial rectus muscle on the right side.

▶ There is no ethmoid or right maxillary sinus disease. There is no orbital abscess or fluid collection.

Differential Diagnosis

▶ Dysthyroid orbitopathy (Graves ophthalmopathy)
▶ Orbital infection
▶ Lymphoproliferative disorders, including lymphoma
▶ Other inflammatory disorders, such as Wegener's granulomatosis or sarcoidosis

Teaching Points

▶ Orbital pseudotumor is an idiopathic inflammatory process involving the orbit, due to infiltration of inflammatory cells.
▶ The most common presentation is acute or subacute orbital pain, often worse with ocular motion. Other symptoms include swelling, redness, proptosis, limited eye motion, and diplopia. Decreased vision can occur.
▶ It is bilateral in 25% of cases.
▶ It can involve any component of the orbit. Involvement of extraocular muscles or the lacrimal gland is most common. It may also cause thickening of the sclera and involve the retro-orbital fat. It may present as a focal or infiltrative orbital mass, and mimic tumors or aggressive infection. Bony erosion is very uncommon. Sometimes it is a diagnosis of exclusion.
▶ If there is intracranial involvement in the cavernous sinus and orbital apex (Tolosa-Hunt syndrome), cranial nerve palsies may result.
▶ Dysthyroid orbitopathy (Graves ophthalmopathy) is another cause of extraocular muscle enlargement. Involvement is often bilateral and most cases are painless. The enlargement of extraocular muscles predominantly involves the muscle belly and spares the tendons. Most patients have hyperthyroidism.
▶ Orbital infections may mimic orbital pseudotumor but are often associated with adjacent sinusitis or have a history of orbital trauma or surgery. They may include subperiosteal or orbital abscess.

Management

▶ Systemic corticosteroids and occasionally intraorbital steroid injections are used for treatment. In refractory cases, immunosuppressive chemotherapy or radiotherapy has been used. The disease may recur after cessation of treatment.

Further Reading

Gordon LK. Orbital inflammatory disease: a diagnostic and therapeutic challenge. *Eye (Lond).* 2006;20:1196-1206.
Weber AL, Romo LV, Sabates NR. Pseudotumor of the orbit. Clinical, pathologic, and radiologic evaluation. *Radiol Clin North Am.* 1999;37:151-168.

History

▶ 69-year-old man with severe blurry vision after blunt facial trauma

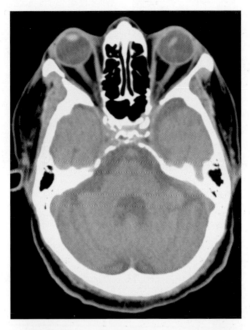

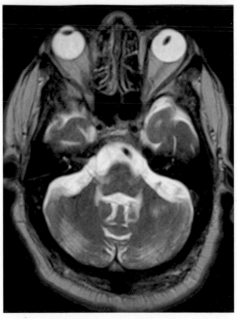

Case 136   Dislocation of the Lens

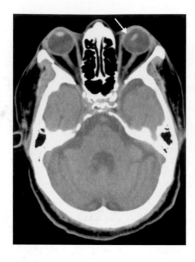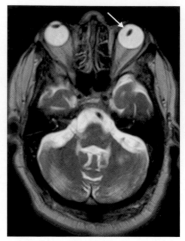

Findings

▶ Axial CT and T2-weighted MRI images show posterior dislocation of the left ocular lens (arrow).

Differential Diagnosis

▶ Traumatic lens dislocation
▶ Connective tissue disorders such as Marfan syndrome, Ehlers-Danlos syndrome, homocystinuria, and hyperlysinuria
▶ Hereditary ectopia lentis

Teaching Points

▶ Penetrating and blunt traumatic forces can cause deformity of the globe with partial or complete rupture of the zonular attachments of the lens, with resultant dislocation.
▶ Trauma is the most common cause of lens dislocation, but not all lens dislocations are traumatic. Connective tissue disorders can manifest as lens dislocation. It is estimated that 80% of Marfan syndrome patients will develop lens dislocation. Suspicion of a nontraumatic etiology should be high in cases of bilateral dislocation.
▶ Blurry vision and diplopia are the most common manifestations. Angle-closure glaucoma and corneal injury can ensue, especially with anterior dislocation. Sometimes the dislocated lens will induce inflammation in the vitreous, with risk of retinal damage.
▶ Posterior dislocation of the lens is much more common. Anterior dislocation is uncommonly seen, in which case the depth of the anterior chamber will be shallow on cross-sectional imaging.
▶ In all cases of orbital trauma, including those with lens dislocation, look carefully for intraocular foreign bodies. MRI is contraindicated in cases of intraocular metallic foreign body.

Management

▶ The lens is surgically extracted in some but not all cases. However, if inflammation occurs, the lens is extracted along with vitrectomy.

Further Reading

Kubal WS. Imaging of orbital trauma. *Radiographics.* 2008;28:1729-1739.
Tonini M, Krainik A, Bessou P, et al. How helical CT helps the surgeon in oculo-orbital trauma. *J Neuroradiol.* 2009;36:185-198.

History

▶ 64-year-old man with diplopia and headaches

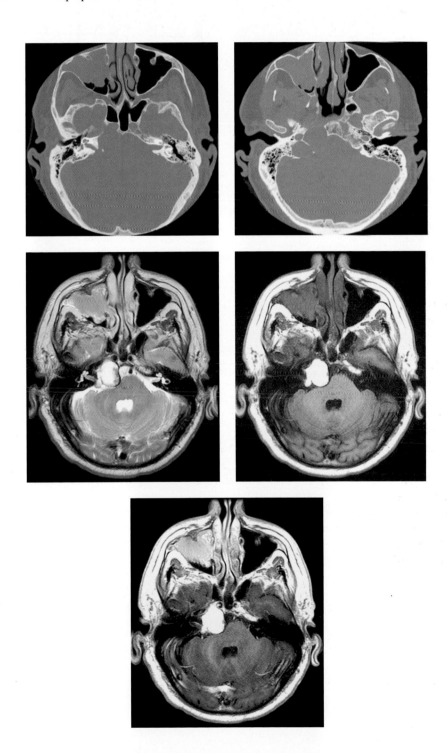

Case 137 Cholesterol Granuloma

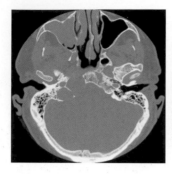 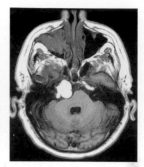

Findings

▶ There is an expansile lesion in the right petrous apex.
▶ There is thinning and remodeling of the bone, with a sharp zone of transition and sclerotic margin.
▶ On MRI the lesion demonstrates fairly homogeneous hyperintense signal on T1-weighted images and no enhancement.
▶ The opacified right maxillary sinus is incidental.

Differential Diagnosis

▶ Congenital cholesteatoma
▶ Trapped proteinaceous fluid in petrous air cell
▶ Mucocele of petrous air cell
▶ Metastasis
▶ Multiple myeloma

Teaching Points

▶ Cholesterol granulomas are slow-growing lesions that result from a chronic inflammatory reaction to cholesterol crystals in the mastoid or middle ear.
▶ The cause of cholesterol granulomas remains a subject of debate. Theories include negative pressure in mastoid air cells causing epithelial hemorrhage, with reaction to blood breakdown causing the chronic inflammation, as well as exposure of marrow spaces in the petrous apex leading to hemorrhage.
▶ Headache, tinnitus, hearing loss, and cranial neuropathies are usual presenting symptoms. Cholesterol granulomas can also be incidentally discovered on imaging studies.
▶ On CT they appear as a well-defined, expansile mass in the petrous apex. Overlying bone may be paper-thin and there is a lack of normal bone trabeculae. They typically lack features of aggressive bone destruction.
▶ On MR imaging, cholesterol granulomas are hyperintense on both T1- and T2-weighted images. A rim of signal loss in the lesion (secondary to hemosiderin) is common.

Management

▶ Treatment of cholesterol granulomas is surgical, with the goal of connecting the obstructed mastoid air cells with the pneumatized portions of the mastoid. In asymptomatic patients with little expansion of the bone, following the lesion with CT or MRI may be appropriate.

Further Reading

Glastonbury CM. The vestibulocochlear nerve, with an emphasis on the normal and diseased internal auditory canal and cerebellopontine angle. In: Swartz JD, Loevner LA. *Imaging of the Temporal Bone*, 4th ed. New York: Thieme, 2009:528-532 .

Mosnier I, Cyna-Gorse F, Grayeli AB, et al. Management of cholesterol granulomas of the petrous apex based on clinical and radiologic evaluation. *Otology Neurotology.* 2002;23:522-528.

History

▶ 45-year-old with facial swelling, pain, and fever

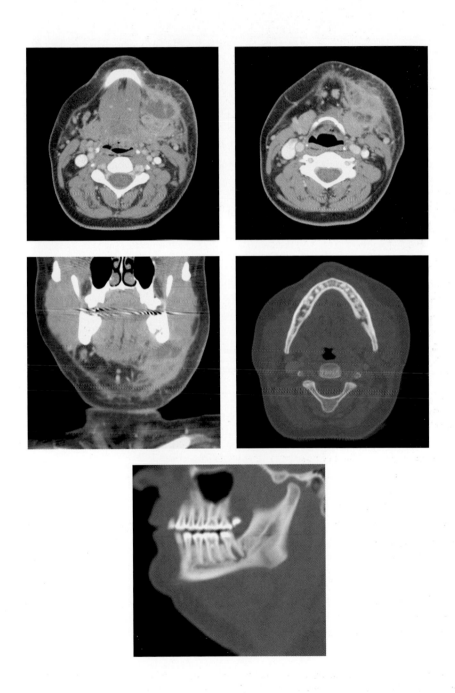

Case 138 Submandibular Abscess

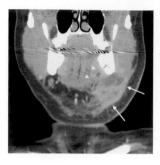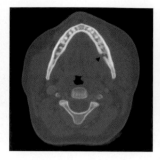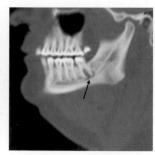

Findings

▶ There is a well-defined, rim-enhancing, low-attenuation collection in the left submandibular space.
▶ There are secondary inflammatory changes, including stranding in the adjacent fat and thickening of the platysma (white arrows).
▶ There is lucency surrounding the roots of the second left mandibular molar (black arrow) with breakthrough of the medial cortex (black arrowhead).
▶ Note the mylohyoid (white arrowheads) on the coronal images, which separates the sublingual and submandibular spaces. The site of cortical breakthrough lies below the insertion of this muscle on the mandible.

Differential Diagnosis

▶ Ranula, infected
▶ Lymphangioma
▶ Submandibular gland neoplasm

Teaching Points

▶ Inflammatory disease involving the submandibular space and/or sublingual space is most commonly the result of spread of infection from dental disease. Other etiologies include secondary infection from penetrating trauma, submandibular gland obstruction, or suppurative adenitis of submandibular lymph nodes. Up to 20% of cases have no identifiable etiology.
▶ Careful evaluation of the mandible and teeth helps identify the source. Early in the disease, the region of cortical disruption in the mandible can be very small and the adjacent subperiosteal abscess can be subtle.
▶ Coronal images are helpful in identifying small abscesses and in determining the location of the infection. Sublingual space infections lie above the attachment of the mylohyoid muscle to the mandible, whereas submandibular infections are below.
▶ The canines, premolars, and first molars have their roots above the mylohyoid insertion, so infections from these teeth tend to affect the sublingual space. The second and third molars have the tips of the roots inferior to the mylohyoid insertion, making extension into the submandibular space the more common route of spread.
▶ Infections can involve both submandibular and sublingual spaces as well, and it is important to remember that they communicate over the posterior free edge of the mylohyoid.

Management

▶ Management includes antibiotics as well as abscess drainage.
▶ Small subperiosteal abscesses can be drained with tooth extraction or root canal, whereas larger abscesses usually need surgical drainage.

Further Reading

Smoker WK. The oral cavity. In: Som PM, Curtin HD. *Head and Neck Imaging*, 4th ed. Philadelphia: Mosby, 2003:1398-1403.

History

▶ 20-year-old man with hearing loss after a motor vehicle collision

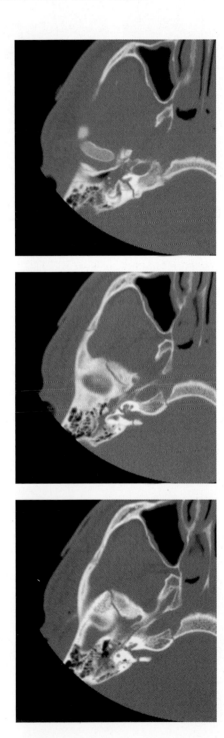

Case 139 Temporal Bone Fracture, Transverse

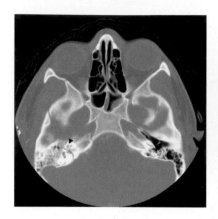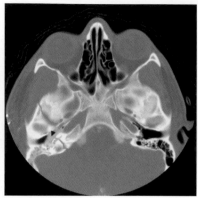

Findings

▶ There is a transverse fracture of the right temporal bone. The fracture extends through the internal auditory canal and otic capsule, coursing through the basal turn of the cochlea.

▶ The patient developed a CSF leak, and subsequent CT cisternography demonstrates high-density contrast extending from the IAC into the cochlea and middle ear (arrowheads).

Differential Diagnosis

▶ Longitudinal temporal bone fracture

Teaching Points

▶ Traditionally, temporal bone fractures are classified as longitudinal, transverse, or mixed. Longitudinal fractures are the most common, with transverse fractures the least common, occurring in 5% to 20% of cases.

▶ Transverse temporal bone fractures that involve the otic capsule have a high incidence of sensorineural hearing loss.

▶ Facial nerve paresis occurs in about 50% of transverse temporal bone fractures and 20% of longitudinal fractures. Paresis can be immediate or, more commonly, delayed.

▶ CSF leak occurs in approximately 15% of temporal bone fractures. Most commonly, the site of the leak is the tegmen tympani or mastoid.

Management

▶ CSF leaks need to be surgically repaired if they persist for greater than 2 weeks or if the leak is a delayed leak to prevent meningitis, which is the major complication.

▶ Patients with early, severe facial paresis likely benefit from early surgical intervention to decompress the nerve, or if it is severed, to perform a sural nerve autograft.

Further Reading

Wang EY, Shatzkes D, Swartz JD. Temporal bone trauma. In: Swartz JD, Loevner LA. *Imaging of the Temporal Bone*, 4th ed. New York: Thieme, 2009:416-440.

History

▶ 54-year-old Chinese man with nasal obstruction and ear pain

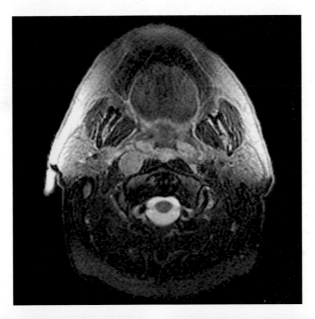

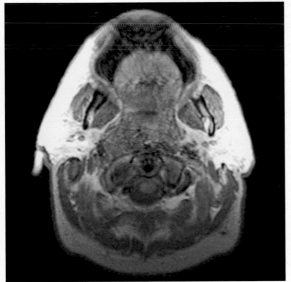

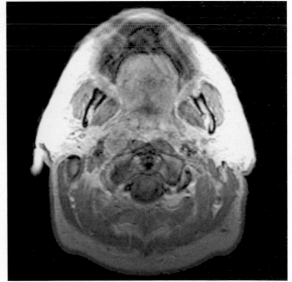

Case 140   Nasopharyngeal Carcinoma (NPC)

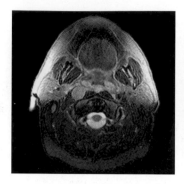
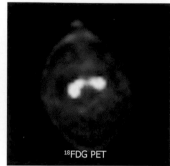

Findings

► There is bulky abnormal nasopharyngeal tissue crossing the midline. It is hyperintense to muscle on T2-weighted images and hypointense on T1-weighted images, and it enhances.

► There is a discrete round mass in the right retropharynx, consistent with an enlarged node of Rouvier.

► The PET study shows avid ^{18}fluorodeoxyglucose uptake.

Differential Diagnosis

► Lymphoma

► For extensive masses, other skull base malignancies may produce a similar appearance.

Teaching Points

► NPC is a rare malignant squamous cell neoplasm arising from the epithelium of the nasopharynx. It represents 95% of nasopharyngeal malignancies in adults.

► NPC is uncommon in the United States but common in southeast China. This neoplasm has been linked to Epstein-Barr virus infection and salt-preserved food.

► Common presenting symptoms include neck mass, epistaxis, and hearing loss. The mass may obstruct the eustachian tube, and attention should be focused on the nasopharynx in any adult with serous otitis media.

► MRI is generally preferred over CT since it provides better evaluation of local spread.

► On MRI the neoplasm is usually slightly hypoenhancing and relatively hypointense on T2-weighted images when compared to normal mucosa.

► Local spread, especially to regional lymph nodes, is common at the time of presentation. Lymphatic spread usually occurs first to retropharyngeal lymph nodes.

► Imaging features of importance for primary tumor staging are:
  ▪ Extension to the oropharynx
  ▪ Extension through pharyngobasilar fascia into the parapharyngeal space
  ▪ Bone invasion (clivus, vertebrae, or paranasal sinuses)
  ▪ Extension to cranial nerves, skull base, orbit, masticator space, infratemporal fossa, or hypopharynx

Management

► ^{18}FDG PET with CT is recommended for patients with any form of regional spread in order to identify metastases.

► Radiation therapy +/- chemotherapy is the treatment of choice for NPC.

Further Reading

Glastonbury CM. Nasopharyngeal carcinoma: the role of magnetic resonance imaging in diagnosis, staging, treatment, and follow-up. *Top Magn Reson Imag.* 2007;18;225-235.

History

▶ 53-year-old woman with bilateral mixed hearing loss

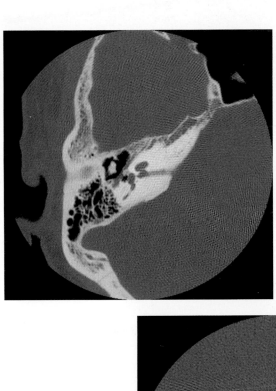
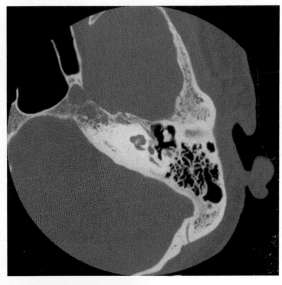
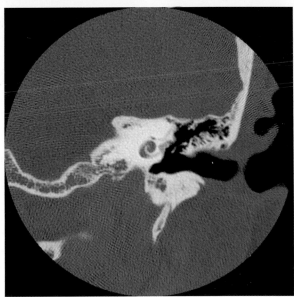

Case 141   Fenestral Otosclerosis

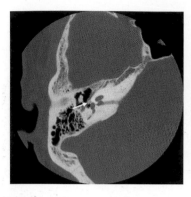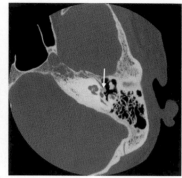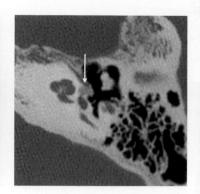

Findings

▶ There is a focal area of demineralization immediately anterior to the oval window bilaterally (arrows), consistent with an otosclerosis plaque.

▶ The magnified view in particular demonstrates the focal nature of this region of bone demineralization.

Differential Diagnosis

▶ Rarely, focal demineralization due to other processes, such as sarcoid, syphilis, or tympanosclerosis, could have a similar appearance.

Teaching Points

▶ Otosclerosis (also known as otospongiosis) is a disease of unknown etiology marked by proliferation and demineralization of portions of the otic capsule.

▶ Otosclerosis is inherited as an autosomal dominant condition with variable penetrance.

▶ The early signs of otosclerosis can be subtle; high-resolution, bone detail CT images are needed for confident diagnosis. Classically, the bone anterior to the oval window (fissula antefenestram) is involved. Mineralized plaques can encroach upon the stapes in the oval window.

▶ The other common form of otosclerosis is retrofenestral (or cochlear) ostosclerosis, where the areas of demineralization in the cochlear capsule are present, typically anterior to the oval window and surrounding the turns of the cochlea.

▶ It is important to ascertain the status of the stapes footplate (oval window) and round window prior to surgical intervention. The location of the facial nerve and the integrity of its osseous covering should be verified.

Management

▶ Stapedectomy and placement of a stapes prosthesis is typical management for otosclerosis. Sodium fluoride treatment has also been shown to have some benefit.

Further Reading

Naumann IC, Porcellini B, Fisch U. Otosclerosis: incidence of positive findings on high-resolution computed tomography and their correlation to audiological test data. *Ann Oto Rhinol Laryngol.* 2005;114:709-716.

Swartz JD, Mukherji SK. The inner ear and otodystrophies. In: Swartz JD, Loevner LA. *Imaging of the Temporal Bone*, 4th ed. New York: Thieme, 2009:382-388.

History

▶ 49-year-old with ear pain and headache

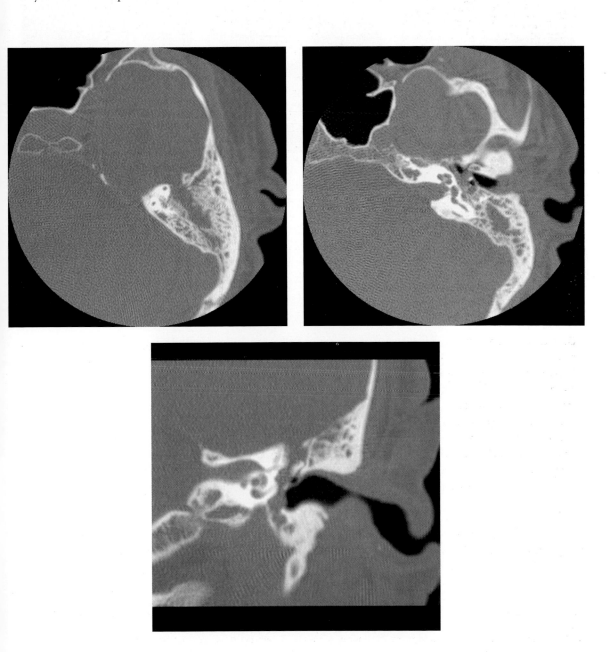

Case 142   Coalescent Mastoiditis

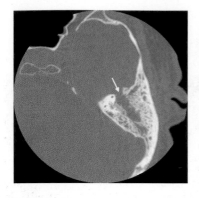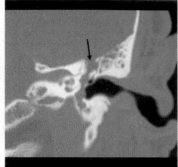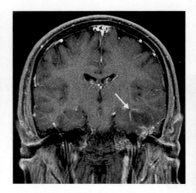

Findings

▶ There is opacification of the left middle ear and mastoid.

▶ There is destruction of bony septations in the mastoid (white arrow). On coronal images there is erosion of the tegmen tympani (black arrow).

▶ Additional MR images demonstrate a rim-enhancing collection in the left temporal lobe (arrow) with surrounding edema. There is restricted diffusion within the collection. The mucosa in the left middle ear and mastoid enhances as well.

Differential Diagnosis

▶ Simple otomastoiditis

Teaching Points

▶ Coalescent mastoiditis is a complication of acute otomastoid inflammatory disease. The diagnosis on CT is established by the presence of bone resorption.

▶ The bone changes are best identified on high-resolution temporal bone CT.

▶ Early in the disease, the bone resorption can be subtle and is easiest to identify by carefully comparing one side to the other.

▶ Intracranial complications of coalescent mastoiditis are present in up to 25% of patients and may be clinically occult. Complications include meningitis, cerebral abscess, subperiosteal abscess, empyema, and dural sinus thrombosis. Pre- and post-contrast MRI and MRV (or contrast-enhanced CT if the patient cannot have an MRI) are necessary to identify these complications.

Management

▶ Aggressive antibiotic therapy and surgical debridement are performed.

Further Reading

Swartz JD. The middle ear and mastoid. In: Swartz JD, Loevner LA. *Imaging of the Temporal Bone*, 4th ed. New York: Thieme, 2009:80-94.
Zevallos JP, Vrabec JT, Williamson RA, et al. Advanced pediatric mastoiditis with and without intracranial complications. *Laryngoscope.* 2009;119:1610-1615.

History

▶ 6-year-old boy with epistaxis and nasal obstruction

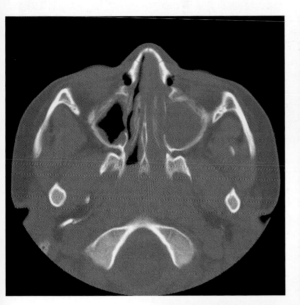

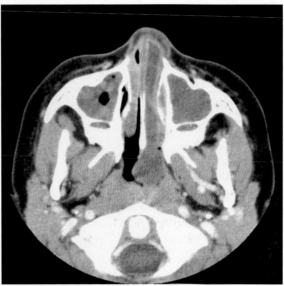

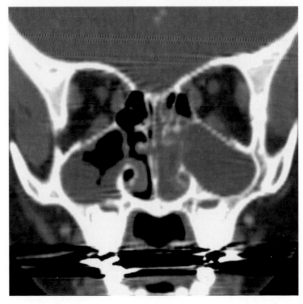

Case 143 Antrochoanal Polyp

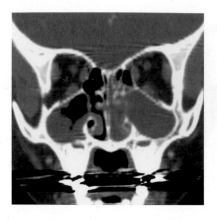

Findings

- Axial CT and coronal reformations demonstrate complete opacification of the left maxillary sinus and a lobular mass extending into the nasal cavity and nasopharynx.
- There is widening of the sinus ostium but no bone destruction.

Differential Diagnosis

- Inverting papilloma
- Mucocele
- Allergic fungal sinusitis
- Sinonasal neoplasm

Teaching Points

- Antrochoanal polyps are inflammatory polyps or retention cysts masses that extend across the maxillary sinus ostium or an accessory ostium into the nasal cavity and nasopharynx.
- Patients present with symptoms of sinus obstruction. The mass may become quite large and become visible in the nares or oropharynx.
- On CT, the infundibulum or an accessory ostium is expanded. There is osseous remodeling but no bone destruction.
- The central attenuation matches that of fluid or mucin.
- MRI is usually not needed but when performed will show hyperintense signal on T2-weighted images and peripheral enhancement of the mucosa on postcontrast T1-weighted images.

Management

- Endoscopic resection

Further Reading

Maldonado M, Martinez A, Alobid I, et al. The antrochoanal polyp. *Rhinol.* 2004;43:178-182.

History

▶ 58-year-old woman with left ear fullness and conductive hearing loss

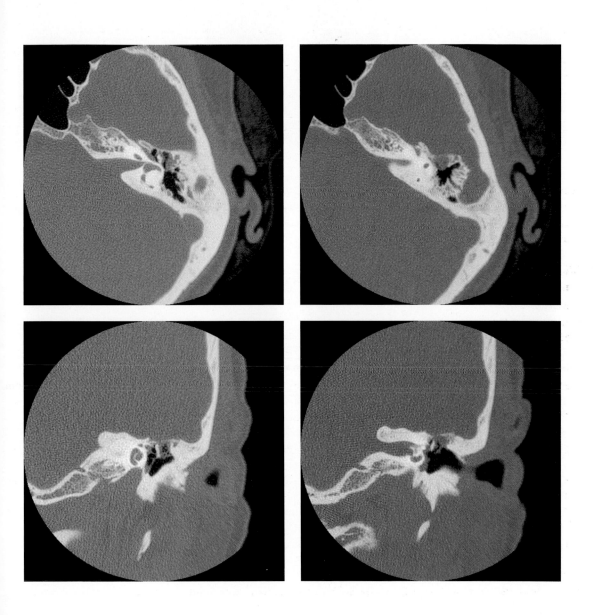

Case 144 Cholesteatoma (Acquired Pars Flaccida Type)

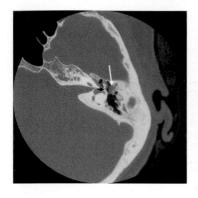 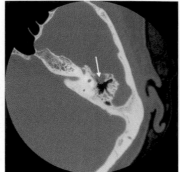 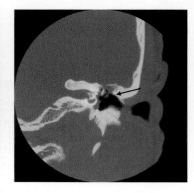

Findings

▶ There is abnormal soft tissue in Prussak's space and the epitympanum (white arrows).
▶ There is erosion of the scutum (black arrow), body, and short process of the incus (short arrow).
▶ The tympanic membrane is thickened and retracted, and ossicles are displaced medially.

Differential Diagnosis

▶ Chronic otitis media with bone erosion

Teaching Points

▶ Cholesteatomas are non-neoplastic but locally aggressive masses that occur when squamous epithelium becomes trapped and proliferates, most commonly within the middle ear.
▶ The presence of abnormal soft tissue in the middle ear with bone erosion is the hallmark of cholesteatoma. Cholesteatomas most commonly extend superior and posterior in Prussak's space, although anterior-superior, anterior, medial, and posterior extension can occur.
▶ Ossicle erosion is present in 70% of pars flaccida and 90% of pars tensa cholesteatomas.
▶ When ossicle erosion is absent, it is not possible to distinguish between granulation tissue and cholesteatoma by CT.
▶ When evaluating patients with cholesteatoma, assess the:
  ▪ Integrity of the ossicles
  ▪ Integrity of the tegmen tympani
  ▪ Integrity of the facial nerve canal
  ▪ Integrity of the bony labyrinth (particularly the horizontal semicircular canal)
  ▪ Presence of extension of cholesteatoma into surgical blind spots, such as the sinus tympani
▶ Recent studies suggest that diffusion-weighted imaging (DWI) may distinguish recurrent cholesteatomas (hyperintense on DWI) from granulation tissue.

Management

▶ Treatment of cholesteatoma is surgical, with a 5% to 10% recurrence rate. Surgical approaches include removing all remnants of the cholesteatoma via mastoidectomy. Ossicular reconstruction may be necessary as well if ossicular erosion has occurred.

Further Reading

Swartz JD. The middle ear and mastoid. In: Swartz JD, Loevner LA. *Imaging of the Temporal Bone*, 4th ed. New York: Thieme, 2009:115-136.

History

► 84-year-old with altered mental status

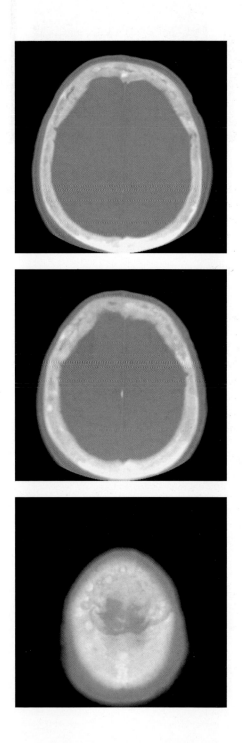

Case 145 Paget's Disease

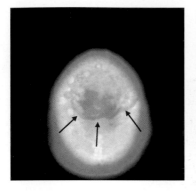 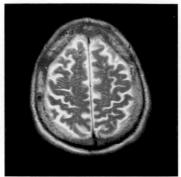 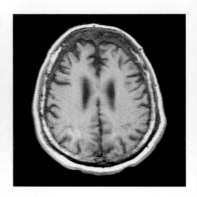

Findings

► CT images with bone windowing demonstrate a large zone of abnormal mixed increased and decreased density in the frontal bone. This area has a sharp, geographic zone of transition (arrows).
► The mixed osteolytic and osteoblastic processes produce a "cotton wool" appearance.
► T1-weighted MRI demonstrates abnormal hypointense signal in the marrow space. There is heterogeneous signal on T2-weighted images.

Differential Diagnosis

► Fibrous dysplasia
► Metastasis
► Multiple myeloma
► Hyperparathyroidism

Teaching Points

► Paget's disease is a chronic disorder characterized by abnormal bone turnover. It occurs most commonly in older adults and is four times more common in men than women.
► It has distinct phases, each with a distinct imaging appearance:
  ▪ Early osteolytic phase: sharply demarcated areas of radiolucency, also known as osteoporosis circumscripta
  ▪ Mixed lytic and blastic phase: mosaic pattern of mixed radiolucency and sclerosis
  ▪ Osteoblastic phase: increasingly sclerotic bone with thickening of cortical bone and trabeculae
  ▪ Remodeling: inactive phase with gradual remodeling to lamellar bone
► Involvement of the skull base leads to a softening of the bone and basilar invagination.
► Involvement of the temporal bone can cause mixed hearing loss, and in the osteolytic phase can be confused with otosclerosis or fibrous dysplasia of the temporal bone.
► Malignant transformation to osteosarcoma occurs in up to 1% of patients with Paget's disease.

Management

► Paget's disease can be entirely asymptomatic and detected only incidentally on imaging studies done for other reasons (as in this case).
► Treatment in symptomatic patients consists of calcitonin and bisphosphonates.

Further Reading

Davidson HC, Harnsberger HR. The temporal bone. In: Som PM, Curtin HD. *Head and Neck Imaging*, 4th ed. Philadelphia: Mosby, 2003:968-969.
Swartz JD, Mukherji SK. The inner ear and otodystrophies. In: Swartz JD, Loevner LA. Imaging of the Temporal Bone, 4th ed. New York: Thieme, 2009:369-375.

▶ 3-year-old with bilateral hearing loss

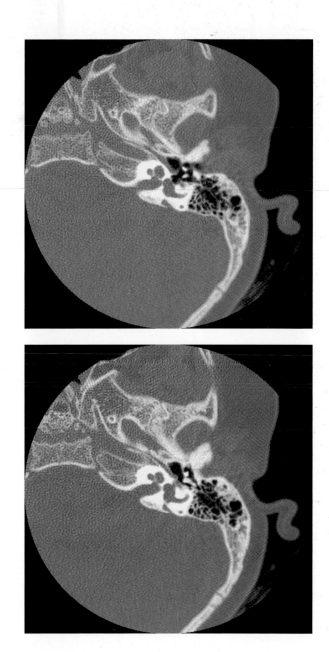

Case 146 Incomplete Partition Type II (Classic Mondini Malformation)

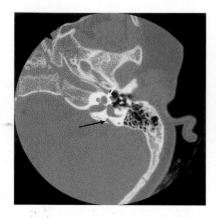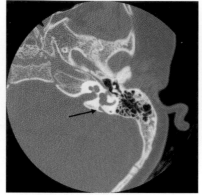

Findings

- ▸ The vestibular aqueduct is enlarged (black arrows).
- ▸ The cochlea is abnormal, with a bulbous appearance to the apical turn, which is fused with the middle turn (white arrow). The modiolus is deficient.
- ▸ The semicircular canals are normal in appearance, but the vestibule is mildly dilated.

Differential Diagnosis

- ▸ Enlarged vestibular aqueduct syndrome
- ▸ Incomplete partition type I

Teaching Points

- ▸ The malformation that Mondini originally described consists of an enlarged vestibular aqueduct, normal basal turn of the cochlea with cystic middle/apical turns (1.5 turns instead of the usual 2.5), and an enlarged vestibule. The term "Mondini malformation" is out of favor due to inconsistent application in the medical literature, in favor of incomplete partition type II (IP type II).
- ▸ In contrast, IP type I is a more severe malformation that consists of a cystic cochlear chamber with absence of the modiolus and interscalar septa as well as enlargement of the vestibule.
- ▸ There is likely overlap and a continuum of IP type II with the enlarged vestibular aqueduct syndrome, which is differentiated from IP type II by a more normal-appearing cochlea (although deficiency of the modiolus is common) and vestibule.
- ▸ Patients with any of these entities present with sensorineural hearing loss.

Management

- ▸ Cochlear implantation is beneficial in patients with IP type II, unlike patients with IP type I or common cavity malformations. Newer types of "modiolar-hugging" cochlear implants make surgery safer in patients with a deficient modiolus.

Further Reading

Sennaroglu L, Saatci I. A new classification for cochleovestibular malformations. *Laryngoscope.* 2002;112:2230-2241.

Swartz JD, Mukherji SK. The inner ear and otodystrophies. In: Swartz JD, Loevner LA. *Imaging of the Temporal Bone*, 4th ed. New York: Thieme, 2009:317-330.

History

► Previously healthy man status post trauma, presenting with swelling, pain, and marked decrease in visual acuity

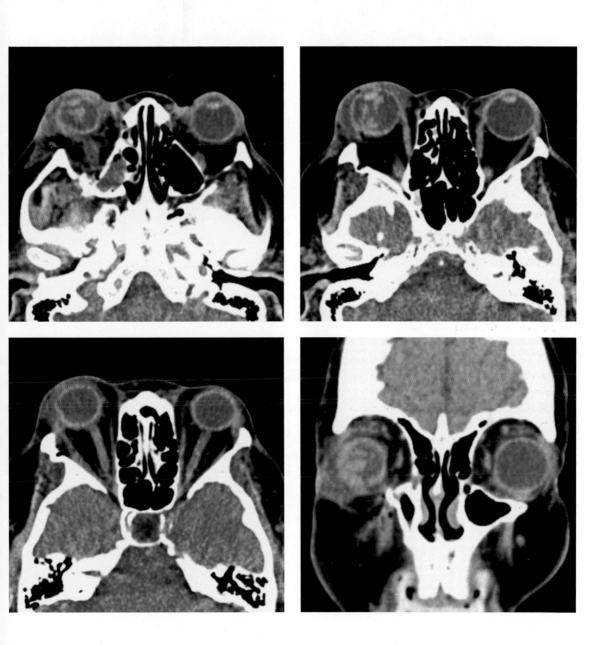

Case 147 Ocular Globe Rupture

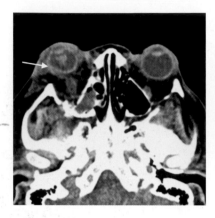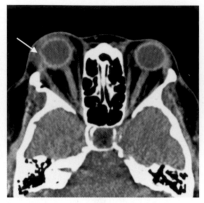

Findings

▶ CT images demonstrate right periorbital swelling and contour deformity of the right globe (arrows).

▶ There is high-attenuation material within the right globe, in keeping with intraocular hemorrhage.

Differential Diagnosis

▶ Nontraumatic vitreous hemorrhage

▶ Ocular neoplasms such as melanoma and retinoblastoma

▶ Perfluoropropane gas injected into vitreous for treatment of retinal detachment

Teaching Points

▶ Ocular globe rupture refers to full-thickness scleral or corneal injury of the eye by blunt or penetrating trauma.

▶ Signs and symptoms include pain, ecchymosis and swelling, decreased visual acuity, irregular pupils, and low intraocular pressure.

▶ In blunt injury, the most common site of rupture is at the attachment of the extraocular muscles and corneoscleral junction, since the sclera is thinnest in these areas.

▶ The best signs of globe rupture are contour deformity and volume reduction of the globe. Other findings that could be seen are vitreous hemorrhage, intraocular foreign bodies, and sometimes lens dislocation (not necessarily a sign of globe rupture).

▶ A deep anterior chamber has been described as a sign of occult globe rupture, secondary to leakage of vitreous posteriorly.

▶ Displaced orbital fractures can stretch or deform the globe without rupture.

▶ The sensitivity of CT for detecting globe rupture is only 70% to 75%, so patients with high clinical suspicion of globe rupture may be surgically explored.

Management

▶ Treatment often includes surgical repair. In very severe cases, enucleation is occasionally performed.

Further Reading

Arey ML, Mootha VV, Whittemore AR, et al. Computed tomography in the diagnosis of occult open-globe injuries. *Ophthalmology.* 2007;114:1448-1452.

Kubal WS. Imaging of orbital trauma. *Radiographics.* 2008;28:1729-1739.

History

▶ 12-year-old patient presenting with redness around right eye, pain, and blurry vision

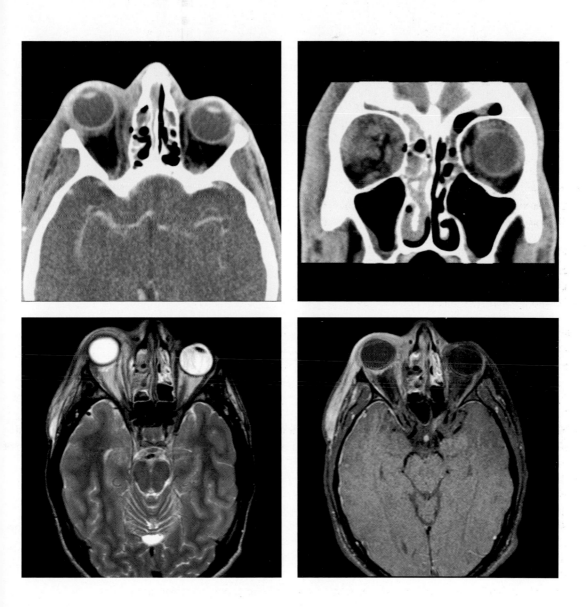

Case 148 Subperiosteal Orbital Abscess

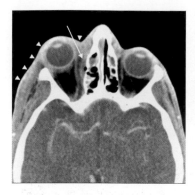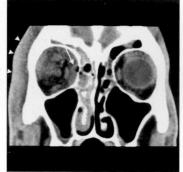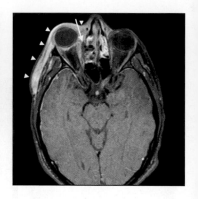

Findings

- ▶ Axial and coronal contrast-enhanced CT images show a small rim-enhancing collection containing a small bubble of gas in the extraconal space, medial to the medial rectus muscle, and adjacent to the lamina papyracea (arrow).
- ▶ There is ethmoid and right frontal sinus opacification.
- ▶ Axial T2-weighted MRI images show hyperintense material within a rim-enhancing collection, consistent with fluid. There is proptosis and extensive periorbital and right facial swelling and enhancement (arrowheads).

Differential Diagnosis

- ▶ Orbital hematoma
- ▶ Other orbital abscess
- ▶ Congenital lesions such as dermoid cyst or lymphatic malformation

Teaching Points

- ▶ Subperiosteal orbital abscess is a collection of purulent material between the orbital wall and periorbita.
- ▶ The disease may be rapidly progressive, with increased pressure and optic nerve compromise that can lead to loss of vision.
- ▶ Almost all patients will have infectious disease of the adjacent paranasal sinus. Extension from the ethmoid sinuses to the medial orbit is most common site. Occasionally there will be a superiorly or laterally located subperiosteal abscess extending from the frontal sinus. In some cases, the orbital disease may be the first presenting sign of sinusitis, especially in children.
- ▶ Initially, the collection may appear phlegmonous without a well-defined hypodense central portion on CT or fluid on MRI. Detection of abnormal extraconal tissue adjacent to the bone in an acu1tely presenting patient with sinus disease is an early clue.
- ▶ On imaging, assess for proptosis and also the extent of disease in the orbit. Also look on multiplanar CT or MRI for intracranial extension of infection, evaluating for signs of epidural abscess, subdural empyema, and cavernous sinus thrombosis.

Management

- ▶ These abscesses require urgent antibiotic treatment and sometimes patients also need surgical drainage. Often patients will undergo endoscopic or open sinus surgery as well.

Further Reading

Pereira FJ, et al. Computed tomographic patterns of orbital cellulitis due to sinusitis. *Arq Bras Oftalmol.* 2006;69:513-518.
Rahbar R, et al. Management of orbital subperiosteal abscess in children. *Arch Otolaryngol Head Neck Surg.* 2001;127:281-286.

History

▶ 14-year-old girl with headaches

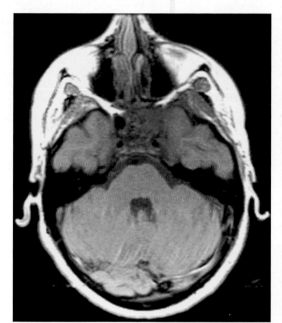 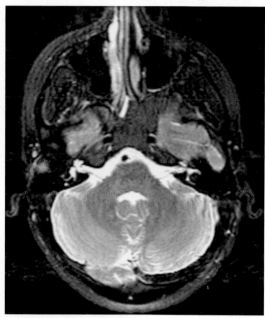

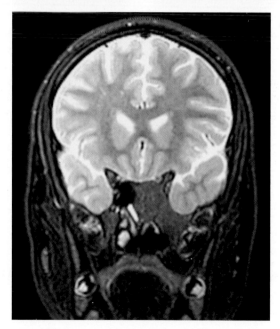

Case 149 Fibrous Dysplasia

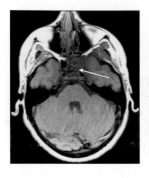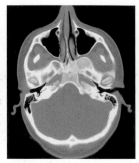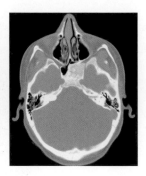

Findings

▸ There is abnormal hypointense signal in the central skull base on T1-weighted and fat-suppressed T2-weighted images (arrow). On the T2-weighted images, the area of signal decrease is largely homogeneous. Note that the process involves the left pterygoid plates and basisphenoid.

▸ The left sphenoid sinus is not aerated.

▸ CT demonstrates a geographic region of "ground-glass" density in the area corresponding to the abnormality on MRI.

Differential Diagnosis

▸ Paget's disease
▸ Osteoma
▸ Ossifying fibroma
▸ Metastasis/myeloma
▸ Chordoma

Teaching Points

▸ Fibrous dysplasia is a developmental bone abnormality with a variety of imaging appearances. Fibrous dysplasia can be asymptomatic or produce symptoms due to bone enlargement (cranial neuropathy, cosmetic or functional deformity).

▸ Cortical bone is preserved, and the marrow space is expanded and replaced with fibro-osseous tissue. Although classically this expanded space has a "ground-glass" appearance on CT, lytic, sclerotic, or mixed patterns can be seen.

▸ Fibrous dysplasia can be confusing when seen on MRI. In general, the lesions are low signal on T1- and T2-weighted images, but heterogeneity in the lesion can lead to the erroneous conclusion that the lesion represents an aggressive process.

▸ There is usually irregular enhancement of fibrous dysplasia, further confusing the imaging appearance on MRI.

▸ Clinically, fibrous dysplasia is most commonly monostotic. Involvement of more than one site (polyostotic fibrous dysplasia) occurs in 25% of patients and is more commonly symptomatic, often in childhood.

▸ The McCune-Albright syndrome is a form of polyostotic fibrous dysplasia that also has multiple café-au-lait spots and endocrine dysfunction.

▸ Rarely, fibrous dysplasia can undergo malignant transformation.

Management

▸ Fibrous dysplasia is usually not treated. If symptoms of cranial neuropathy, functional impairment, or cosmetic deformity are present, decompression and/or resection can be considered.

Further Reading

Davidson HC, Orrison WW, Glastonbury CM, Moore KR. The skull base. In: Orrison WW. *Neuroimaging*. Philadelphia: Saunders, 2000:990-991.

Kransdorf MJ, Moser RP, Gilkey FW. Fibrous dysplasia. *Radiographics*. 1990;10:519-537.

History

▶ 69-year-old woman with a palpable mass in her left neck

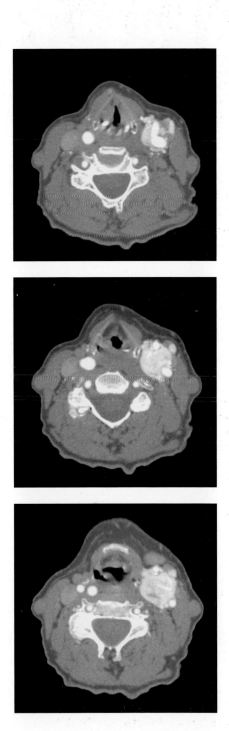

Case 150 Carotid Body Paraganglioma

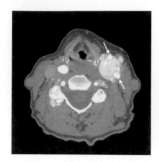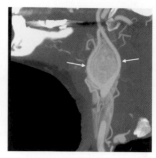

Findings

- ▶ Axial images from a CT angiogram demonstrate an intensely enhancing mass at the carotid bifurcation.
- ▶ The mass splays the internal and external carotid arteries (arrows).
- ▶ Even in this early arterial phase there is marked enhancement of the mass.

Differential Diagnosis

- ▶ Schwannoma
- ▶ Glomus vagale
- ▶ Lymphadenopathy
- ▶ Aneurysm

Teaching Points

- ▶ Carotid body tumors are paragangliomas that arise at the carotid bifurcation. They are the most common of the head and neck paragangliomas. Histologically, they are indistinguishable from other glomus tumors, so it is the location between internal and external carotid arteries that labels the lesion.
- ▶ Paragangliomas are a family of neoplasms, usually benign, that arise from clusters of neuroendocrine cells that form part of both sympathetic and parasympathetic nervous systems. Rarely these tumors secrete catecholamines.
- ▶ In sporadic cases, the incidence of bilateral paragangliomas is as high as 15%. Paragangliomas can be familial, and here the incidence of multiple paragangliomas exceeds 50%. There is an association with multiple endocrine neoplasia syndrome type II.
- ▶ Other paragangliomas of the head and neck include:
  - ▪ Glomus vagale, arising along the vagus nerve medial to the carotid
  - ▪ Glomus jugulare, arising in the jugular fossa
  - ▪ Glomus tympanicum, arising in the middle ear
- ▶ Glomus tumors are hypervascular and demonstrate characteristic early and intense enhancement.
- ▶ Discreet flow voids in the mass can be identified on MR imaging in most lesions over 1.5 cm in size. Slower-flowing vessels may be hyperintense. The combination gives some paragangliomas a "salt-and-pepper" appearance.
- ▶ Similarly, on CT angiography small vessels in the mass can usually be identified.
- ▶ There can be areas of cystic change within the lesion, but this should not be a dominant feature.

Management

- ▶ The management of carotid body tumors is surgical. Preoperative embolization can be performed to decrease operative blood loss. For patients who cannot undergo surgery, radiotherapy is an alternative treatment choice.

Further Reading

Rao AB, Koeller KK, Adair CF. Paragangliomas of the head and neck. *Radiographics.* 1999;19:1605-1632.
Som PM, Curtin HD. Parapharyngeal and masticator space lesions. In: Orrison WW. *Neuroimaging.* Philadelphia: Saunders, 2000:1966-1972.

History

▶ 8-month-old girl with right neck mass

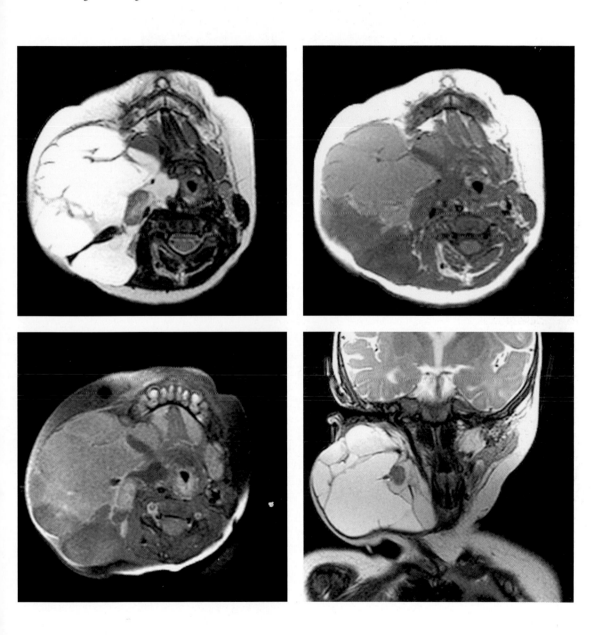

Case 151 Lymphangioma

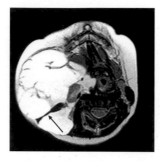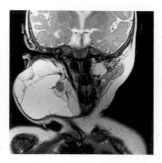

Findings

▶ There is a large, multi-septated mass in the right neck.
▶ The signal intensity within the lesion on T1-weighted images is slightly brighter than simple fluid. It is hyperintense on T2-weighted images. There is little postcontrast enhancement.
▶ The mass involves multiple spaces in the neck and envelops neck structures such as the sternocleidomastoid muscle (arrow).

Differential Diagnosis

▶ Branchial cleft cyst
▶ Thyroglossal duct cyst
▶ Cystic metastasis
▶ Abscess

Teaching Points

▶ Lymphangiomas are congenital malformations that result from the abnormal development of the primordial venous and lymphatic channels of the neck. These malformations can have both cystic and solid vascular components.
▶ There are multiple classification schemes for these lesions. One divides them into four subtypes: cystic hygroma, capillary lymphangioma, cavernous lymphangioma, and vasculolymphatic malformation. These can be thought of as a spectrum of the same process; frequently multiple subtypes can be found in the same lesion.
▶ Lymphangiomas can enlarge because of hemorrhage into the cystic components or due to hypertrophy of lymphoid tissue contained in the lesions during an upper respiratory infection.
▶ The typical lymphangioma is multi-septated and involves multiple compartments in the neck. The posterior cervical space is the one most commonly involved, but lymphangiomas can occur with any space in the neck. Fluid–fluid levels may be present, and enhancing components are not unusual.
▶ The primary role of imaging (best done with MRI) is to evaluate the full extent of the lesion. The laterality of the lesion (unilateral vs. bilateral) and involvement of suprahyoid structures and infrahyoid structures affects the recurrence rate and difficulty of treatment.

Management

▶ Surgical excision can be performed, but the recurrence rate is high and surgical cure of large lesions is difficult. Percutaneous sclerotherapy with such agents as doxycycline has been used with success. Small lesions occasionally regress spontaneously.

Further Reading

Perkins JA, Manning SC, Tempero RM, et al. Lymphatic malformations: Review of current treatment. *Otol Head Neck Surg.* 2010;142:796-803.
Som PM, Smoker WRK, Curtin HD, et al. Congenital lesions. In: Som PM, Curtin HD. *Head and Neck Imaging*, 4th ed. Philadelphia: Mosby, 2003:1848-1852.

History

▶ 49-year-old woman with anterior neck mass

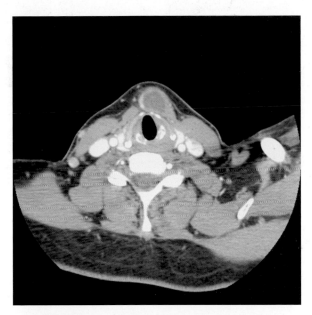

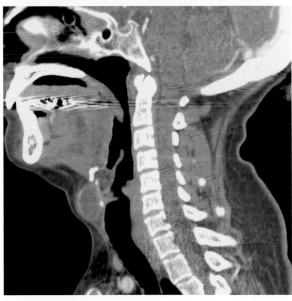

Case 152 Thyroglossal Duct Cyst

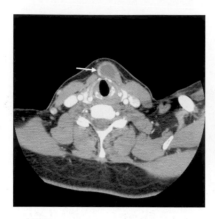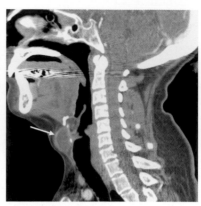

Findings

▶ Well-defined low-attenuation anterior neck mass, deep to the strap muscles, abutting both the hyoid and left thyroid lamina

▶ A small focus of higher-attenuation material along the right side of the lesion (arrow) represents ectopic thyroid tissue.

Differential Diagnosis

▶ Metastatic cancer in lymph node (e.g., papillary thyroid cancer)

▶ Abscess

Teaching Points

▶ Thyroglossal duct cysts are remnants of the thyroglossal duct and can be found anywhere along the path of descent of the embryologic thyroid from the foramen cecum in the tongue base to the thyroid bed. About half are located at the level of the hyoid bone, and are usually paramedian.

▶ Thyroglossal duct cysts are congenital but can enlarge if they become infected or during an upper respiratory infection. They are the most common congenital neck cysts.

▶ Ectopic thyroid tissue is commonly associated with the lesion, and the thyroid bed should be inspected to ensure thyroid gland is present.

▶ Rarely, thyroid cancer can occur in thyroglossal duct cyst, most commonly papillary thyroid cancer.

Management

▶ Thyroglossal duct cysts are treated by surgical removal. The Sistrunk procedure removes the cyst and a portion of the hyoid bone and results in a recurrence rate of under 4%.

Further Reading

Som PM, Smoker WRK, Curtin HD, et al. Congenital lesions. In: Som PM, Curtin HD. *Head and Neck Imaging*, 4th ed. Philadelphia: Mosby, 2003:1840-1847.

History

▶ 34-year-old woman with blurry vision

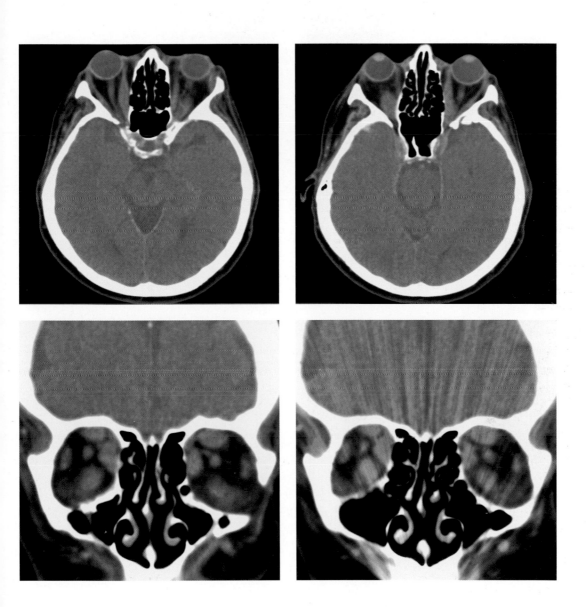

Case 153   Dysthyroid Ophthalmopathy

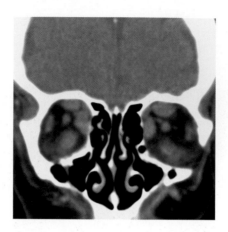

Findings

► The axial and coronal CT images show enlargement of the inferior, medial, and superior rectus muscles in the orbits. The lateral rectus and oblique muscles are relatively spared.
► On the axial images, the enlargement of the muscles can be seen to involve the belly of the muscles. The tendons are relatively spared.
► There is mild proptosis.

Differential Diagnosis

► Idiopathic inflammatory orbital disease (orbital pseudotumor)
► Neoplasm (e.g., lymphoma or metastases)
► Infectious myositis and other inflammatory disorders such as sarcoidosis or Wegener's granulomatosis

Teaching Points

► Dysthyroid ophthalmopathy (thyroid-associated orbitopathy or Graves ophthalmopathy) is an autoimmune inflammatory disorder associated with thyroid disease.
► Most, but not all, patients have hyperthyroidism. Occasionally the orbital manifestations clinically precede thyroid disease. Patients may present with blurry vision, restricted gaze, and proptosis, but the process is usually painless. Optic nerve compression or severe stretching may lead to vision loss.
► It is bilateral in 90% of patients and more common in females.
► Enlargement of the extraocular muscles, proptosis, and/or increased orbital fat are the main imaging findings. A useful mnemonic is I'M SLO, indicating the prevalence order of extraocular muscle involvement: inferior > medial > superior > lateral > obliques.
► Enlargement of extraocular muscles involves the muscle belly and typically spares the tendons.

Management

► Many cases are self-remitting. Treatment includes corticosteroids, and corneal care in patients with significant proptosis. In more severe cases, radiation therapy or surgical decompression of the orbit is performed.

Further Reading

Parmar H, Ibrahim M. Extrathyroidal manifestations of thyroid disease: thyroid ophthalmopathy. *Neuroimaging Clin North Am.* 2008;18:527-536.
Weber AL, Dallow RL, Sabates NR. Graves' disease of the orbit. *Neuroimaging Clin North Am.* 1996;6:61-72.

History

▶ 46-year-old woman with headaches

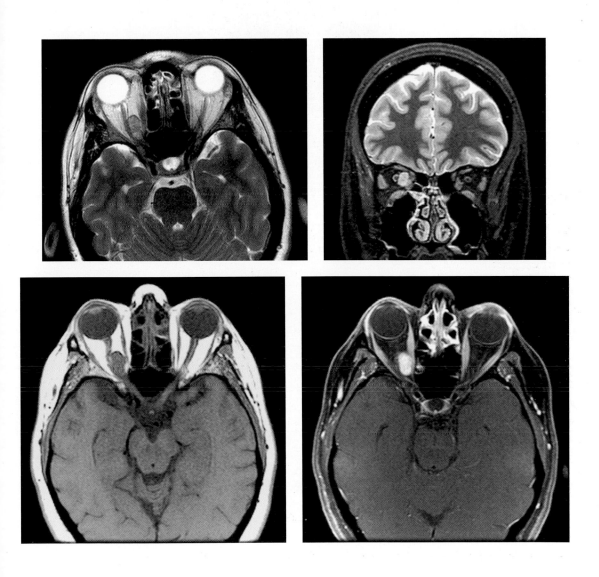

Case 154   Orbit Hemangioma

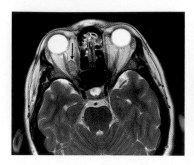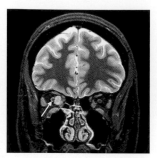

Findings

▶ There is a well-defined intraconal mass in the right orbit, between the medial rectus muscle and optic nerve. It displaces the optic nerve laterally but the nerve does not appear primarily involved (white arrow).

▶ The mass has increased signal relative to muscle on axial T2-weighted and coronal STIR images. The lesion is iso-intense on T1 images. It homogeneously enhances after intravenous contrast administration.

▶ On the axial T2-weighted images, there is a pseudocapsule (black arrow) visible around the anterior half of the lesion. The appearance of this pseudocapsule is due to chemical shift artifact, so it is not visible on STIR or fat-suppressed T2 sequences.

Differential Diagnosis

▶ Schwannoma
▶ Meningioma
▶ Lymphoma
▶ Metastasis
▶ Venous varix

Teaching Points

▶ Cavernous hemangiomas are mass-like vascular malformations. The latest terminology for vascular lesions of the orbit renames these lesions as "encapsulated venous malformations," reflecting their venous origin and the nondistensibility that distinguishes them from a venous varix.

▶ They are the most common orbital masses in adults.

▶ They can be incidentally found, or the patient may present with proptosis or vision loss.

▶ Although not neoplasms, cavernous hemangiomas can become larger over time, and may increase their rate of growth during pregnancy.

▶ On CT, these lesions are well-defined, homogeneous, soft-tissue-attenuation masses.

▶ On MRI, they are hyperintense on T2-weighted images and iso-intense on T1-weighted images, and show striking enhancement.

▶ Cavernous hemangiomas are slow-flowing lesions, and angiography is not usually warranted.

Management

▶ If incidentally found, or if symptoms are minimal, hemangiomas can be observed over time. If the lesion needs to be treated because of proptosis or vision loss, surgical excision is the preferred method; when excised, there is a very low incidence of recurrence.

Further Reading

Bilaniuk LT. Orbital vascular lesions. Role of imaging. *Radiol Clin North Am*. 1999;37:169-183.

Harris GJ. Orbital vascular malformations: a consensus statement on terminology and its clinical implications. Orbital Society. *Am J Ophthalmol*. 1999;127:453-455.

History

▶ Hearing loss after cochlear implantation

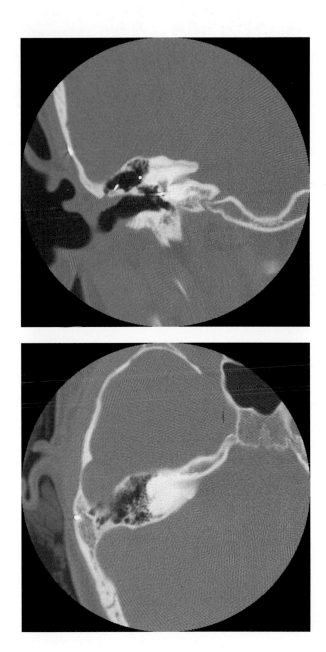

Case 155   Labyrinthitis Ossificans

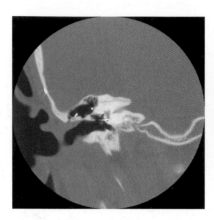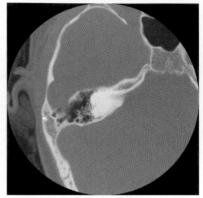

Findings

▶ There has been prior placement of a cochlear implant. There is abnormal ossification that obliterates the semicircular canals and the majority of the cochlea.

Differential Diagnosis

▶ Labyrinthitis ossificans
▶ Cochlear hypoplasia/aplasia

Teaching Points

▶ Labyrinthitis ossificans is the end stage of labyrinthitis. There are a number of causes of labyrinthitis, including viral, bacterial, autoimmune, toxic, and post-traumatic. They all can lead to labyrinthitis ossificans.
▶ The clinical symptom of hearing loss occurs early in the course of labyrinthitis, with the radiographic signs of ossification occurring late. Gadolinium-enhanced MRI, however, can show labyrinthine enhancement in the early stages of the disease.
▶ Unilateral ossification is typical for infections that arise from middle ear disease, whereas ossification after meningitis can be bilateral.
▶ Early labyrinthitis ossificans commonly affects the basal turn of the cochlea.
▶ Thin, heavily T2-weighted images can be used to identify the fibrous as well as osseous components to the process.
▶ In the key differential consideration, cochlear dysplasia, the outline of the otic capsule is reduced or deformed. Labyrinthitis ossificans preserves the outline of the otic capsule.

Management

▶ Labyrinthitis ossificans is an important finding to recognize in patients undergoing evaluation for cochlear implantation. It will often cause the surgeon to alter the approach or device.

Further Reading

Casselman JW, Kuhweide R, Ampe W, et al. Pathology of the membranous labyrinth: comparison of T1- and T2-weighted and gadolinium-enhanced spin-echo and 3DFT-CISS imaging. *AJNR Am J Neuroradiol.* 1993;14:59-69.
Swartz JD, Mukherji SK. The inner ear and otodystrophies. In: Swartz JD, Loevner LA. *Imaging of the Temporal Bone,* 4th ed. New York: Thieme, 2009:349-356.

History

▶ 4-year-old with unilateral nasal obstruction

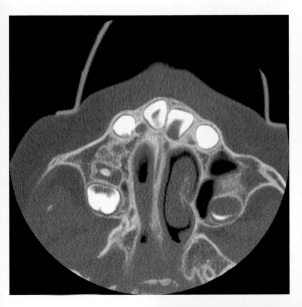 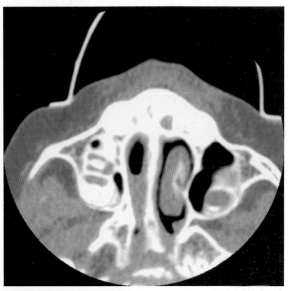

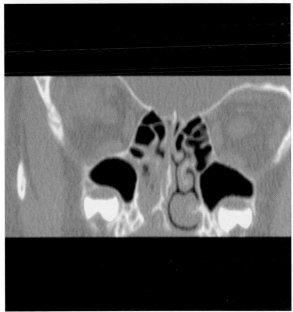

Case 156   Unilateral Choanal Atresia

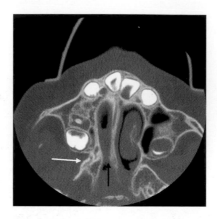

Findings

▸ The posterior right nasal cavity is obstructed (black arrow). There is thickening and medial deviation of the posterior maxilla and pterygoid plates (white arrow), which creates a narrowed bony opening that is further obstructed by soft tissue.

▸ Coronal images demonstrate asymmetry of the palate and a thickened inferior vomer.

Differential Diagnosis

▸ Deviated nasal septum
▸ Choanal stenosis

Teaching Points

▸ Choanal atresia is a congenital disorder in which the posterior nasal passage fails to fully open and is obstructed by osseous or soft tissue.

▸ When bilateral, this results in severe respiratory distress and cyanosis in infancy, since infants are obligate nose-breathers.

▸ Unilateral atresia accounts for 50% to 60% of choanal atresia cases and tends to present later in life than the bilateral form. Although other congenital anomalies, including CHARGE syndrome (coloboma or microphthalmos, heart anomalies, atresia of the choanae, developmental/growth delay, genitourinary anomalies, and ear anomalies) can occur in patients with unilateral atresia, it is commonly an isolated anomaly. Bilateral atresia has associated anomalies in 75% of patients.

▸ Essentially all patients with choanal atresia have abnormalities of the adjacent pterygoid plates and vomer. There is debate about the existence of purely membranous choanal atresia.

▸ The role of imaging is to evaluate the extent of anatomic abnormalities and exclude other causes of nasal obstruction. Suctioning of the nasal cavity immediately prior to CT scanning allows better depiction of the true thickness of soft tissue abnormality.

Management

▸ Patients who have severe respiratory compromise related to bilateral atresia usually undergo urgent surgery. Unilateral atresia, without respiratory compromise, is electively repaired.

Further Reading

Brown OE, Pownell P, Manning SC. Choanal atresia: a new anatomic classification and clinical management applications. *Laryngoscope*. 1996;106:97-101.

Robson CS, Hudgins PA. Pediatric airway disease. In: Som PM, Curtin HD. *Head and Neck Imaging*, 4th ed. Philadelphia: Mosby, 2003:1538-1540.

History

▶ 25-year-old man with conductive hearing loss one year after trauma

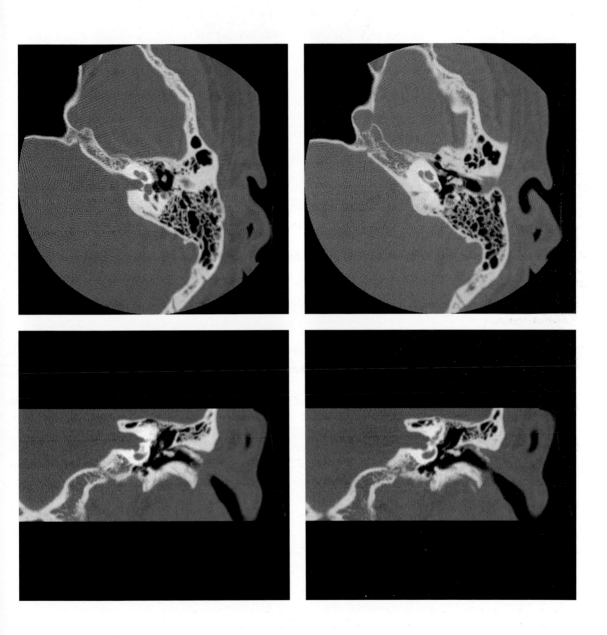

Case 157 Dislocation of Incus

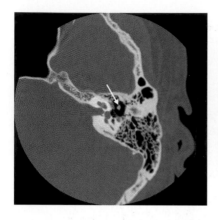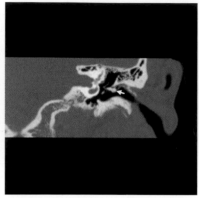

Findings

▶ Axial temporal bone images demonstrate absence of the incus in the epitympanum with disruption of the incudomalleolar joint, leaving only the head of the malleus visible (arrow). A normal-appearing stapes suprastructure is present.

▶ Coronal images demonstrate the incus deforming the tympanic membrane (arrow). The incudostapedial joint is intact.

Differential Diagnosis

▶ The images are diagnostic of incus dislocation. Other patterns of ossicle disruption include incudostapedial subluxation, malleoincudal subluxation, stapes fracture, and malleus fracture.

Teaching Points

▶ The incus is the ossicle most vulnerable to traumatic dislocation because it is not as firmly held in place as the stapes and malleus.

▶ Fractures of ossicles are much less common than dislocation.

▶ Clinically, patients present with post-traumatic conductive hearing loss.

Management

▶ Ossicular reconstruction can restore the conductive chain from the tympanic membrane to the oval window. The integrity of the stapes is important in deciding the type of ossicular reconstruction needed.

Further Reading

Meriot P, Veillon F, Garcia JF, et al. CT appearance of ossicular injuries. *Radiographics*. 1997;17:1445-1454.

Wang EY, et al. Temporal bone trauma. In: Swartz JD, Loevner LA. *Imaging of the Temporal Bone*, 4th ed. New York: Thieme, 2009:427-432.

History

▶ 70-year-old man with 2-month history of anosmia. Now presenting with diplopia

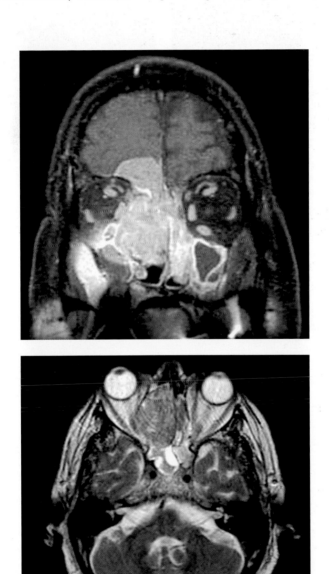

Case 158 Olfactory Neuroblastoma (Esthesioneuroblastoma)

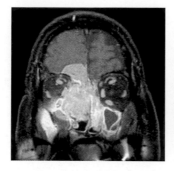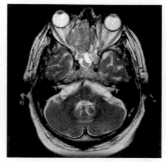

Findings

▶ Postcontrast T1-weighted MR demonstrates a large enhancing mass spanning the cribriform plate, entering the anterior cranial fossa, filling the upper sinonasal cavity, and entering the medial orbit.

▶ The mass is relatively hypointense on T2-weighted images.

▶ There is obstruction of the maxillary and sphenoid sinuses.

Differential Diagnosis

▶ Squamous cell carcinoma

▶ Lymphoma

▶ Adenocarcinoma

▶ Adenoid cystic carcinoma

▶ Melanoma

▶ Meningioma

▶ Sarcoma (esp. rhabdomyosarcoma)

▶ Metastatic neoplasm

Teaching Points

▶ Olfactory neuroblastoma is an aggressive neuroectodermal neoplasm with histology similar to other neural crest neoplasms but arising from olfactory epithelium in the cribriform plate.

▶ Patients present with anosmia, nasal stuffiness, pain, and epistaxis.

▶ These masses typically span the cribriform plate, but they may lie solely in the anterior cranial fossa or the upper nasal cavity.

▶ On CT, the mass is typically of higher attenuation than muscle. There may or may not be bone destruction.

▶ On MR, the mass is of intermediate signal intensity on T1-weighted images and relatively low signal intensity on T2-weighted images. Heterogeneous enhancement is typical.

▶ The imaging appearance does not usually permit differentiation from other sinonasal neoplasms. However, the presence of peripheral cystic foci suggests olfactory neuroblastoma.

▶ Spread to the dura, subarachnoid space, or cerebral parenchyma is possible.

Management

▶ Craniofacial resection and adjuvant radiation therapy are standard therapy for tumors with intracranial or orbital extension. Endoscopic resection with radiation is performed in patients with more limited disease.

Further Reading

Loevner LA, Sonners AI. Imaging neoplasms of the paranasal sinuses. *Magn Reson Imaging Clin North Am.* 2002;10:467-493.
Parmar H, Gujar S, Shah G, et al. Imaging of the anterior skull base. *Neuroimaging Clin North Am.* 2009;19:427-439.

History

▶ 18-year-old man with epistaxis

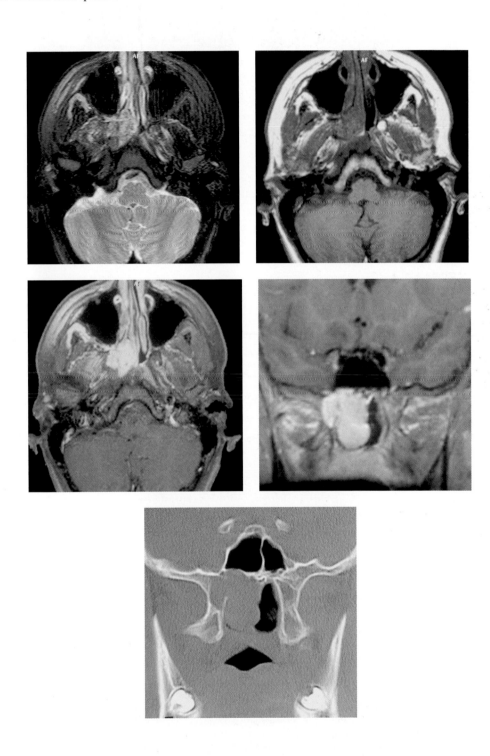

Case 159 Juvenile Nasopharyngeal Angiofibroma

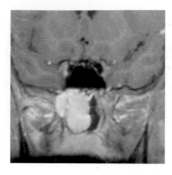 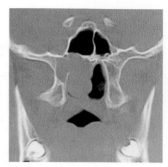

Findings

- MRI demonstrates a lobular, homogeneously enhancing mass in the posterior right nasal cavity.
- There is extension into the medial aspect of the pterygopalatine fossa (PPF) best demonstrated on axial T1-weighted images.
- On coronal CT, there is erosion into the sphenoid bone at the base of the pterygoid plates.

Differential Diagnosis

- Rhabdomyosarcoma
- Squamous cell carcinoma
- Lymphoma
- Inverted papilloma
- Invasive fungal infection
- Sinonasal polyp

Teaching Points

- Juvenile nasopharyngeal angiofibroma is an aggressive vascular neoplasm thought to arise from myofibroblasts along the rim of the sphenopalatine foramen. It occurs almost exclusively in young males.
- Common presenting symptoms include epistaxis and nasal obstruction.
- The mass protrudes into the nasopharynx and extends into the PPF. The PPF extension results in replacement of the normal fat at that site and is well demonstrated on CT or MRI. This feature differentiates juvenile angiofibroma from nonaggressive sinonasal processes (e.g., polyp).
- On CT, erosion of the adjacent sphenoid bone is often present. With expansion of the PPF, bowing of the posterior wall of the maxillary sinus may be present.
- On MRI the mass is homogeneously and intensely enhancing. MRI is best able to demonstrate extension into the skull base.
- Angiography is not needed for preoperative diagnosis, but the tumor will demonstrate intense vascular blush. Supply is primarily from the internal maxillary artery and its branches but can also derive from small branches of the cavernous internal carotid artery.

Management

- Preoperative particle embolization reduces intraoperative blood loss.
- Surgical resection is the treatment of choice, with the approach depending on location and size. Despite resection, recurrence occurs in as many as 50% of patients.

Further Reading

Das S, Kirsch CFE. Imaging of lumps and bumps in the nose: a review of sinonasal tumors. *Cancer Imag.* 2005;5:167-177.

History

▶ Patient 1: 34-year-old with vision loss after motor vehicle accident

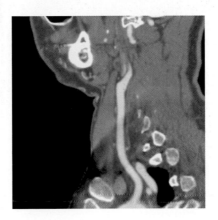

▶ Patient 2: 47-year-old with neck pain and dizziness after chiropractic manipulation

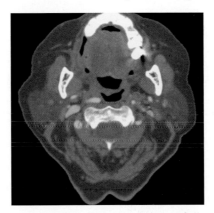

▶ Patient 3: 22-year-old with spontaneous neck pain

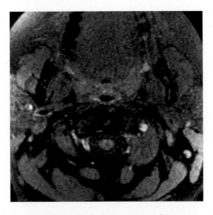

T1-weighted with fat saturation

Case 160 Arterial Dissection

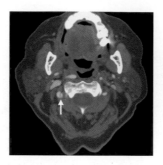

Findings

► Patient 1: Curved reformatted CT angiogram demonstrates tapered occlusion of the left internal carotid artery (ICA).
► Patient 2: Axial CT angiogram reveals an intimal flap within the right vertebral artery (arrow).
► Patient 3: Fat-saturated axial T1-weighted image demonstrates crescentic T1 hyperintense intramural hematoma adjacent to the attenuated left vertebral artery lumen.

Differential Diagnosis

► Atherosclerotic disease
► Vasospasm
► Vasculitis

Teaching Points

► Arterial dissection represents intimal injury with intramural hematoma formation.
► Dissections are often caused by blunt neck trauma but may be spontaneous or appear to result from rapid head movement. Persons with connective tissues diseases (e.g., fibromuscular dysplasia) have a higher risk.
► Arterial dissection may occur at any age and is an important cause of acute infarction in young patients. Presentations include neck pain, intracranial ischemia, Horner syndrome or cranial nerve palsies, subarachnoid hemorrhage (with intracranial extension).
► Arterial dissection can have a variable angiographic appearance:
  ▪ Tapered occlusion or stenosis
  ▪ Intimal flap
  ▪ Irregular or beaded luminal narrowing
► CT and MR angiography are first-line tests that perform reasonably well, but there is significant variation in reported sensitivity (50–100%) and specificity (30–100%).
► Intramural hematoma in acute or subacute dissection may be detected on MRI as crescentic T1 hyperintensity along the vessel wall.
► Catheter angiography is the gold standard but is reserved for equivocal CT or MRI or for planned treatment.

Management

► The natural history of dissection is often benign (most dissections demonstrate recanalization with healing), and anticoagulation or antiplatelet therapy may suffice for extradural dissection.
► Severe stenosis (especially with clinical or imaging evidence of hypoperfusion), recurrent ischemic events on medical management, or intradural dissection may require endovascular therapy (coil occlusion or stenting).

Further Reading

Dziewas R, Konrad C, Dragner B, et al. Cervical artery dissection—clinical features, risk factors, therapy and outcome in 126 patients. *J Neurol.* 2003;250:1179-1184.
Provenzale JM. Dissection of the internal carotid and vertebral arteries: imaging features. *AJR Am J Roentgenol.* 1995;165:1099-1104.

History

▶ 2-year-old with fever and torticollis

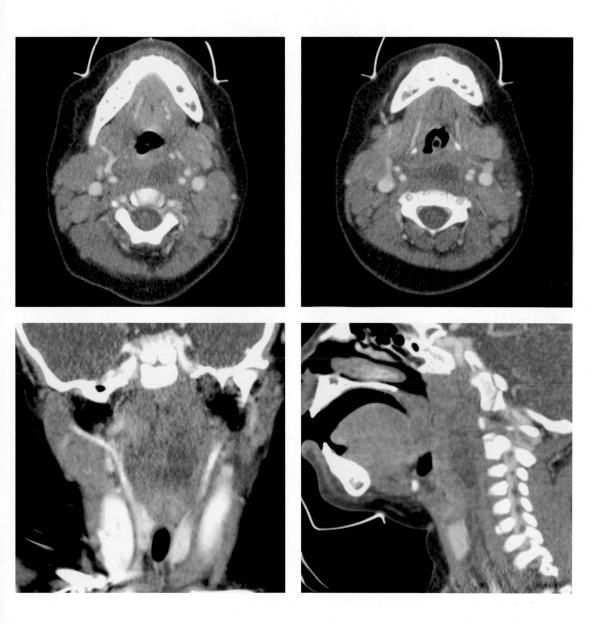

Case 161 Retropharyngeal Abscess

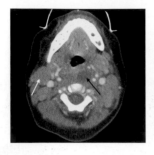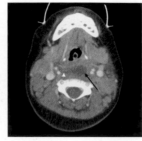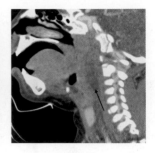

Findings

▶ There is a retropharyngeal fluid collection (black arrows) that exerts mass effect on the pharynx. The collection has a faint rim of enhancement.

▶ Adjacent retropharyngeal edema is present (arrowhead).

▶ Reactive lymphadenopathy is present (white arrow).

Differential Diagnosis

▶ Retropharyngeal edema

▶ Suppurative lymphadenitis

▶ Peritonsillar abscess

▶ Retropharyngeal neoplasm (especially metastatic squamous cell carcinoma in adults)

Teaching Points

▶ Retropharyngeal abscesses are most commonly seen in children under the age of 6.

▶ The road to developing a retropharyngeal abscess usually starts with an infection in the tonsil, pharynx, or sinus.

 ▪ The retropharyngeal nodes serve as a primary drainage pathway for this region and the retropharyngeal nodes become secondarily infected, resulting in suppurative adenitis.

 ▪ If not treated, the suppurative retropharyngeal lymph nodes can then break into the retropharyngeal space, leading to the development of a frank abscess in the retropharyngeal space.

▶ Secondary infection of the retropharyngeal space from discitis/osteomyelitis or penetrating trauma can also occur.

▶ The retropharyngeal space communicates with the mediastinum via the "danger space." Consequently, imaging of retropharyngeal inflammatory disease should include at least the upper chest to search for this life-threatening complication.

▶ Other complications of retropharyngeal inflammatory disease include vertebral osteomyelitis, discitis, and involvement of the carotid arteries or jugular vein.

▶ It is important to distinguish a retropharyngeal abscess from retropharyngeal edema and suppurative adenopathy of the retropharyngeal nodes, as neither is treated surgically. In general, if the enhancement and fluid collection is confined laterally in the region of the lateral retropharyngeal lymph nodes, suppurative adenopathy is the diagnosis.

Management

▶ Treatment involves antibiotics with or without drainage surgically.

▶ Suppurative lymphadenopathy, without a frank retropharyngeal abscess, is now primarily managed with antibiotics.

▶ A frank retropharyngeal abscess is usually drained, with smaller abscesses treated transorally and larger ones via a conventional open drainage.

Further Reading

Mukherji SK. Pharynx. In: Som PM, Curtin HD. *Head and Neck Imaging*, 4th ed. Philadelphia: Mosby, 2003:1503-1504.

Page NC, Bauer EM, Lieu JE. Clinical features and treatment of retropharyngeal abscess in children. *Otolaryngol Head Neck Surg.* 2008;138:300-306.

History

▶ Newborn with a lump over the upper nose

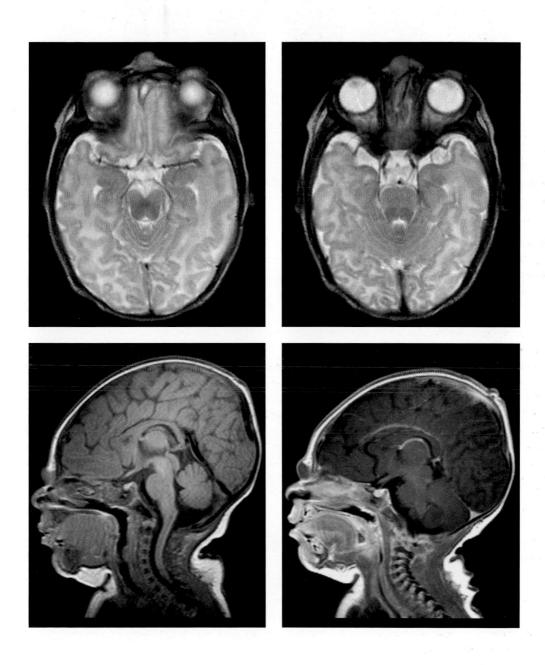

Case 162 Nasal Glioma

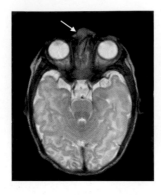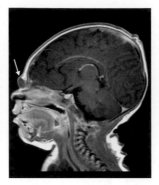

Findings

- ▶ There is a nodular mass along the dorsum and bridge of the nose, which is iso-intense to gray matter on T2- and T1-weighted images (arrows).
- ▶ No CSF or other connection is seen with the intracranial cavity.
- ▶ There is no postcontrast enhancement within the mass.

Differential Diagnosis

- ▶ Frontoethmoidal cephalocele
- ▶ Dermoid or epidermoid cyst
- ▶ Hemangioma
- ▶ Nasal polyp (if intranasal)

Teaching Points

- ▶ A nasal glioma is a developmental heterotopia of neuroglial tissue within the nasal cavity or along the dorsum of the nose, without any CSF connection to the brain. There may uncommonly be a thin fibrous connection through the cribriform plate region. Nasal gliomas are not neoplasms; hence the term "glioma" is a misnomer.
- ▶ Nasal gliomas may occur along the dorsum of the nose and glabella (extranasal glioma), at the medial canthus, or as a nasal cavity mass (intranasal glioma). Intranasal gliomas usually present with nasal obstruction.
- ▶ MRI is the preferred modality for evaluating masses of the nasal dorsum, medial canthus region, and nasal cavity. On imaging, nasal gliomas appear as nonenhancing soft tissue masses, without a CSF connection to the intracranial cavity.
- ▶ Use of CT for primary assessment may be confusing since, in the young infant, the unossified structures in the frontonasal region may lead to a false impression of bony dehiscence. Additionally, the presence of nasal secretions may mimic a mass on CT.
- ▶ The lack of a CSF connection distinguishes them from a cephalocele and is one of the most important aspects of the imaging evaluation for surgical planning.
- ▶ Dermoid cysts of this region have fatty content within them. Epidermoids often have restricted diffusion.
- ▶ Nasal gliomas may have a rim of surrounding nasal mucosa that enhances but lack the more extensive enhancement of hemangiomas.

Management

- ▶ Treatment is surgical resection.

Further Reading

Hedlund G. Congenital frontonasal masses: developmental anatomy, malformations, and MR imaging. *Pediatr Radiol.* 2006;36:647-662.
Khanna G, Sato Y, Smith RJH, et al. Causes of facial swelling in pediatric patients: correlation of clinical and radiologic findings. *Radiographics.* 2006;26:157-171.

History

▶ 39-year-old man with left retro-orbital pain and periorbital edema. He has a remote history of closed head injury

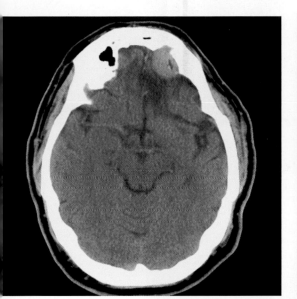
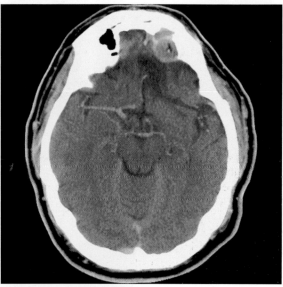
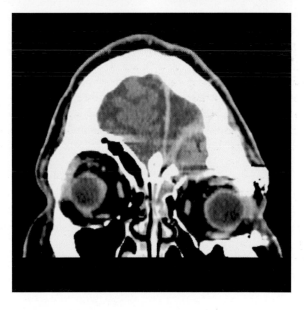

Case 163 Mucocele

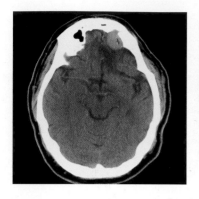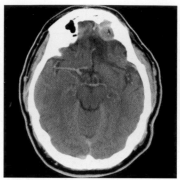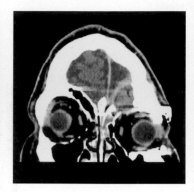

Findings

▶ Axial CT shows a high-attenuation, rim-enhancing, extra-axial mass in the left anterior cranial fossa.
▶ Coronal reformations show the mass to be in contiguity with a defect in the posterior wall of the left frontal sinus.
▶ There is left frontal lobe encephalomalacia. There is left orbital deformity consistent with old fractures.

Differential Diagnosis

▶ Pyogenic mucocele
▶ Sinonasal neoplasm
▶ Fungal sinusitis

Teaching Points

▶ Mucoceles are a benign but locally aggressive process in which a mucus-laden sac fills and expands a paranasal sinus.
▶ Mucoceles occur as result of sinus obstruction. While the cause is often unknown, they can result from prior trauma, surgery, or neoplasm.
▶ The frontal sinus is the most common site.
▶ CT will show an expanded sinus with remodeling of the sinus walls. The wall may be severely thinned or eroded. The contents have an attenuation of 10 to 18 HU but may be of higher attenuation as water content diminishes.
▶ On MRI, the contents have variable signal characteristics depending on water, protein, blood, and mineral content.
▶ On MRI, mucoceles show only thin peripheral enhancement, and this helps to distinguish them from enhancing neoplasms.

Management

▶ Surgical exenteration and obliteration of the involved sinus

Further Reading

Eggsbo HB. Radiological imaging of inflammatory lesions in the nasal cavity and paranasal sinuses. *Eur Radiol.* 2006;16:872-888.
Lloyd G, Lund VJ, Savy L, et al. Optimum imaging for mucoceles. *J Laryngol Otol.* 2000;114:233-236.

6-year-old with hearing loss in the left ear

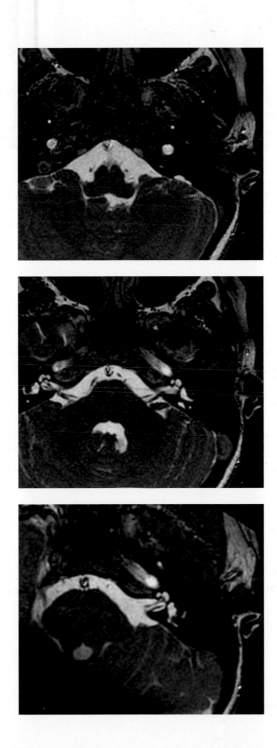

Case 164 Enlarged Vestibular Aqueduct Syndrome

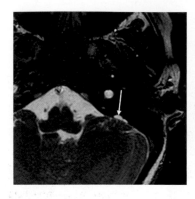 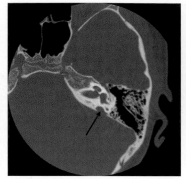 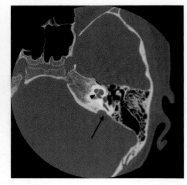

Findings

▶ 3D T2-weighted images demonstrate an enlarged endolymphatic sac and duct (white arrow).
▶ There is subtle asymmetry of the modiolus, which is deficient.
▶ CT images demonstrate an enlarged vestibular aqueduct (black arrow) and slightly dilated apical turn of the cochlea, with deficiency of the modiolus (arrowhead).
▶ The semicircular canals and vestibule are normal in appearance.

Differential Diagnosis

▶ Incomplete partition type II
▶ Incomplete partition type I

Teaching Points

▶ The vestibular aqueduct is considered enlarged when it measures more than 1.5 mm at the midpoint from the common crus and the external aperture.
▶ In this developmental abnormality, the enlarged aqueduct is usually accompanied by deficiency of the modiolus. It is the mildest form of the recognized cochlear dysplasias.
▶ The enlarged vestibular aqueduct syndrome is a common cause of hearing loss. Although the enlarged vestibular aqueduct syndrome is congenital, the hearing loss can present at any age.
▶ Enlarged vestibular aqueduct syndrome is associated with Pendred's syndrome. Pendred's syndrome is an autosomal recessive genetic disorder of the pendrin gene (chromosome 7q31), and affected individuals have enlarged vestibular aqueducts and goiter.

Management

▶ Patients are generally advised against playing contact sports as even minor head injury is thought to be able to precipitate hearing loss. Patients with enlarged vestibular aqueduct syndrome are offered testing for the pendrin gene. Cochlear implantation is beneficial in patients when hearing loss occurs.

Further Reading

Sennaroglu L, Saatci I. A new classification for cochleovestibular malformations. *Laryngoscope.* 2002;112:2230-2241.
Swartz JD, Mukherji SK. The inner ear and otodystrophies. In: Swartz JD, Loevner LA. *Imaging of the Temporal Bone*, 4th ed. New York Thieme, 2009:317-330.

History

▶ 15-year-old girl with prominent left skull since birth

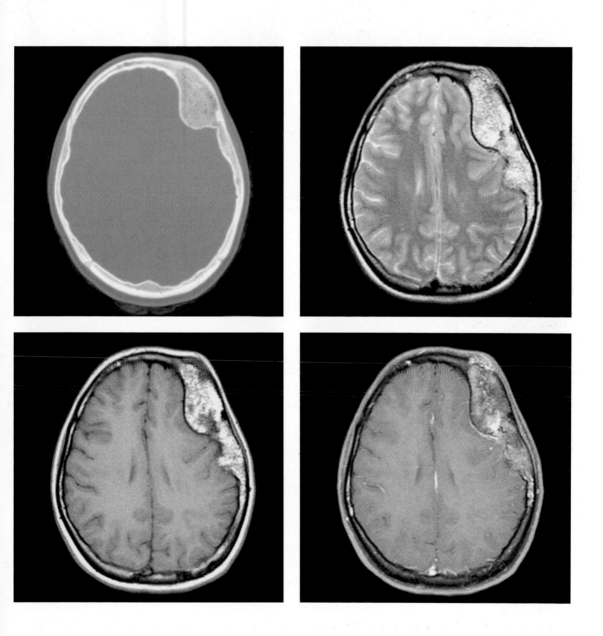

Case 165   Hemangioma of the Calvarium

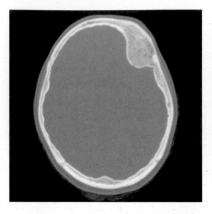 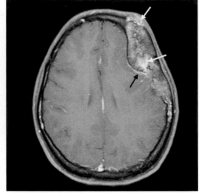

Findings

- CT demonstrates a well-defined intraosseous lesion involving the left frontal and parietal bones. It expands the diploic space. Internally, there is a characteristic trabecular pattern to the lesion.
- On MRI the lesion has predominantly high signal intensity on T2-weighted images. T1-weighted images show extensive fat within the lesion. There is heterogeneous enhancement. There is an enhancing soft tissue component to the lesion (white arrows) and accompanying dural enhancement (black arrow).

Differential Diagnosis

- Fibrous dysplasia
- Intraosseous meningioma

Teaching Points

- Osseous hemangiomas are benign, slow-growing tumors composed of vascular spaces lined by endothelium. After the vertebral bodies, the calvarium is the most common location. These lesions are generally painless and present incidentally or as palpable masses.
- Calvarial hemangiomas have a characteristic radiographic and CT appearance with a well-marginated lucent area containing radial ("sunburst") or web-like ("honeycomb") trabecular thickening.
- Lytic areas with extra-osseous extension may be present, most often in the outer table.
- These lesions, like other osseous hemangiomas, often contain a large proportion of fat. Presence of fat on the MR helps distinguish the hemangiomas from the other entities in the differential diagnosis.
- Calvarial hemangiomas are usually very vascular, so suggesting the diagnosis preoperatively can be helpful prior to surgical intervention.

Management

- Although these tumors can be watched, deformity and growth may necessitate removal. Hemangiomas are more vascular than other fibrovascular lesions of the skull, making complete removal the usual treatment (as opposed to simply recontouring the external surface of the skull).

Further Reading

Lloret I, Server A, Taksdal I. Calvarial lesions: A radiological approach to diagnosis. *Acta Radiologica*. 2009;50:531-542.
Politi M, Romeike BFM, Papanagiotou P, et al. Intraosseous hemangioma of the skull with dural tail sign: radiologic features with pathologic correlation. *AJNR Am J Neuroradiol*. 2005;26:2045-2052.

▶ 36-year-old woman with progressive facial nerve paralysis

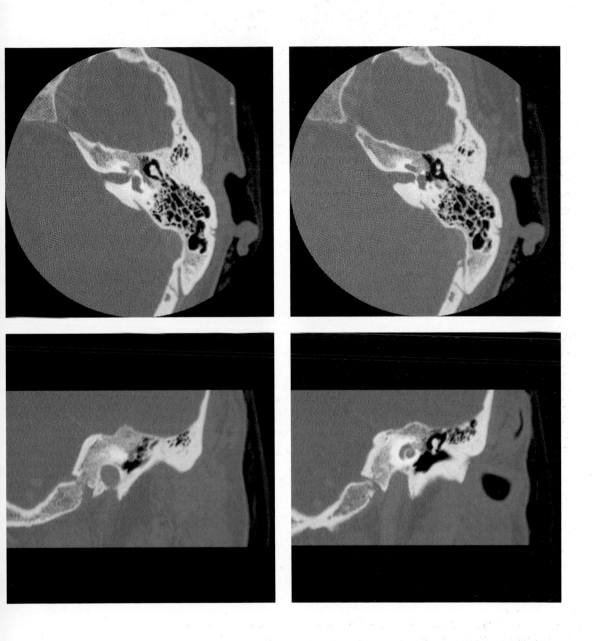

Case 166 Venous Vascular Malformation of the Facial Nerve (Ossifying Hemangioma of Temporal Bone)

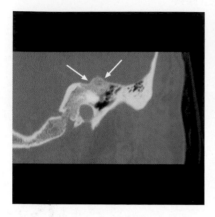 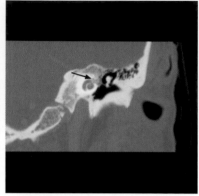

Findings

▸ There is a sharply marginated, calcified temporal bone lesion arising in the region of the geniculate ganglion that contains bone spicules (white arrows).

▸ The lesion also involves the cochlea (black arrow).

Differential Diagnosis

▸ Meningioma
▸ Fibrous dysplasia
▸ Facial nerve schwannoma

Teaching Points

▸ These venous malformations arise along the course of the facial nerve (most commonly at the geniculate ganglion). The lesions characteristically contain bone spicules, which are different from the amorphous or punctuate calcifications found in fibrous dysplasia or meningiomas.
▸ Slowly progressive facial nerve paralysis is the usual clinical presentation.
▸ At surgery, the lesion can usually be dissected from the facial nerve, unlike schwannomas.

Management

▸ Surgical removal is the usual treatment. This can often be accomplished without having to sacrifice the facial nerve.

Further Reading

Curtin HD, Jensen JE, Barnes L, et al. "Ossifying" hemangiomas of the temporal bone. *Radiology*. 1987;164:831-835.

History

▸ 10-year-old girl with incidental findings on a routine dental x-ray

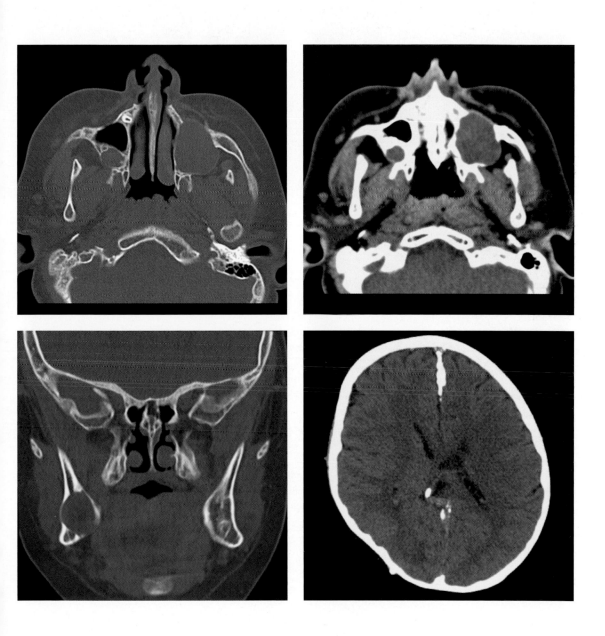

Case 167   Basal Cell Nevus Syndrome (Gorlin Syndrome)

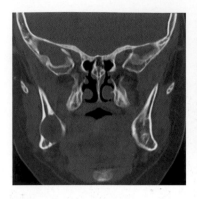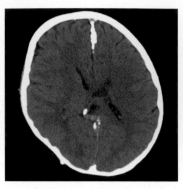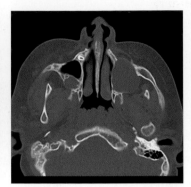

Findings

▶ CT scan images of the face demonstrate multiple expansile cyst-like lesions in the maxilla and mandible with smooth borders.

▶ Noncontrast CT of the head shows extensive dural calcifications, which is abnormal at this age.

Differential Diagnosis

▶ Nonsyndromic odontogenic keratocyst
▶ Dentigerous cysts
▶ Ameloblastoma
▶ Cherubism
▶ Giant cell tumor

Teaching Points

▶ Basal cell nevus syndrome (also known as Gorlin syndrome or nevoid basal cell carcinoma syndrome) is a syndrome due to mutations in the PTCH tumor suppressor gene, and manifests as multiple jaw cysts (odontogenic keratocysts), dural calcifications, and multiple basal cell carcinomas.

▶ Between 3% and 20% of basal cell nevus syndrome patients will have a medulloblastoma in the cerebellum. Other commonly associated features include fused or bifid ribs, kyphoscoliosis, macrocephaly, palmar/plantar pits, and ovarian fibromas.

▶ Patients may present with jaw pain, jaw deformity, or incidental findings on dental examination, or may even present with symptoms of medulloblastoma before the jaw abnormalities are discovered.

▶ Odontogenic keratocysts are expansile cysts in the jaws with scalloped borders. They may have areas of higher attenuation within them due to proteinaceous content or hemorrhage. They may displace or resorb the roots of the nearby teeth, and they may destroy the overlying bone. They may occur sporadically or in association with Gorlin syndrome.

Management

▶ Patients need periodic dermatologic screening and treatment for basal cell carcinoma. MRI examinations may be performed to assess for medulloblastoma or to assess perineural spread of aggressive basal cell carcinomas.

▶ The odontogenic keratocysts can be surgically excised, but there is a very high rate of recurrence and new cyst formation.

Further Reading

Kimonis VE, Mehta SG, Digiovanna JJ, et al. Radiological features in 82 patients with nevoid basal cell carcinoma (NBCC or Gorlin) syndrome. *Genet Med.* 2004;6:495-502.

Manfredi M, Vescovi P, Bonanini M, et al. Nevoid basal cell carcinoma syndrome: a review of the literature. *Int J Oral Maxillofac Surg.* 2004;33:117-124.

History

▶ 2-year-old boy with periorbital swelling and redness

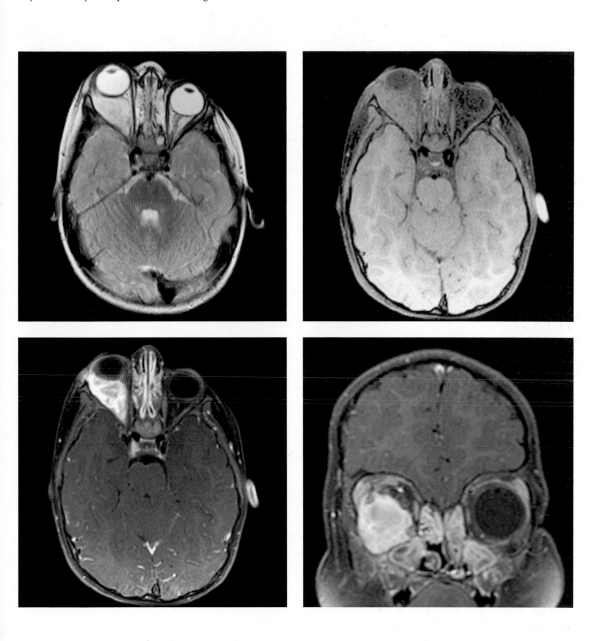

Case 168 Rhabdomyosarcoma

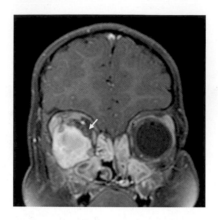

Findings

- ► There is a large, enhancing, intraorbital mass on the right, producing marked proptosis.
- ► It is hyperintense on T2-weighted images and iso-intense on T1-weighted images.
- ► The mass displaces the optic nerve medially (arrow).

Differential Diagnosis

- ► Optic glioma
- ► Lymphoma
- ► Metastasis (e.g., neuroblastoma)
- ► Langerhans cell histiocytosis

Teaching Points

- ► Rhabdomyosarcoma is a malignant neoplasm arising from primitive mesenchyme with a differentiation resembling that of striated muscle. It is the most common soft tissue sarcoma in children.
- ► It is divided into four subtypes based on histologic features: embryonal, botryoid, alveolar, and pleomorphic. Embryonal rhabdomyosarcoma is the most common form, especially in the head and neck.
- ► The most common sites in the head and neck are the orbit, nasopharynx, middle ear and mastoid, nasal cavity, and paranasal sinuses.
- ► Orbital rhabdomyosarcomas have an especially good prognosis, with a 94% 3-year survival for local disease. Involvement of parameningeal sites, such as the nasal cavity, paranasal sinuses, infratemporal fossa, nasopharynx, and middle ear, carries a worse prognosis, with 3-year survival of about 65%.
- ► At any site in the head and neck, these enhancing tumors are often rapidly growing and infiltrative, with a propensity for bone invasion (best demonstrated on CT) and spread through neural foramina (best demonstrated on MR).
- ► This diagnosis should be considered for any aggressive mass found in the common locations in a child.

Management

- ► Treatment consists of chemotherapy, radiation, and surgery.

Further Reading

Eskey CJ, Robson CD, Weber AL. Imaging of benign and malignant soft tissue tumors of the head and neck. *Radiol Clin North Am.* 2001;38:1091-1104.
Karcioglu ZA, Hadjistilianou D, Rozans M, et al. Orbital rhabdomyosarcoma. *Cancer Control.* 2004;11:328-333.

History

► 27-year-old woman with decreased vision in the left eye and pain behind the eye

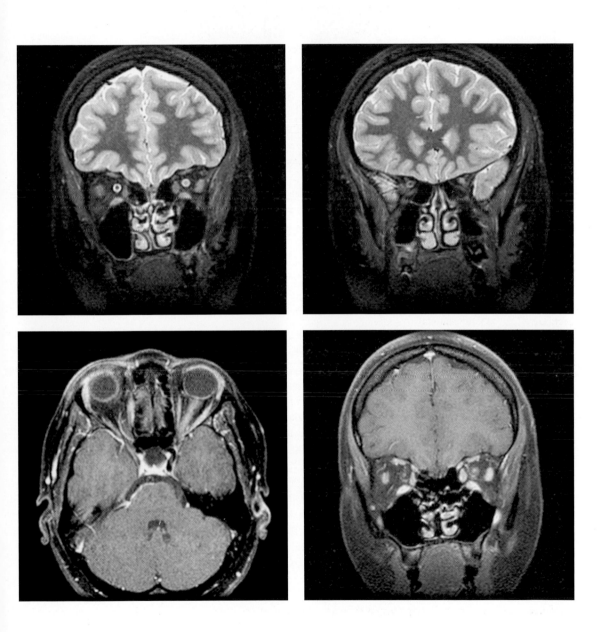

Case 169   Optic Neuritis

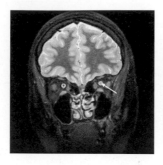 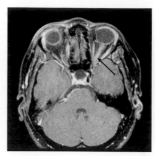

Findings

▶ On the coronal T2-weighted images, there is abnormal increased signal in the substance of the left optic nerve (white arrow).
▶ On postcontrast T1-weighted images, there is abnormal enhancement of the left optic nerve (black arrow).

Differential Diagnosis

▶ Other inflammatory optic nerve disease (Lyme disease, syphilis, varicella, sarcoid)
▶ Leukemia/lymphoma
▶ Optic glioma
▶ Ischemic optic neuropathy
▶ Radiation-induced optic neuropathy

Teaching Points

▶ Optic neuritis is a demyelinating disorder of the optic nerve. Patients present with vision loss and eye pain.
▶ Patients with typical signs and symptoms of optic neuritis do not need imaging of the orbits. If clinical features are atypical, orbit MRI (with 2- to 3-mm-thick coronal sections with fat suppression) is useful in excluding alternative pathology.
▶ Optic neuritis produces hyperintense signal within the optic nerve on T2-weighted images. In the acute phase, abnormal enhancement is also present. The optic nerve is little, if at all, enlarged.
▶ The primary role of MRI in optic neuritis is to evaluate the brain for the presence of white matter lesions. If one or more white matter lesions are present, 72% of patients develop multiple sclerosis (MS). If there are no white matter lesions, 25% develop MS.
▶ The imaging appearance of idiopathic optic neuritis caused by a primary demyelinating disorder can be indistinguishable from optic neuritis caused by other inflammatory or infectious etiologies.
▶ MS patients presenting with optic neuritis tend to have a better overall prognosis and a more benign course.
▶ Optic neuritis accompanied by acute transverse myelitis of the spinal cord is known as Devic's disease or neuromyelitis optica.

Management

▶ In the acute phase, intravenous steroids result in quicker recovery of vision and a decreased 2-year incidence of MS. Immunomodulatory therapy reduces the incidence of MS and active plaques.

Further Reading

Optic Neuritis Study Group. The 5-year risk of MS after optic neuritis: Experience of the Optic Neuritis Treatment Trial. *Neurology.* 1997;49:1404-1413.
Osbourne BJ, Volpe NJ. Optic neuritis and risk of MS: Differential diagnosis and management. *Cleveland Clin J Med.* 2009;76:181-190.
Ramsaransing GS, De Keyser J. Benign course in multiple sclerosis: a review. *Acta Neurol Scand.* 2006;113:359-369.

History

▶ 86-year-old man with rigors and ear pain

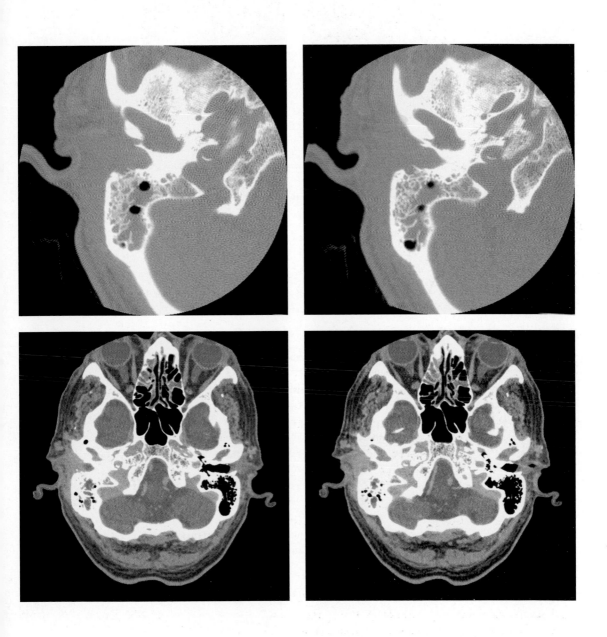

Case 170 Malignant Otitis Externa

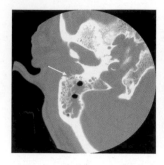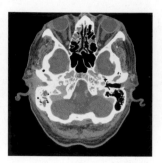

Findings

▶ There is marked soft tissue swelling in the right external auditory canal. Note the difference compared to the left external canal.

▶ There is subtle erosion of the osseous external auditory canal on the right (arrow), seen best on the high-resolution temporal bone CT.

▶ Fluid is present in the right mastoid.

▶ The sigmoid sinus enhances normally.

Differential Diagnosis

▶ Neoplasm involving the external auditory canal (e.g., squamous cell carcinoma or other skin cancer)

▶ Mastoiditis with secondary involvement of the external canal

Teaching Points

▶ Malignant otitis externa is a serious infection of the external auditory canal that usually occurs in diabetics or individuals with impaired immune systems.

▶ Clinically, patients present with severe otalgia and otorrhea.

▶ *Pseudomonas aeruginosa* is the most common organism cultured in malignant otitis externa, particularly in the diabetic population.

▶ From the external canal, infection can spread into the mastoid, skull base, dural sinuses, meninges, and brain.

▶ Cranial neuropathies can also develop. The facial nerve is the most commonly affected, followed by cranial nerves IX, X, and XI within the jugular foramen.

▶ High-resolution temporal bone CT is useful in confirming the diagnosis and in demonstrating erosion of the osseous margins of the external canal in malignant otitis externa. However, CT may not show bone erosion early in the disease process.

▶ If CT is equivocal, bone scan can be helpful in identifying the bone involvement.

▶ MRI is useful to demonstrate cranial nerve involvement and intracranial extension.

Management

▶ Malignant otitis externa is treated with a combination of long-term intravenous antibiotics, topical antibiotics, and local cleaning/débridement.

Further Reading

Castillo M, Jewells VL, Buchman C. The external auditory canal and pinna. In: Swartz JD, Loevner LA. *Imaging of the Temporal Bone*, 4th ed. New York: Thieme, 2009:36-37.

Sudhoff H, Rajagopal S, Mani N, Moumoulidis I, et al. Usefulness of CT scans in malignant external otitis: effective tool for the diagnosis, but of limited value in predicting outcome. *Eur Arch Otorhinolaryngol.* 2008;265:53-56.

History

▶ 7-year-old boy with decreased vision

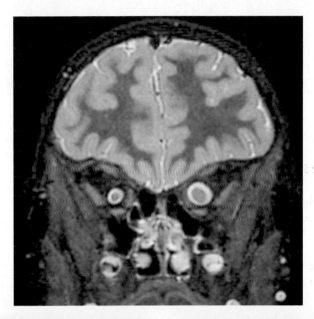

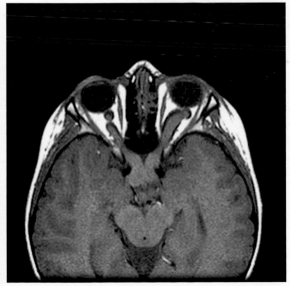

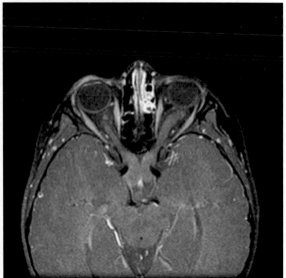

Case 171 Optic Glioma

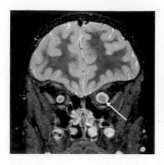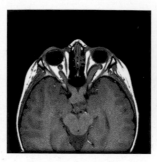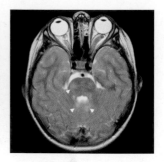

Findings

- ▶ MRI shows abnormal, fusiform enlargement of the left optic nerve, optic chiasm, optic tracts, and the intracranial right optic nerve. The coronal STIR image best shows the left optic nerve enlargement (white arrow).
- ▶ There is no enhancement of the optic nerves.
- ▶ Axial T2-weighted image of the brain shows hyperintense signal in the deep cerebellum and right pons, consistent with hamartomatous changes common in neurofibromatosis type 1 (arrowheads).

Differential Diagnosis

- ▶ Optic nerve sheath meningioma
- ▶ Optic neuritis (atypical)

Teaching Points

- ▶ Optic gliomas are astrocytomas of the optic nerve. When associated with neurofibromatosis type 1 (NF-1), they are almost always pilocytic astrocytomas. When not associated with NF-1, they may be pilocytic or fibrillary astrocytomas.
- ▶ Optic gliomas can occur anywhere along the visual pathways, from the optic nerve to the optic tracts.
- ▶ Optic gliomas are found in 15% to 20% of patients who have NF-1. 30% to 40% of patients with optic glioma have NF-1.
- ▶ Optic gliomas associated with NF-1 tend to have a less aggressive course, and spontaneous regression can occur with no treatment.
- ▶ Optic gliomas have a varied imaging appearance. The tumors can demonstrate intense enhancement, focal enhancement, or no enhancement. Cystic areas may be present.
- ▶ Calcification is rare in optic gliomas, and it helps to distinguish them from optic nerve sheath meningiomas.
- ▶ "Kinking" of the optic nerve is commonly seen in optic gliomas but is not a specific finding. A kinked optic nerve without enlargement of the nerve should not be used to make a diagnosis of optic glioma.

Management

- ▶ Optic glioma is a presumptive diagnosis in patients with NF-1 and optic nerve enlargement, and no biopsy is needed. Treatment is delayed as long as possible because of the good prognosis, indolent course, and frequent spontaneous regression.
- ▶ For patients without NF-1, biopsy is typically required to confirm the diagnosis. Surgical debulking, radiation, and/or chemotherapy are used for treatment. Chemotherapy is used to delay radiation therapy in younger patients.

Further Reading

Listernick R, Ferner RE, Liu GT, et al. Optic pathway glioma in neurofibromatosis-1: controversies and recommendations. *Ann Neurol.* 2007;61:189-198.

Zimmerman RA, Bilaniuk LT, Savino PJ. Visual pathways. In: Som PM, Curtin HD. *Head and Neck Imaging*, 4th ed. Philadelphia: Mosby, 2003:742-744.

History

▶ 55-year-old man with left cheek numbness. He has a history of squamous cell carcinoma of the left cheek removed eight months earlier

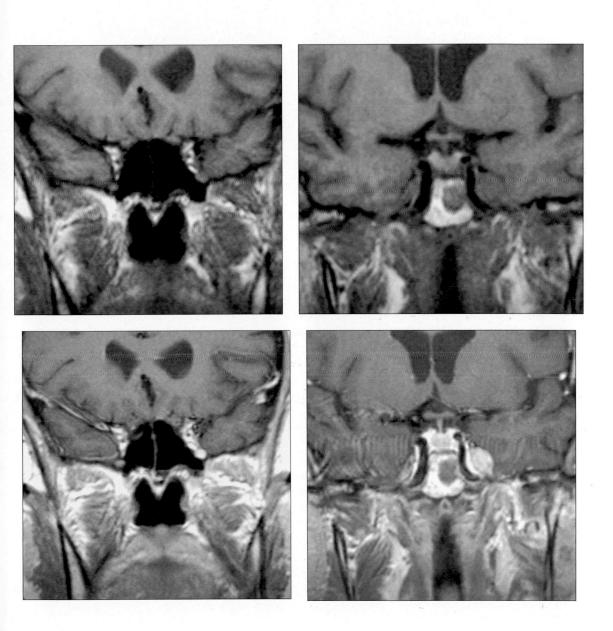

Case 172 Perineural Spread of Neoplasm (Squamous Cell Cancer)

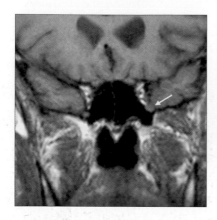 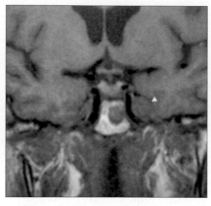

Findings

▶ Coronal T1-weighted MRI shows abnormal enlargement and enhancement of the left second division of the trigeminal nerve within the foramen rotundum (arrow).

▶ There is soft tissue filling a portion of Meckel's cave (arrowhead).

Differential Diagnosis

▶ Nerve sheath tumor

▶ Inflammatory neuropathy

Teaching Points

▶ Head and neck neoplasms have a distinct propensity for perineural spread. Squamous cell carcinoma, basal cell carcinoma, adenoid cystic carcinoma, and mucoepidermoid carcinoma all frequently display this biologic behavior.

▶ The trigeminal nerve and facial nerves are the most frequently involved. Tumor can spread both anterograde toward the face and retrograde toward the brain stem.

▶ Perineural spread of tumor can be asymptomatic and thus must be actively searched for in patients with head and neck tumors.

▶ The new onset of facial weakness or numbness in patient with a head and neck neoplasm should prompt a detailed evaluation for perineural tumor spread.

▶ Evaluation for perineural spread of tumor is best done with MRI and should include thin, high-resolution images that cover the entire course of the nerve in question, from the face to the brain stem.

▶ Imaging features of perineural spread of tumor include abnormal enlargement of the nerve, erosion or widening of the foramina, loss of fat planes around nerves, and abnormal enhancement of the nerve. Denervation atrophy of muscles supplied by the involved nerve can also be identified on imaging studies.

Management

▶ Perineural spread of tumor is a poor prognostic sign. Aggressive surgical resection of the involved nerve and postoperative radiation can be performed. Definitive treatment guidelines have not been established.

Further Reading

Ginsberg LE. Imaging of perineural tumor spread in head and neck cancer. In: Som PM, Curtin HD. *Head and Neck Imaging*, 4th ed. Philadelphia: Mosby, 2003:865-885.

Mendenhall WM, Amdur RJ, Williams LS, et al. Carcinoma of the skin of the head and neck with perineural invasion. *Head Neck*. 2002;24:78-83.

History

▶ 5-year-old boy with leukocoria and strabismus

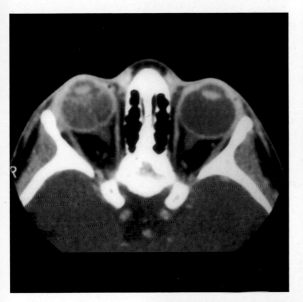
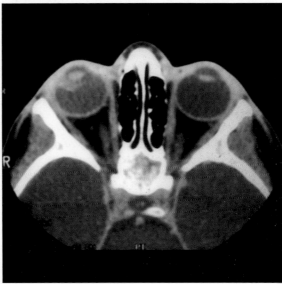
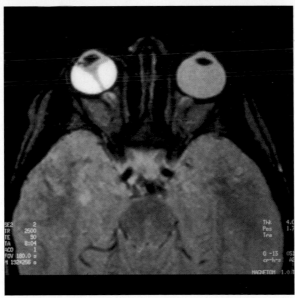

Case 173 Persistent Hyperplastic Primary Vitreous (PHPV)

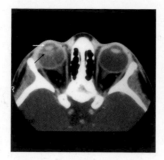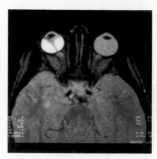

Findings

► Axial CT images demonstrate abnormal increased density of the vitreous humor in the right eye, with a more focal region of soft tissue attenuation immediately posterior to the lens (black arrow).

► The abnormal material extends as a band from the posterior lens to the optic nerve head.

► The right eye is slightly smaller than the left, and the anterior chamber is shallow (white arrow).

► These findings are also well seen on the proton-density MRI image.

Differential Diagnosis

► The imaging appearance is diagnostic of PHPV. The differential diagnosis for leukocoria is:
  ▪ Retinoblastoma
  ▪ Chronic retinal detachment
  ▪ Coats' disease
  ▪ Toxocariasis
  ▪ Retinopathy of prematurity

Teaching Points

► PHPV is a developmental anomaly of the eye in which there is failure of the primary vitreous to regress. The result is abnormal soft tissue along the canal that extends from the lens to the optic nerve head (Cloquet's canal).

► PHPV is the second most common cause of leukocoria after retinoblastoma.

► Imaging features include:
  ▪ A small eye (microphthalmia)
  ▪ Shallow anterior chamber
  ▪ Abnormal soft tissue behind the lens (retrolental mass)
  ▪ Funnel-shaped soft tissue that extends from the lens to the optic nerve head
  ▪ Hyperintense vitreous on T1-weighted MR
  ▪ Fluid–fluid levels in the vitreous

► The majority of retinoblastomas will contain calcification, which is lacking in PHPV. The smaller size of the affected eye and characteristic tissue extending from the lens to the optic nerve head also suggest PHPV as the diagnosis.

► Rarely, PHPV is bilateral. In these cases, there is often an underlying retinal dysplasia.

Management

► Treatment consists of removal of the cataractous lens and any abnormal vascular/fibrotic tissue in the eye. With treatment, many patients are now able to gain functional vision in the affected eye.

Further Reading

Mafee MF. The Eye. In: Som PM, Curtin HD. *Head and Neck Imaging*, 4th ed. Philadlephia: Mosby, 2003:484-491.

Schulz E, Griffiths B. Long-term visual function and relative amblyopia in posterior persistent hyperplastic primary vitreous (PHPV). *Strabismus*. 2006;14:121-125.

Images reprinted from Belden CJ. MR Imaging of the Globe and Optic Nerve. Magnetic Resonance Imaging Clinics of North America 2002;10(4):663-678, with permission from Elsevier.

History

► 73-year-old man with enlarging anterior neck mass after subtotal thyroidectomy

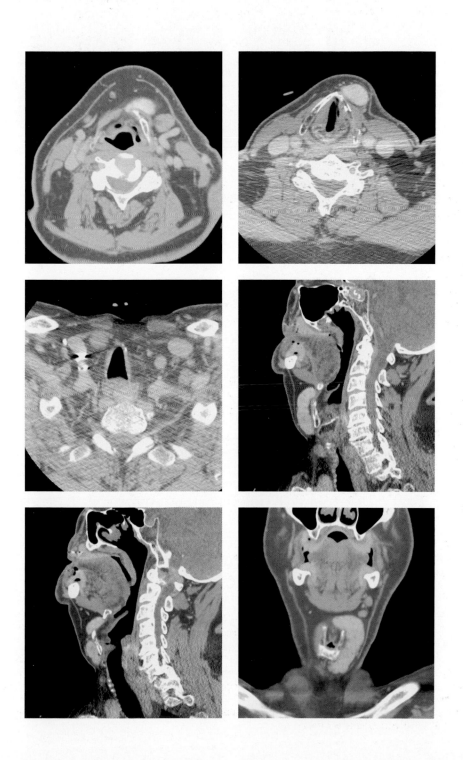

Case 174 Ectopic Thyroid

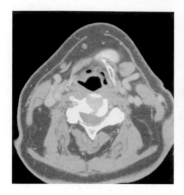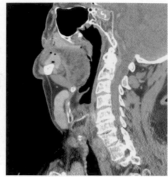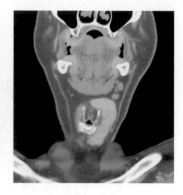

Findings

- ▶ A well-defined enhancing mass extends from the inferior hyoid to the cricothyroid junction.
- ▶ The mass is predominantly to the left of midline and overlies the strap muscles.
- ▶ The thyroid gland is absent.

Differential Diagnosis

- ▶ Thyroid carcinoma
- ▶ Vascular malformation (e.g., hemangioma, venous vascular malformation)

Teaching Points

- ▶ Embryologically, the thyroid stalk connects the foramen cecum in the tongue base to the aortic arch. Thyroid tissue moves down the stalk until it reaches the region in front of the trachea in the seventh week.
- ▶ Ectopic thyroid tissue can be found along this track in up to 10% of adults, but most rests are small and of no clinical significance.
- ▶ The most common site for ectopic thyroid is in the tongue base, and frequently in this location the ectopic tissue is the only functioning thyroid tissue. Prior to removal of a high-density tongue base mass, a search should be made to be sure it is not the patient's only functioning thyroid tissue.
- ▶ When ectopic thyroid is in the neck, it is commonly near or just off midline, and it may extend to the hyoid bone in the midline (as in this case).
- ▶ The diagnosis is easier to make on CT than MRI because of the high attenuation of the gland.
- ▶ Carcinoma can arise in ectopic thyroid tissue. The ectopic tissue can also increase in size after thyroidectomy, if the patient develops goiter, or at puberty.

Management

- ▶ Ectopic thyroid tissue does not need to be treated unless symptomatic.
- ▶ If symptoms arise from a lingual thyroid, either surgical excision or iodine-131 ablation can be performed.
- ▶ Cervical transplantation of thyroid tissue is an option for patients with lingual thyroid as their only functioning thyroid tissue.

Further Reading

Mussak EN, Kacker A. Surgical and medical management of midline ectopic thyroid. *Otolaryngol Head Neck Surg.* 2007;136:870-872.
Som PM, Smoker WRK, Curtin WD, Reidenberg JS, Laitman J. Congenital lesions. In: Som PM, Curtin HD. *Head and Neck Imaging,* 4th ed. Philadelphia: Mosby, 2003:1840-1847.

History

▶ 64-year-old man with red middle ear mass

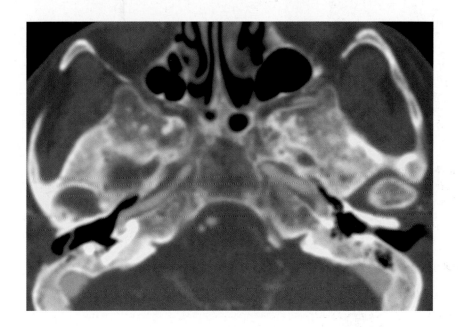

Case 175 Aberrant Internal Carotid Artery

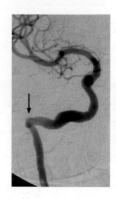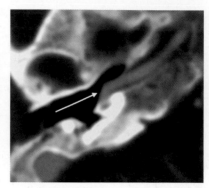

Findings

▶ CT angiography demonstrates a vessel that travels anteriorly within the medial aspect of the right middle ear cavity (white arrow). There is absence of the bony plate that normally separates the petrous internal carotid artery (ICA) from the tympanic cavity.

▶ On digital subtraction angiography, the course of the distal right cervical ICA is more lateral than normal, with a "reverse 7" appearance (black arrow). The caliber of the distal cervical and petrous ICA is smaller than normal.

Differential Diagnosis

▶ While the imaging appearance is diagnostic of this entity, differential diagnosis for a pulsatile red middle ear mass includes:
  ▪ Glomus tympanicum
  ▪ Dehiscent jugular bulb

Teaching Points

▶ The aberrant ICA is a rare vascular variant resulting from agenesis of the distal cervical ICA.

▶ There is compensatory enlargement of the inferior tympanic branch of the ascending pharyngeal artery, which is often taken to be the cervical ICA. With cervical ICA agenesis, enlarged inferior tympanic and caroticotympanic arteries reconstitute the proximal petrous ICA within the middle ear.

▶ The aberrant ICA is usually asymptomatic and found incidentally on imaging performed for other reasons. Occasionally, it may produce pulsatile tinnitus or hearing loss or is found on otoscopy as a pulsatile retrotympanic mass.

▶ The abnormal course of the artery may be seen with noncontrast skull base CT or CT angiography.

▶ Catheter angiography is no longer needed to establish the diagnosis. The AP view demonstrates a more lateral course at the skull base and the lateral view a more posterior course than expected.

▶ Aberrant ICA is associated with a persistent stapedial artery in one third of cases.

Management

▶ Middle ear surgery for a presumed paraganglioma, without preoperative recognition of this variant, carries a risk of catastrophic hemorrhage.

Further Reading

Lo WW, Solti-Bohman LG, McElveen JT, Jr. Aberrant carotid artery: Radiologic diagnosis with emphasis on high-resolution computed tomography. *Radiographics.* 1985;5:985-993.
Windfuhr JP. Aberrant internal carotid artery in the middle ear. *Ann Otol Rhinol Laryngol Suppl.* 2004;192:1-16.

History

▶ 6-year-old with congenital aural atresia

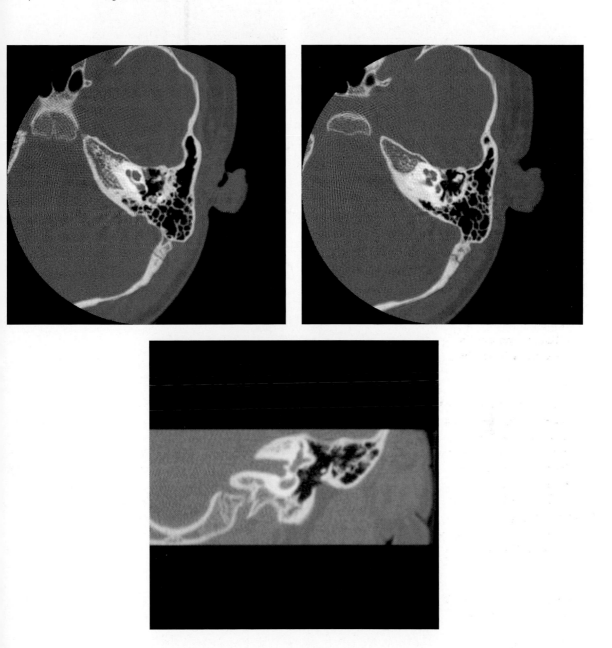

Case 176 External Auditory Canal Atresia

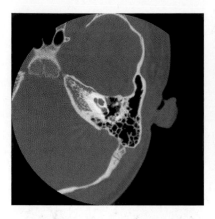 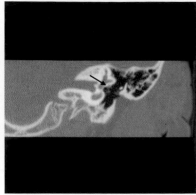

Findings

▶ There is membranous external canal atresia with a narrowed tympanic annulus, best seen on the coronal image.
▶ The middle ear is well pneumatized.
▶ There is abnormal fusion of the malleus and incus, confirmed at surgery.
▶ The facial nerve is in a normal anatomic position (arrow).

Differential Diagnosis

▶ The images are diagnostic for external canal atresia.

Teaching Points

▶ The external auditory canal (EAC) arises from portions of the first and second branchial arches. EAC atresia and stenosis is commonly seen with microtia, with more severe atresia associated with more severe microtia.
▶ When describing EAC atresia, it is important to note the size of the middle ear and mastoid, position of the facial nerve, whether the atresia is bony or membranous, and ossicular anomalies.
▶ Ossicular abnormalities occur in 54% of patients with EAC atresia.
▶ Cholesteatomas can occur in patients with EAC atresia.

Management

▶ Surgical repair of the atresia (atresiaplasty) is performed by drilling out the temporal bone, forming a new EAC. A tympanic membrane is created from temporalis fascia and the ossicles are freed from the atresia plate, if adherent. Overall, when there are favorable anatomic features, the surgery is successful in 75% of patients. If repair is not performed, due to either an aberrant facial nerve or small middle ear cavity, an osseointegrated cochlear stimulator can be used.

Further Reading

Castillo M, Jewells VL, Buchman C. The external auditory canal and pinna. In: Swartz JD, Loevner LA. *Imaging of the Temporal Bone*, 4th ed. New York: Thieme, 2009:27-33.

History

▶ 18-month-old with speech difficulty and floor of mouth mass

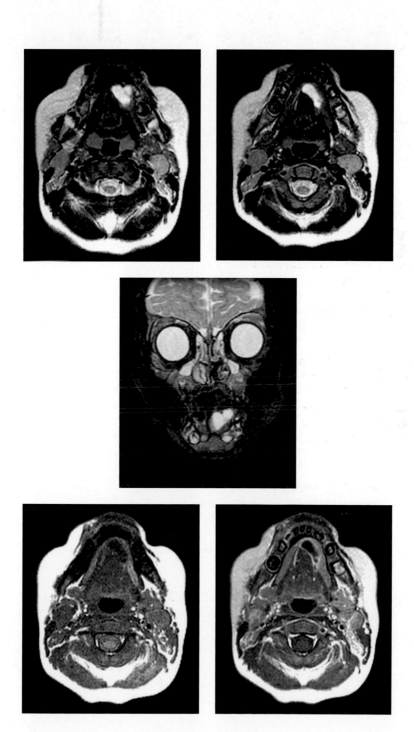

Case 177 Ranula, Simple

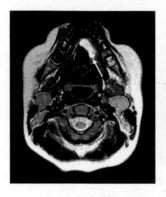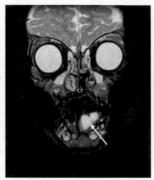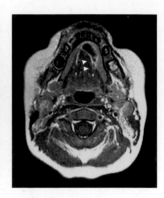

Findings

- There is a well-defined mass within the left sublingual space (arrows) that extends to the midline anteriorly. Note that the collection is lateral to the genioglossus muscle (arrowheads).
- On T1- and T2-weighted images the mass has internal signal characteristics similar to those of CSF. There is a thin rim of enhancement, shown on the postcontrast axial T1-weighted image.
- There is no extension into the submandibular space, best demonstrated on the coronal STIR sequence.

Differential Diagnosis

- Epidermoid or dermoid
- Lymphangioma
- Abscess

Teaching Points

- A ranula is a mucous retention cyst that involves the sublingual salivary gland.
- Most commonly, a ranula presents as a unilocular cyst involving the sublingual space, lateral to the genioglossus muscle.
- A ranula that extends through or over the posterior free edge of the mylohyoid muscle is termed a "plunging" or "diving" ranula.
  - Plunging ranulas form when a simple ranula (which has a true epithelial lining) ruptures, forming a mucocele that is rapidly contained by an inflammatory response.
  - These can present as masses in the submandibular space.
- Ranulas can look identical to epidermoids in the sublingual space. Dermoids should have demonstrable fat by imaging.
- The presence of multiple loculations or fluid–fluid levels would suggest a lymphangioma rather than a ranula.

Management

- The treatment for ranulas is transoral surgical removal of the sublingual gland and evacuation of the ranula on the affected side. This approach is used for both simple and plunging ranulas, and there is a low incidence of recurrence (<3%).

Further Reading

Patel MR, Deal AM, Shockley WW. Oral and plunging ranulas: What is the most effective treatment? *Laryngoscope.* 2009;119:1501-1509.
Som PM, Brandwein MS. Salivary glands: anatomy and pathology. In: Som PM, Curtin HD. *Head and Neck Imaging*, 4th ed. Philadlephia: Mosby, 2003:2063-2066.

History

▶ 53-year-old woman with proptosis and decreased vision in the right eye

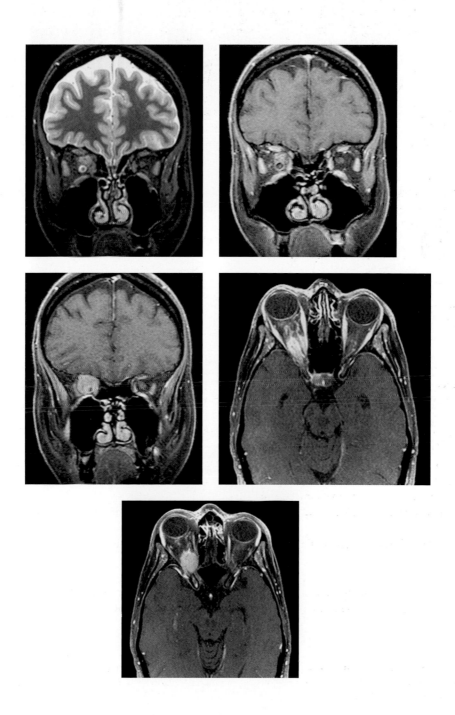

Case 178   Optic Nerve Sheath Meningioma

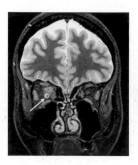 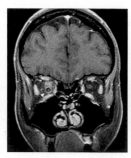 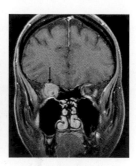

Findings

▶ There is a mass surrounding the right optic nerve that causes mild proptosis.
▶ Coronal post-gadolinium, fat-suppressed T1 images demonstrate circumferential enhancement around the optic nerve (arrowhead). The right optic nerve can be identified as a structure separate from the mass (white arrow).
▶ The mass is iso-intense to muscle on coronal STIR images and demonstrates uniform enhancement (black arrow).
▶ The optic sheath between the globe and tumor is dilated.

Differential Diagnosis

▶ Optic glioma
▶ Inflammatory pseudotumor
▶ Lymphoma
▶ Metastasis

Teaching Points

▶ Meningiomas of the optic nerve typically present with painless proptosis and unilateral decrease in vision. There is a 4:1 female:male predominance.
▶ Optic nerve sheath meningiomas should be searched for in any patient presenting with unilateral vision loss, optic atrophy or disc pallor, or low-tension glaucoma.
▶ An intraconal orbital mass that surrounds or partially surrounds the optic nerve is a common appearance and is usually readily apparent on CT or MR imaging.
▶ Some optic nerve meningiomas are thin, circumferential tumors and have a "tram-track" appearance on CT or MRI. This variation can be difficult to distinguish from inflammatory disease of the optic nerve sheath (e.g., sarcoidosis and Wegener's granulomatosis).
▶ On CT, up to 50% of optic nerve sheath meningiomas have calcification. Widening of the optic canal and adjacent bony hyperostosis may be present.
▶ Optic nerve sheath meningiomas are optimally imaged with MRI using thin, high-resolution T1-weighted, fat-suppressed T2-weighted, and fat-suppressed postcontrast T1-weighted images.

Management

▶ Stereotactic radiation is the treatment that is most likely to result in preservation of functional vision, and is the preferred therapy if useful vision remains. Surgery is used if vision is poor, to address intracranial tumor extension, or for biopsy if the diagnosis is in question.

Further Reading

Turbin RE, Thompson CR, Kennerdell JS, et al. A long-term visual outcome comparison in patients with optic nerve sheath meningioma managed with observation, surgery, radiotherapy, or surgery. *Ophthalmology.* 2002;109:890-899.
Zimmerman RA, Bilaniuk LT, Savino PJ. Visual pathways. In: Som PM, Curtin HD. *Head and Neck Imaging*, 4th ed. Philadelphia: Mosby, 2003:744-746.

History

▸ 14-month-old girl with neck swelling for 2 months

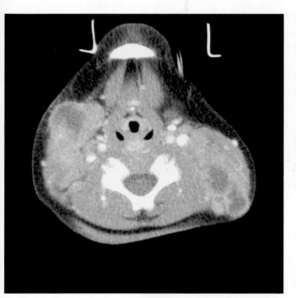
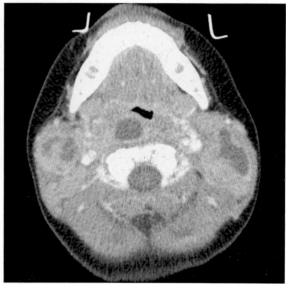

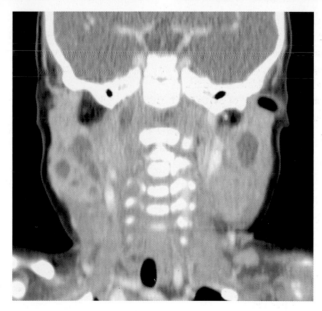

Case 179 Inflammatory Adenitis, Mycobacterium Avium Complex

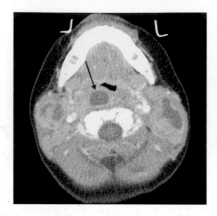 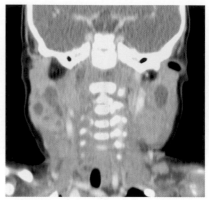

Findings

- ▶ There are several rim-enhancing, thick-walled, low-attenuation fluid collections in the neck bilaterally, including the retropharyngeal space (arrow).
- ▶ The lesions lie along major lymph node chains.
- ▶ There is minimal reticulation in the surrounding fat, and there are none of the typical inflammatory features seen in pyogenic adenitis.

Differential Diagnosis

- ▶ Other bacterial or fungal lymphadenitis
- ▶ Partially treated suppurative adenitis
- ▶ Cystic neoplasm (e.g., squamous cell carcinoma)

Teaching Points

- ▶ Adenitis caused by atypical mycobacterium can occur in young children with no evidence of prior or currently active tuberculous infection. Children with atypical mycobacterium infection often have normal immune systems. Standard PPD testing is positive in 50% or less.
- ▶ Painless adenopathy with a lack of associated inflammatory findings is the typical history.
- ▶ Lymph nodes vary in appearance, from centrally necrotic with thick, enhancing rims to simple lymph node enlargement without abnormal enhancement.
- ▶ The presence of superimposed inflammatory changes suggests bacterial superinfection or fistula formation.
- ▶ Calcification can occur in affected lymph nodes.
- ▶ In adults, the imaging appearance of atypical inflammatory adenitis is difficult to differentiate from necrotic lymphadenopathy related to metastatic squamous cell cancer.

Management

- ▶ Treatment of atypical mycobacterial lymphadenitis can be difficult. Surgical removal of the affected lymph nodes is generally performed, and has a better cosmetic result than incision and drainage. Antibiotic treatment with multiple agents, sometimes up to 6 months, may be necessary for complete treatment.

Further Reading

Som PM, Brandein MS. Lymph nodes. In: Som PM, Curtin HD. *Head and Neck Imaging*, 4th ed. Philadelphia: Mosby, 2003:1893-1894.
Wolinsky E. Mycobacterial lymphadenitis in children: a prospective study of 105 nontuberculous cases with long-term follow-up. *Clin Infect Dis.* 1995;20:954-963.

History

▶ 74-year-old woman with red mass behind eardrum, hearing loss, and pulsatile tinnitus

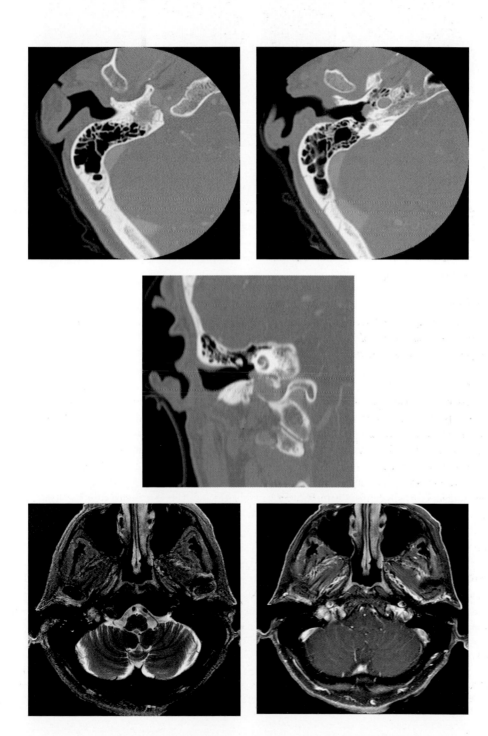

Case 180 Glomus Jugulotympanicum

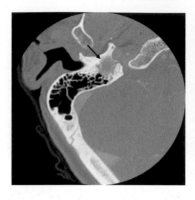 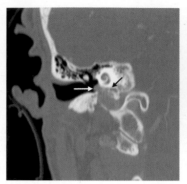 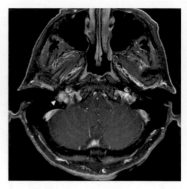

Findings

- Axial CT images through the temporal bone demonstrate bone erosion around the jugular foramen (black arrow).
- There is a small mass in the hypotympanum (white arrow). The carotid canal is separate from the lesion.
- MR images demonstrate a mass in the jugular foramen and middle ear (arrowhead). Tiny flow voids can be seen in the lesion on the precontrast T1- and T2-weighted images.

Differential Diagnosis

- Glomus tympanicum
- Aberrant carotid artery
- Meningioma of jugular foramen
- Schwannoma of jugular foramen
- Pseudolesion (normal jugular bulb)

Teaching Points

- Glomus jugulotympanicum tumors are paragangliomas that arise from small clusters of neuroendocrine cells along the nerves of Arnold and Jacobson in the middle ear and adjacent to the jugular fossa.
- They often present with pulsatile tinnitus. On otoscopy, a red mass is visible in the middle ear.
- Glomus jugulotympanicum tumors are benign neoplasms but are often locally aggressive and produce a permeative pattern of bone destruction around the jugular foramen.
- It is important to distinguish a glomus jugulotympanicum from simple glomus tympanicum since the surgical approach is different. When the mass is limited to the middle ear and there is an intact osseous plate at the lateral aspect of the jugular foramen, it is a glomus tympanicum. When the mass involves the jugular plate and foramen, it represents a glomus jugulotympanicum.

Management

- Small simple glomus tympanicum tumors may be removed using a transtympanic approach without embolization. Glomus jugulotympanicum tumors require a skull base resection, often with preoperative embolization. Larger lesions may require a partial resection with postoperative radiotherapy. Radiotherapy can also be used as a palliative measure for older patients.

Further Reading

Moonis G, Kim A, Bigelow D, et al. Temporal bone vascular anatomy, anomalies, and disease, with an emphasis on pulsatile tinnitus. In: Swartz JD, Loevner LA. *Imaging of the Temporal Bone*, 4th ed. New York: Thieme, 2009:276-286.
Remley KB, Coit WE, Harnesberger HR, et al. Pulsatile tinnitus and the vascular tympanic membrane: CT, MR, and angiographic findings. *Radiology.* 1990;174:383-389.

History

▶ 65-year-old man with nasal congestion

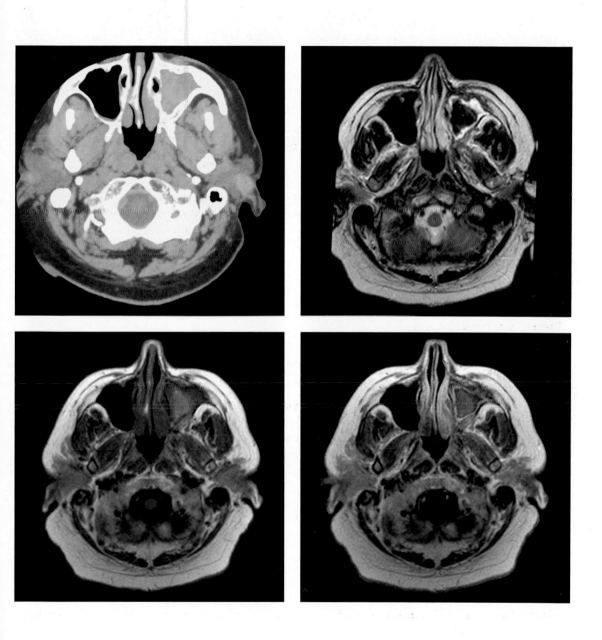

Case 181 Allergic Fungal Sinusitis

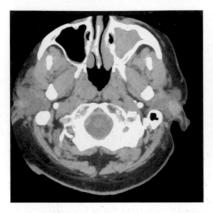 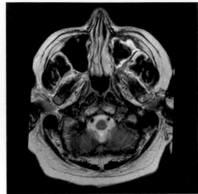

Findings

▶ CT demonstrates complete opacification of the left maxillary sinus by heterogeneous high-attenuation material. There is marked thickening of the sinus walls.

▶ On MR imaging the material centrally within the sinus is markedly hypointense on T2-weighted images and hyperintense on T1-weighted images.

▶ There is peripheral sinus enhancement, but the bulk of the material is non-enhancing.

Differential Diagnosis

▶ Chronic sinusitis with inspissated secretions

▶ Fungal mycetoma

▶ Trauma and sinonasal blood

Teaching Points

▶ Allergic fungal sinusitis is a chronic inflammatory condition characterized by a hypersensitivity reaction to colonization of the sinus by fungi, often *Aspergillus*.

▶ Patients are usually immunocompetent adults who present with nasal congestion, headache, or nasal discharge.

▶ CT of the sinuses is marked by sinus opacification with high-attenuation material or frank calcification. As with any chronic inflammatory condition, there is reactive thickening and sclerosis of sinus walls.

▶ MRI is warranted when a more invasive process is suspected. MRI has superior ability to detect intracranial, orbital, and other soft tissue extension.

▶ T2-weighted images may deceptively show absence of signal within the sinus due to the high mineral content (calcium, iron, manganese) and low water content of the material. Signal on T1-weighted images is heterogeneous and variably hyper- to hypointense.

▶ While the peripheral sinus mucosa may enhance, the material is largely nonenhancing.

▶ Fungal mycetoma may have a similar imaging appearance but is often a more focal process involving only one sinus.

Management

▶ Treatment consists of endoscopic sinus surgery with removal of the colonized material. Intranasal steroids may help prevent recurrence.

Further Reading

Aribandi M, McCoy VA, Bazan C. Imaging features of invasive and noninvasive fungal sinusitis: A review. *Radiographics*. 2007;27: 1283-1296.

Mafee MF. Imaging of rhinosinusitis and its complications. *Clin Rev Allergy Immunol*. 2006;30:165-186.

History

▶ 12-month-old boy with leukocoria

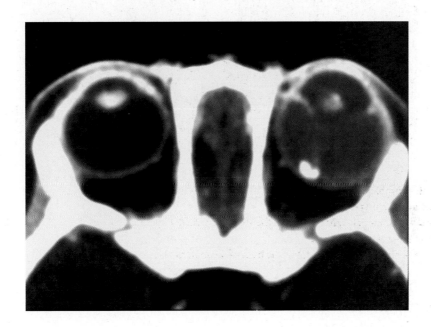

Case 182 Retinoblastoma

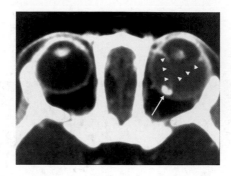

Findings

► Axial CT demonstrates a calcified mass in the left globe (arrow).
► There is an accompanying retinal detachment (arrowheads).
► The globes are of similar sizes.

Differential Diagnosis

► Toxocariasis
► Astrocytic hamartoma
► Persistent hyperplastic primary vitreous (PHPV)

Teaching Points

► Retinoblastoma is a malignant neoplasm of neuroectodermal origin. The average age of diagnosis is 13 months of age, and 90% of patients are under 5 years old.
► It is the most common cause of leukocoria, and patients with retinoblastoma generally present with either leukocoria and/or strabismus.
► The retinoblastoma gene is on chromosome 13q14 (Rb1).
  ▪ Retinoblastoma can be sporadic (two thirds) or inherited (one third).
  ▪ When inherited, the inheritance is autosomal dominant, and 85% of patients will have bilateral retinoblastoma.
  ▪ Patients with familial retinoblastoma have a strong propensity to develop second primary tumors, both inside and outside of the radiation field (up to 50% at 20 years, and 90% at 30 years).
► Calcification occurs in over 90% of retinoblastomas. A calcified ocular mass in a patient under 3 years of age should be considered to be a retinoblastoma until proven otherwise.
► Trilateral and tetralateral retinoblastoma (bilateral retinoblastoma along with retinoblastoma occurring ectopically in the pineal or suprasellar region) can be seen in familial retinoblastoma.
► Retinoblastomas that are confined to the globe have a good overall prognosis, whereas those that extend outside of the globe have nearly 100% 5-year mortality.

Management

► Unilateral retinoblastoma, particularly if small, is now often managed with the goal of salvaging some useful vision in the affected eye. Very small lesions can be treated with local therapy (often laser or cryotherapy).
► Chemotherapy with two or three agents is used for larger lesions.
► Advanced lesions may still require enucleation.

Further Reading

Lin P, O'Brien JM. Frontiers in the management of retinoblastoma. *Am J Ophthalmol.* 2009;148:192-198.
Mafee MF. The eye. In: Som PM, Curtin HD. *Head and Neck Imaging*, 4th ed. Philadelphia: Mosby, 2003:477-484.

History

▶ 33-year-old woman with right shoulder pain and weakness in her right arm that have worsened over last 3 months

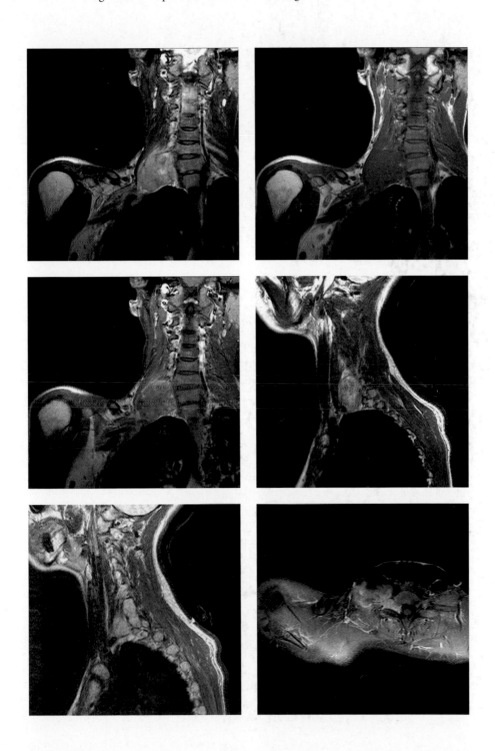

Case 183 Brachial Plexus Neurofibroma

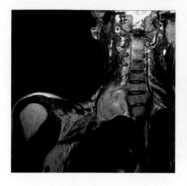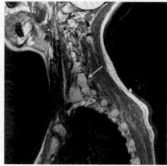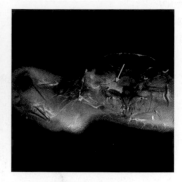

Findings

▶ There is a well-circumscribed, rounded mass along the right brachial plexus. It is hyperintense on T2-weighted images. On postcontrast T1-weighted images it enhances heterogeneously.
▶ The mass extends back along the right C7 and C8 nerve roots with expansion on the respective neural foramina (arrows).
▶ The mass abuts the right subclavian artery without narrowing it.

Differential Diagnosis

▶ Desmoid tumor
▶ Metastatic neoplasm
▶ Lymphoma

Teaching Points

▶ The brachial plexus consists of the C5-T1 nerve roots, which course inferolaterally towards the axilla to innervate the arm. It runs between the anterior and middle scalene muscles and in close approximation to the subclavian artery.
▶ Other than lipomas, neurogenic neoplasms are the most common brachial plexus tumors. They most commonly arise in the nerve roots proximal to the scalene triangle.
▶ Patients commonly present with shoulder pain, arm weakness, and slow-growing neck mass.
▶ Of the neurogenic tumors, neurofibromas are more common than schwannomas. Their imaging appearance is similar. Typical imaging findings are a well-defined, fusiform-shaped mass in the scalene triangle with T2 hyperintensity and enhancement. The degree of enhancement depends on the amount of degeneration and hemorrhage (which are more common in schwannomas).
▶ Malignant nerve sheath tumors account for 14% of the neurogenic tumors and are most common in patients with neurofibromatosis or previous radiation treatment. These tumors differ from benign neurofibromas by having rapid enlargement and irregular margins.
▶ Another common benign process in this region is the desmoid tumor, also known as fibromatosis. These tumors are infiltrative and demonstrate T2 hyperintensity with intense enhancement.

Management

▶ Surgical excision with intraoperative neurophysiological monitoring

Further Reading

Bowen BC, Siedenwurm DJ. Expert Panel on Neurological Imaging. Plexopathy. *AJNR Am J Neuroradiol.* 2008;29:400-402.
Wittenberg KH, Adkins MC. MR imaging of nontraumatic brachial plexopathies: frequency and spectrum of findings. *Radiographics.* 2000;20:1023-1032.

History

► Child with palpable scalp lesion. History of fall from second-story window four months earlier

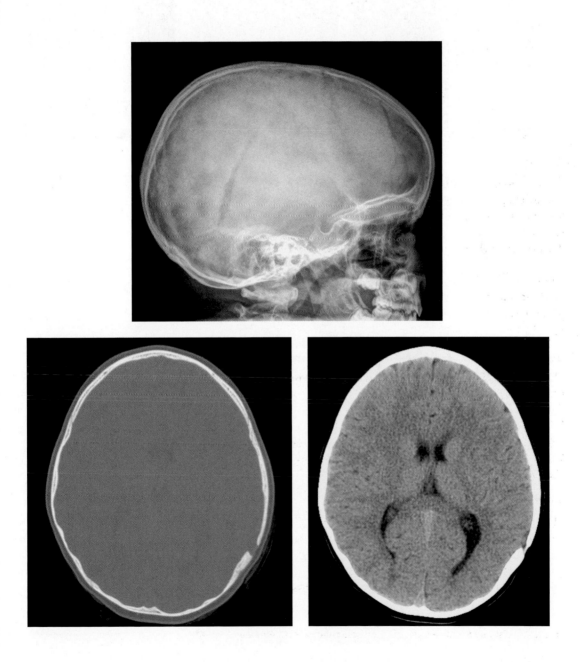

Case 184 Growing Fracture (Leptomeningeal Cyst)

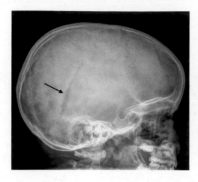 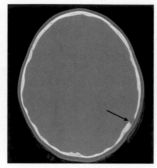 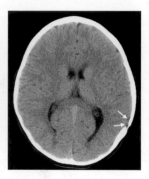

Findings

- ▸ There is a sharply marginated defect in left parietal bone (arrow, plain film and bone window CT).
- ▸ A small extra-axial leptomeningeal cyst is adjacent to the fracture (white arrows).
- ▸ Both bone defect and cyst are at site of prior fracture (prior study not shown).

Differential Diagnosis

- ▸ Unhealed fracture with adjacent encephalomalacia
- ▸ Langerhans cell histiocytosis
- ▸ Metastasis

Teaching Points

- ▸ Growing fracture is a rare complication of skull fracture and is found almost exclusively in children under 3 years old.
- ▸ A tear in the dura mater is a prerequisite for "growing fracture," but an actual cyst is not always present.
- ▸ It can be associated with a cyst or brain tissue extending through the defect.
- ▸ The cyst can extend into the subgaleal space.

Management

- ▸ Surgery is needed to repair the dural tear and prevent recurrence.

Further Reading

Edwards-Brown MK, Hart BL. Traumatic brain injuries in children. In: Orrison WW. Neuroimaging. Philadelphia: Saunders, 2000:1765.

Muhonen MG, Piper JG, Menezes AH. Pathogenesis and treatment of growing skull fractures. *Surg Neurol.* 1995;43:367-373.

History

▶ Small right eye

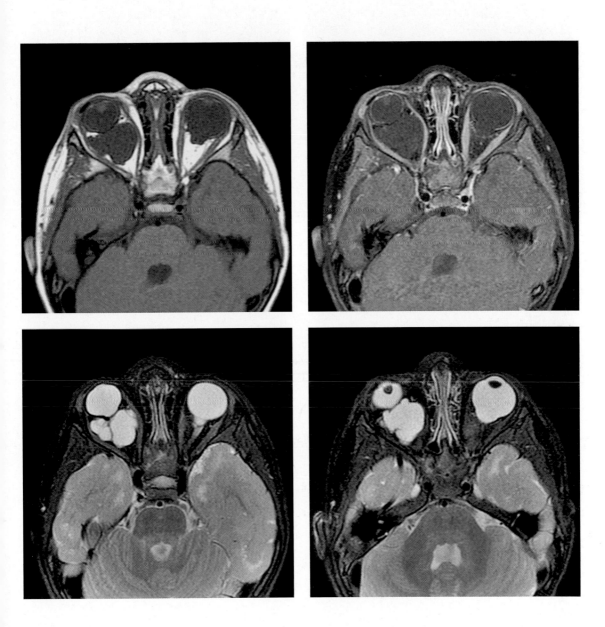

Case 185   Bilateral Coloboma in CHARGE Syndrome

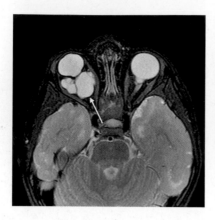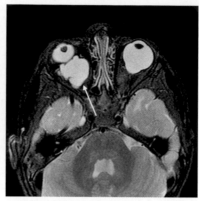

Findings

▶ The right eye is small (microphthalmia) and has a focal change in contour of the posterior pole. There is a lobulated cystic lesion posterior to the right globe (arrow).

▶ The left globe has a focal bulge in the contour of the posterior sclera as well.

▶ There is no abnormal enhancement.

Differential Diagnosis

▶ Lymphangioma of orbit (right orbit)

▶ Staphylomas

Teaching Points

▶ Colobomas are congenital malformations of the eye that result from incomplete or abnormal closure of the fetal optic fissure.

▶ Colobomas can involve the choroid, iris, eyelid, or optic nerve. Imaging is used to evaluate colobomas that involve the choroid or optic nerve most commonly.

▶ Colobomas occur both sporadically or in association with syndromes, most notably the CHARGE syndrome and Aicardi syndrome. They can be unilateral or bilateral, with bilateral involvement more common when associated with syndromes.

▶ Associated imaging features of colobomas include a small globe (microphthalmia) and the frequent occurrence of a cyst posterior to the globe. The cyst is usually related to retinal/vitreous tissue that has passed through the defect in the sclera.

▶ Isolated optic nerve head colobomas result in an unusual-appearing optic nerve head that is termed the "morning glory" anomaly.

▶ Staphylomas are focal contour changes in the globe caused by thinning of the sclera and can be idiopathic or related to collagen-vascular diseases such as rheumatoid arthritis.

Management

▶ There is no specific treatment other than correcting vision with proper refraction. Evaluation for associated brain and systemic findings should be considered, especially for patients with bilateral colobomas.

Further Reading

Maffee MF. The eye. In: Som PM, Curtin HD. Head and Neck Imaging, 4th ed. Philadelphia: Mosby, 2003:463-465.
Onwochei BC, Simon JW, Bateman JB, et al. Ocular colobomata. *Surv Ophthalmol.* 2000;45:175-194.

History

▶ 55-year-old man with decreased peripheral vision in one eye in the past few days

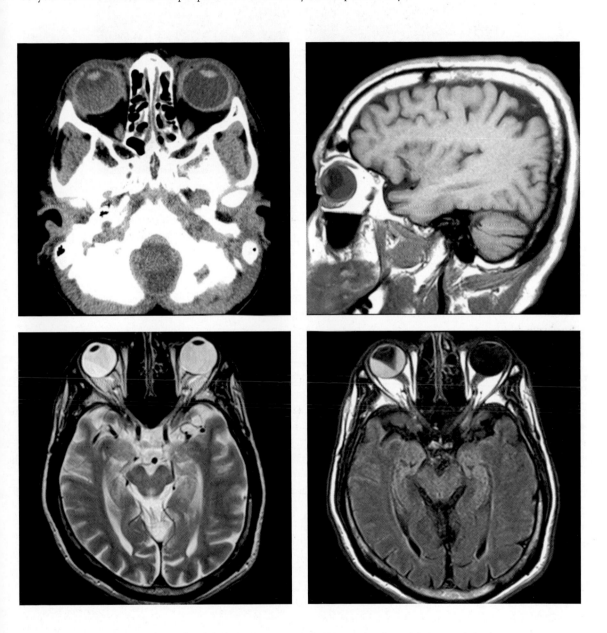

Case 186 Retinal Detachment

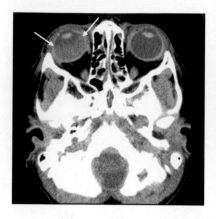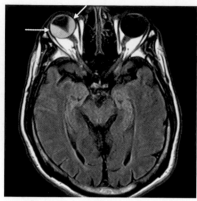

Findings

▶ Axial CT image shows subtle high density in the posterior aspect of the vitreous of the right globe (white arrows).
▶ Sagittal T1-weighted and axial T2-weighted and FLAIR images show V-shaped hyperintensity along the posterior globe with the apex towards the optic disc and its anterior margins at the ciliary bodies.

Differential Diagnosis

▶ Choroidal or hyaloid membrane detachment
▶ Persistent hyperplastic primary vitreous
▶ Coats' disease
▶ Ocular neoplasm

Teaching Points

▶ Retinal detachment occurs when the sensory retina is separated from the retinal pigmented layer, with accumulation of exudative or transudative fluid in the potential subretinal space.
▶ Risk factors for retinal detachment include old age, trauma, prior cataract surgery, high myopia, diabetes mellitus, and inflammatory or neoplastic conditions of the eye.
▶ On imaging, the fluid or blood behind the detached retina can often be visualized on CT or MRI. Fluid content varies, producing variable attenuation on CT and signal intensities on MRI.
▶ In most patients, there is sparing of detachment at the insertion point of the optic nerves, which produces a V-shaped appearance.
▶ Often choroidal detachment can be distinguished from retinal detachment on CT and MRI, since the detached choroid is restricted by the anchoring effect of the vortex veins and does not extend to the region of the optic nerves. If this distinction can be made, it will help with patient management as the treatment differs between these two entities.

Management

▶ Cryopexy and laser photocoagulation may repair small lesions. For most lesions, various surgical procedures such as scleral buckling, pneumatic retinopexy, or vitrectomy are performed.
▶ Intravitreous silicone oil is sometimes injected to provide a mechanical tamponade that helps retinal attachment following retinal detachment repair. The silicone oil will show chemical shift artifact on MRI.

Further Reading

Kubal WS. The pathological globe: clinical and imaging analysis. *Semin Ultrasound CT MR.* 1997;18:423-436.
Mafee MF, Karimi A, Shah JD, et al. Anatomy and pathology of the eye: role of MR imaging and CT. *Neuroimaging Clin North Am.* 2005;15:23-47.

History

▶ 58-year-old woman undergoing elective cerebral angiography

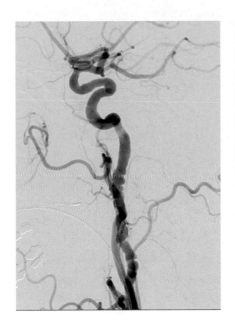
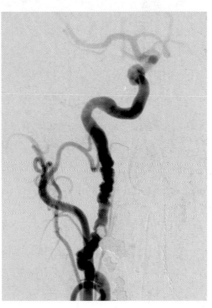

Case 187   Fibromuscular Dysplasia

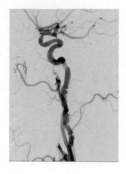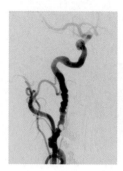

Findings

▶ Injection of the right common carotid artery demonstrates alternating narrowing and dilatation ("string of beads") in the mid-cervical internal carotid artery (ICA).

Differential Diagnosis

▶ Standing waves (normal transient contrast-related vessel wall corrugation)
▶ Arterial dissection
▶ Takayasu arteritis

Teaching Points

▶ Fibromuscular dysplasia (FMD) is a non-inflammatory vasculopathy of unknown cause. It is characterized by fibrous proliferation within the intimal, medial, or adventitial layer of the artery wall. The most common type is medial dysplasia (>90% of affected patients).
▶ The renal and cerebrovascular arteries are most commonly involved, although it can affect any artery, including the vertebral arteries. Renal disease usually presents as hypertension in a young adult. Cerebrovascular involvement is generally asymptomatic. However, it can produce dissection, ischemic stroke, Horner syndrome, and cranial nerve palsy.
▶ Patients with FMD have an increased risk of cerebral aneurysm formation and arterial dissection.
▶ While the characteristic imaging changes may be apparent on CT or MR angiography, catheter angiography remains the diagnostic test of choice.
▶ Angiographic changes typically involve the ICAs (>90%), often bilaterally and in the mid- or distal cervical segments. The imaging appearance is related to the FMD type.
  ▪ Medial dysplasia produces the classic "string of beads" appearance, in which the affected artery demonstrates irregular multifocal narrowing. The "beads" are often larger than the normal lumen diameter.
  ▪ The intimal type (5% of patients) causes long-segment, smooth narrowing. This form is difficult to distinguish from arterial dissection.
  ▪ The adventitial type (<1%) results in focal stenosis with or without aneurysms.

Management

▶ Therapeutic trials are lacking, but antiplatelet medication may decrease the risk of infarction in asymptomatic cerebrovascular FMD.
▶ Treatment of choice for ischemic symptoms is balloon angioplasty. Stenting is reserved for recurrent stenosis or dissection.

Further Reading

Furie DM, Tien RD. Fibromuscular dysplasia of arteries of the head and neck: Imaging findings. *AJR Am J Roentgenol.* 1994;162:1205-1209.
Morris P. Other vascular diseases. In: Morris P. Practical Neuroangiography, 2nd ed. Philadelphia: Lippincott Williams & Wilkins, 2007:405-407.

History

▶ 34-year-old woman with headaches

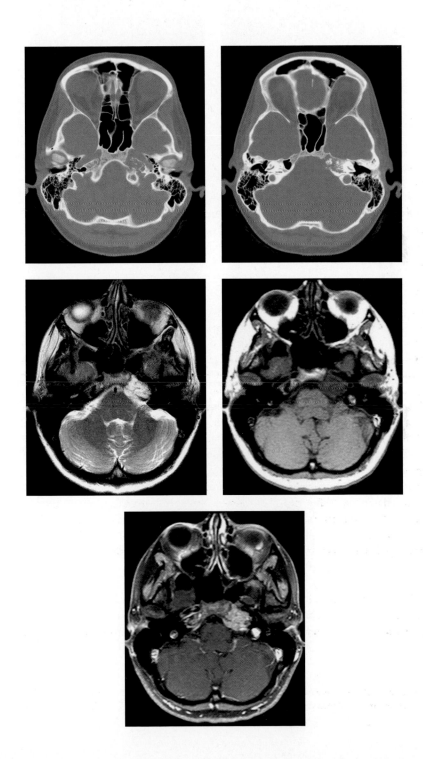

Case 188 Chondrosarcoma, Low-grade Myxoid

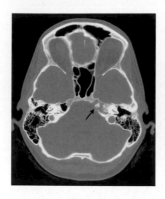 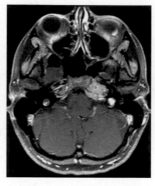

Findings

► CT shows a region of bone destruction along the left petroclival synchondrosis (arrow).
► Calcifications are present in the region of bone destruction, suggesting a chondroid matrix.
► MR shows hyperintense signal on T2-weighted images, hypointense signal on T1-weighted images, and moderate enhancement within the lesion. Enhancing soft tissue extends into the prepontine cistern.

Differential Diagnosis

► Chordoma
► Meningioma
► Myeloma
► Metastasis
► Nasopharyngeal cancer

Teaching Points

► Chondrosarcomas are aggressive malignancies arising from chondroid tissues. They usually present with headaches or symptoms related to cranial nerve palsy (VI, III, V, VII, VIII).
► Chondrosarcomas of the head and neck most commonly arise off midline in the region of the petro-sphenoid or petro-occipital synchondrosis, although occasionally they arise from the spheno-occipital synchondrosis in the midline.
► Location is the most reliable feature distinguishing chondrosarcomas from chordomas. It is very unusual for chordomas to arise off midline.
► Hyperintense signal on T2-weighted images is present in both chordomas and chondrosarcomas but is less common in myeloma, meningiomas, and nasopharyngeal cancer.
► Bone destruction and internal calcification can be seen in both chordomas and chondrosarcomas, but the presence of a chondroid-appearing matrix suggests chondrosarcoma.

Management

► Chondrosarcomas are optimally treated with surgical resection and radiation therapy. Overall patients with chondrosarcoma of the skull base have an excellent prognosis, with >90% 10-year survival common (a much better prognosis than chordomas).

Further Reading

Curtin HD, Rabinov JD, Som PM. Central skull base: embryology, anatomy, and pathology. In: Som PM, Curtin HD. Head and Neck Imaging, 4th ed. Philadelphia: Mosby, 2003:509–520.

History

▸ 36-year-old with decreased vision in left eye

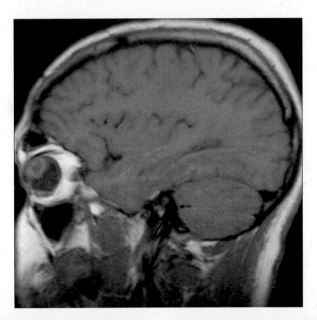

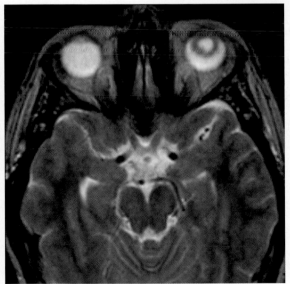

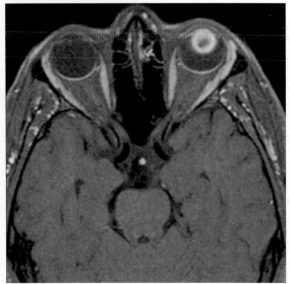

Case 189 Ocular Melanoma

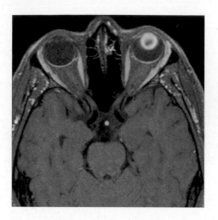

Findings

▶ There is a well-defined left intraocular mass. It abuts both the ciliary body and posterior iris.

▶ The mass has a peripheral zone of enhancement that is iso-intense on precontrast T1-weighted images and hyperintense on T2-weighted images.

Differential Diagnosis

▶ Metastasis

▶ Choroidal hemangioma

▶ Medulloepithelioma

Teaching Points

▶ Ocular melanoma is the most common primary malignant neoplasm of the globe, and most arise from preexisting melanocytic nevi in the globe.

▶ Primary ocular melanomas can arise from the choroid, ciliary body, or iris, with choroidal melanomas being the vast majority.

▶ Ocular melanomas, like melanomas elsewhere in the body, can display bright signal on T1-weighted sequences due to the presence of melanin or blood products.

▶ When they arise from the choroid, exudative retinal detachments frequently accompany the tumor and can lead to a more confusing imaging appearance because the subretinal fluid can be proteinaceous and appear bright on T1-weighted sequences.

▶ Ocular melanoma has a 10-year survival of 50% to 70%, with systemic metastasis being the most common reason for death.

Management

▶ Small tumors may be treated with local radiation, brachytherapy, or thermotherapy. Larger tumors may require enucleation or orbital exenteration. Occasionally, small lesions that might represent either ocular nevus or melanoma can be closely followed for growth.

Further Reading

Maffee MF. Uveal melanoma, choroidal hemangioma, and simulating lesions. Role of MR imaging. *Radiol Clin North Am.* 1998;36:1083-1099.

Mancuso AA, Smith MF, Bhatt D, Verbist BM. Eye: Intraocular neoplastic masses and vascular malformations. In: Mancuso AA, Hanafee WN. Head and Neck Radiology. Philadelphia: Lippincott Williams & Wilkins, 2011:97-104.

History

▶ 18-month-old with a painless lump along the lateral aspect of the orbit for a few months

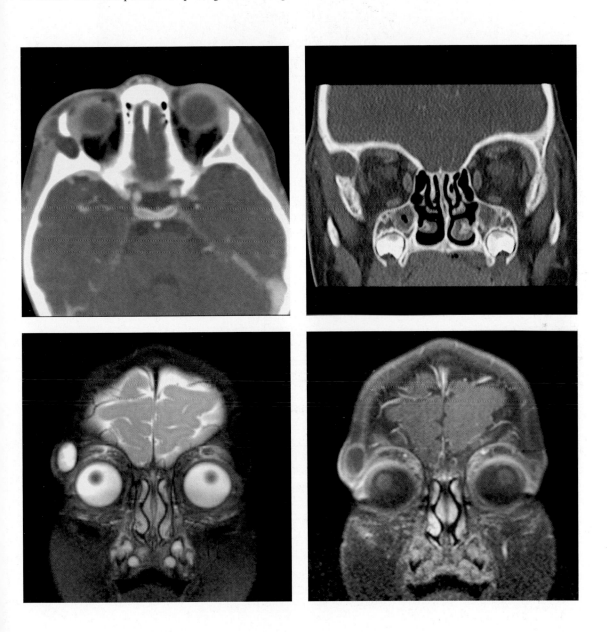

Case 190 Orbital Dermoid

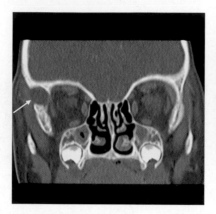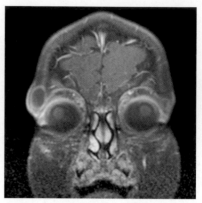

Findings

▶ CT images demonstrate a well-circumscribed, slightly low-attenuation mass along the lateral orbit (white arrow), with smooth remodeling and scalloping of the adjacent orbital wall.

▶ Coronal fat-saturated T2-weighted and postcontrast T1-weighted images show a well-defined T2-hyperintense nonenhancing mass with a thin enhancing rim.

Differential Diagnosis

▶ Lipoma
▶ Epidermoid

Teaching Points

▶ Dermoid and epidermoid inclusion cysts of the orbit are choristomas arising from congenital epithelial remnants. They are the most common orbital masses in children.

▶ They most commonly present later in the first decade as painless masses as they slowly accumulate debris and grow. They may rupture or get infected.

▶ In the orbit they often arise near the developing sutures of the orbital bones. The most common location is the superotemporal orbital-periorbital region.

▶ These lesions appear as well-circumscribed, encapsulated, unilocular cystic masses, and the appearance of the cyst varies depending on its contents. If there is a significant fatty component, they will demonstrate lipid attenuation on CT and the characteristics of fat on MRI. They may show restricted diffusion on diffusion-weighted imaging.

▶ They often smoothly remodel the adjacent bones and may produce thinning or dehiscence.

▶ These lesions generally do not enhance, though they may have thin rim enhancement. Intense irregular enhancement may be a sign of rupture or superimposed infection.

Management

▶ Surgical resection of the entire lesion is often curative.

Further Reading

Chung EM, et al. From the Archives of the AFIP. Pediatric orbit tumors and tumor-like lesions: osseous lesions of the orbit. *Radiographics.* 2008;28:1193-1214.

Pryor SG, et al. Pediatric dermoid cysts of the head and neck. *Otolaryngol Head Neck Surg.* 2005;132:938-942.

History

▶ 6-month-old with a deformed head

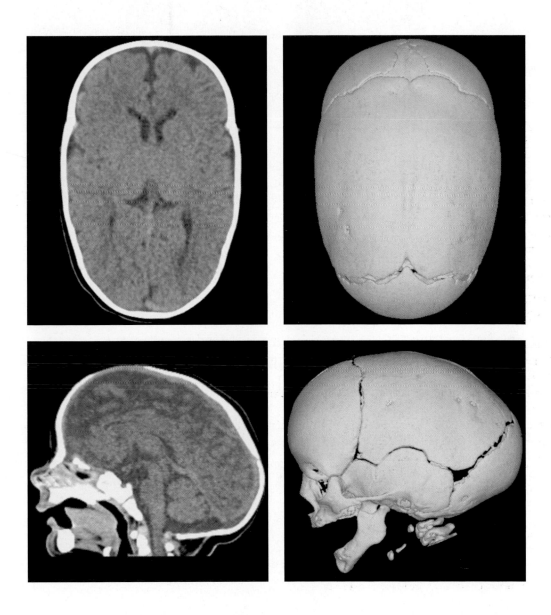

Case 191 Sagittal Craniosynostosis

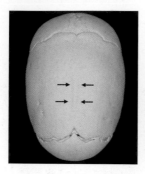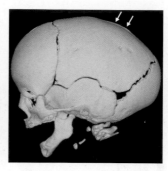

Findings

- There is an abnormally elongated skull (scaphocephaly) with increased anteroposterior diameter of the skull compared to its transverse diameter.
- On the surface-rendered images of the skull there is fusion of the sagittal suture, with slight ectocranial ridging along the course where the suture was located (arrows).

Differential Diagnosis

- Positional or postural plagiocephaly and flattening of the skull
- Secondary craniosynostosis due to arrest of brain growth

Teaching Points

- Craniosynostosis (craniostenosis) refers to a diverse group of disorders with premature fusion of the cranial sutures. They may occur as an isolated finding or as part of a syndrome (syndromic craniosynostosis).
- Patients present with an abnormally shaped head, or with decreased head growth on periodic head circumference measurements.
- Premature fusion of different sutures results in varied skull shapes. As a rule of thumb, after premature fusion of a suture, skull growth stops in the direction perpendicular to the fused suture and the calvarium grows in a direction parallel to the fused suture.
  - Sagittal synostosis: scaphocephaly, dolichocephaly
  - Metopic synostosis: trigonocephaly
  - Unilateral lambdoid or coronal synostosis: plagiocephaly
  - Bilateral lambdoid or coronal synostosis: brachycephaly, turricephaly
- Craniosynostosis can be seen in a large number of congenital syndromes, with more common entities being Crouzon, Pfeiffer, and Apert syndromes.
- There are associated facial, orbital, and ear abnormalities in many syndromic craniosynostosis patients. These patients can also develop hydrocephalus or occasionally have congenital brain anomalies.
- CT is the imaging method of choice in determining the extent of sutural involvement and fusion. 3D shaded surface displays or volume-rendered images are helpful in delineating the involved sutures and craniofacial deformities.

Management

- Major deformities will need surgical correction, sometimes requiring multiple operations. Mild deformities may be helped by head repositioning or by helmets and orthotics.

Further Reading

Blaser SI. Abnormal skull shape. *Pediatr Radiol.* 2008;38:S488-496.
Kotrikova B, et al. Diagnostic imaging in the management of craniosynostoses. *Eur Radiol.* 2007;17:1968-1978.

History

▶ 33-year-old woman with nasal stuffiness

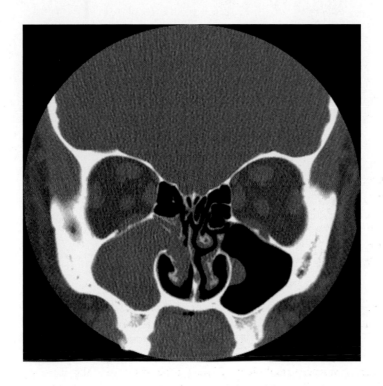

Case 192 Inverted Papilloma

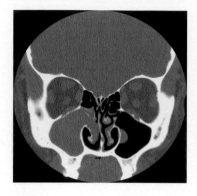 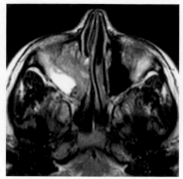 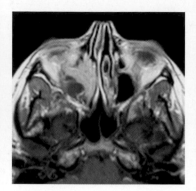

Findings

▶ Direct coronal sections from sinus CT show a lobular mass spanning the right maxillary sinus and lateral nasal cavity. There is complete opacification of the right maxillary sinus.

▶ There is remodeling of the uncinate process and ethmoid bulla with widening of the infundibulum

▶ MRI shows the enhancing mass to be largely hypointense on T2-weighted images and to have a subtly lamellated internal architecture. Much of the maxillary sinus opacification is trapped fluid.

Differential Diagnosis

▶ Antrochoanal polyp

▶ Sinonasal polyposis

▶ Mucocele

▶ Malignant neoplasm (e.g., squamous cell carcinoma, salivary neoplasms)

Teaching Points

▶ Inverted papilloma is a benign neoplasm of the paranasal sinuses and nasal cavities characterized by inversion of the overgrown epithelium into the underlying stroma.

▶ They most commonly arise from the lateral wall of the nasal cavity, near the middle turbinate.

▶ Clinical presentation may include unilateral nasal obstruction, epistaxis, rhinorrhea, pain, and epiphora.

▶ Inverted papillomas are associated with the presence of squamous cell carcinoma in about 10% of cases.

▶ On CT they appear as a soft-tissue-attenuation sinonasal mass, associated with the lateral wall of the nasal cavity, remodeling or eroding adjacent bone.

▶ On MR the pattern of folded epithelium may be apparent, giving the mass a lamellated (or cerebriform) appearance. They are typically iso- to hypointense on T2-weighted images and enhance intensely.

▶ The presence of aggressive bone destruction or metastasis is a clue to malignant transformation.

Management

▶ Given their propensity for malignant transformation, surgical resection (usually endoscopic) is recommended. The relatively high recurrence rate necessitates postsurgical imaging follow-up.

Further Reading

Jeon TY, Kim HJ, Chung SK, et al. Sinonasal inverted papilloma: Value of convoluted cerebriform pattern on MR imaging. *AJNR Am J Neuroradiol.* 2008;29:1556-1560.

Melroy CT, Senior BA. Benign sinonasal neoplasms: a focus on inverting papilloma. *Otolaryngol Clin North Am.* 2006;39:601-610.

Index of Cases

Index